THE BIG BOOK OF

HEALTH

AND

FITNESS

A Practical Guide to Diet, Exercise,
Healthy Aging, Illness Prevention, and Sexual Well-Being

Dr. Philip Maffetone

Skyhorse Publishing

Skyhorse Publishing books may be purchased in bulk at special discounts for sales promotion, corporate gifts, fund-raising, or educational purposes. Special editions can also be created to specifications. For details, contact the Special Sales Department, Skyhorse Publishing, 307 West 36th Street, 11th Floor, New York, NY 10018 or info@skyhorsepublishing.com.

Skyhorse® and Skyhorse Publishing® are registered trademarks of Skyhorse Publishing, Inc.®, a Delaware corporation.

www.skyhorsepublishing.com

10 9 8

Library of Congress Cataloging-in-Publication Data

Maffetone, Philip.

The big book of health and fitness : a practical guide to diet, exercise, sexual well-being, healthy aging, and illness prevention / Philip Maffetone.
    p. cm.
ISBN 978-1-61608-379-3 (pbk. : alk. paper)
1. Health. 2. Physical fitness. 3. Nutrition. 4. Self-care, Health. I. Title.
RA775.M34 2012
613.7--dc23
                                2011035885

Printed in the United States of America

CONTENTS

INTRODUCTION

"Health care" has turned into "health scare." Those with health insurance worry about rising premiums or limited and dropped coverage. Those without insurance keep their fingers crossed that they won't get chronically sick or injured. Guided more by rising costs and administrative duties, doctors are forced to become less personal and more bureaucratic. Emergency rooms have turned into crowded, makeshift physician offices for the uninsured.

How did the health care crisis become so acute in America? And what can you do as an individual not to become a victim of our deeply flawed medical system? After all, one of the main reasons families go into debt, even bankruptcy, is due to hospitalization or long-term care.

What if there is a sensible, cost-effective way to remain healthy, even into old age? And what if this only requires that you learn how to take responsibility for your own health? Because the best alternative to *health scare* is *self-health care*.

It's why I wrote this book.

When I first began my private practice in holistic, complementary medicine in Upstate New York in 1977, the health care landscape was much different than it is today. Patients would come to my clinic with all sorts of common aliments, including fatigue, back pain, asthma and allergies, and intestinal complaints. Most of these problems I treated right there in my office, or in some cases, I would refer a patient to a specialist for further diagnosis, especially with heart or neurological disorders. I would also give each patient a list of specific lifestyle recommendations that matched his or her needs regarding diet, stress, and regular exercise. I believed that the body most often best heals itself once proper nutrients and physical activity are balanced and stress is regulated. Medication or surgery should only be used as the last resort. And I did mean "last."

Once a patient left my office after getting treated and paying me, it was up to that individual to collect from his or her insurance company. Paperwork and bookkeeping were kept at a minimum, especially for me. But as the years went by, the insurance companies, along with a heavy hand from government and lobbyists, began to dictate which therapies would be allowed and even which type of doctors could apply them. Regulations and restrictions increased. Red tape ensnared the system. Costs skyrocketed. Hospital administrators and health insurance company bureaucrats—not doctors—now determined the quality of medical care. Insurance premiums began to soar. As expected, the ranks of the uninsured rapidly began to increase. Ultimately, the health care landscape became so dysfunctional that it contributed significantly to the reason why I decided to leave a successful private practice after twenty years (I continued to privately consult on a limited basis).

While most of the everyday health problems that I used to address with my patients have remained the same, there's one thing that's noticeably different: people no longer fully participate in the process or understanding when it comes to their own health care. Most have forfeited control over their own care to an indifferent Big Brother health care system overseen by MBA grads with their spreadsheets and financial forecasts and not by trained medical professionals.

The centuries-old Hippocratic Oath, handed down by the Greeks, and which required physicians to swear that "I will prescribe regimens for the good of my patients according to my ability and my judgment and never do harm to anyone," has been replaced by the Hypocrisy Oath, which demands that no financial harm should be done that will affect the bottom line of HMOs.

Ironically, people are living longer. That's due to technological advances and better hospital care, not because everyone is truly healthier. While millions are blowing out more candles on their sugar-fortified birthday cakes, their latter years can hardly qualify as healthy, active, and quality living. The average American spends his or her last twelve years in a state of physical and mental dysfunction—often unable to care for himself or herself and draining untold amounts of money for critical life support. As a result of poor diet and lifestyle decisions, many "old age" diseases such as cancer and heart disease have migrated toward middle age, and even all the way to our "overfat" youth where diabetes has become a growing problem.

Today's health care is a huge fiction wrapped inside a much bigger lie. The health industrial complex is a sprawling juggernaut

2

in which providers are for-profit businesses, consumers have been stripped of their freedom, and health care professionals are caught smack in the middle. Despite the fact that most chronic diseases can be prevented, they're not. The reason is that causes of disease are not adequately addressed, and instead, only the symptoms are usually treated. It's a disease-care system that's broken way beyond repair. Now all we can do is wait for the worst to happen—and hope that someday we don't get sick.

But wait for what? Companies sell their unhealthy products to the public with the full knowledge that they will someday lead to chronic sickness and disease. The cycle of ill health is perpetuated. For example, cigarettes—exposed decades ago as a deadly habit—are still being sold despite the surgeon general warning labels and higher taxes. Banning or taxing soft drinks is the current target of health advocates, but the beverage giants such as Coke and Pepsi simply respond by spending more money on advertising and marketing, even going so far as supporting public school projects. Or take the case of unregulated over-the-counter drugs that claim to treat everything from joint pain to insomnia—but also come with a long list of unpleasant side effects. All these products are marketed to consumers in every conceivable way—radio, TV, Internet, magazines, newspapers, billboards—brainwashing almost everyone into eagerly accepting unhealthy food, drink, and pills as the American way.

It's the ideal, profitable business model—sell harmful products to people that will eventually make them sick and then sell them goods and services to keep them alive for many more years but then ultimately claim success because everyone is living longer. Start them early with Juicy Juice and Frosted Flakes as toddlers, fill their bellies with fast food and highly processed packaged fare as teens and adults, and when they are infirmed geriatrics, load them up with Maalox and meds. It's a cradle-to-grave rip-off. And it's no surprise that the top five preventable conditions in the United States are heart disease, cancer, stroke, lung conditions, and diabetes.

We can change all this. We can break free from the devastating ravages of foods that make us sick and the disease-care system that is more interested in its own financial welfare than in genuine and effective health care. And we can do it by assuming greater responsibility for our own health.

In this book, you'll learn all about taking care of your own health. I call this self–health care. You will be able to assess your own signs and symptoms. You will understand how to eliminate common health problems by making appropriate changes with your diet, nutrition, physical activity, or reduction of stress. In doing so, you'll reduce your risk of future disease. Or more accurately, you'll outlive cancer, heart disease, Alzheimer's, and most of the other preventable conditions.

But what does "outlive" really mean? One doesn't actually prevent or entirely elimi-

3

LET THE FACTS SPEAK

By 2035, government health care spending—driven by rising medical costs and an aging population—is projected to account for almost 40 percent of the federal budget.

An estimated fourteen million Americans are struggling with medical bills that they believe were sent in error to collection agencies, according to the Commonwealth Fund, a nonprofit health care research group.

About one hundred thousand Americans a year are killed by infections acquired in hospitals; many of these superbugs are resistant to multiple antibiotics. Methicillin-resistant *Staphylococcus aureus*, or MRSA, now kills more Americans each year than AIDS.

More than a quarter of U.S. children and teens are taking a medication regularly, according to Medco Health Solutions, the nation's largest pharmacy-benefit manager with sixty-five million members.

For over-the-counter pain relief, thirty-three million Americans regularly use non-steroidal anti-inflammatory drugs, also known as NSAIDs—aspirin, ibuprofen (Advil, Motrin), naproxen sodium (Aleve).

NSAIDs account for about 16,500 deaths annually; the culprit is usually ulcer-related complications associated with the drug's continued use.

Americans will keep growing fatter until 42 percent of the nation is considered obese, according to a 2010 published study by researchers at Harvard University; the team also found that an American adult has a 2 percent chance of becoming obese in any given year.

Americans now consume an average of thirty-three pounds of cheese a year—that is three times the 1970 amount; in fact, cheese has become the largest source of saturated fat in the nation's diet, which comes as good news to Dairy Management, a marketing creation of the United States Department of Agriculture, that has spent millions of dollars on research to support a national advertising campaign promoting the notion that people could lose weight by consuming more dairy products.

Each year, the average American consumes 140 pounds of high-fructose sweeteners, including corn-based sweeteners.

In the United States, the mean average weight is now 194.7 pounds for men and 164.7 pounds for women, according to the National Center for Health Statistics at the Centers for Disease Control and Prevention.

INTRODUCTION

Almost 10 percent of the world's population was obese in 2008, according to studies published by the medical journal *The Lancet*, while Americans grew fatter at a faster pace than residents of any other wealthy nation since 1980.

Obesity-related diseases account for nearly 10 percent of U.S. medical spending, or an estimated $147 billion a year.

Diabetes is reaching epidemic proportions and is one of the fastest-growing diseases in the United States; it currently affects about twenty-six million Americans.

The costs for cancer care topped $124 billion in 2010 in the United States.

Based on studies by the Organization for Economic Co-operation and Development and the World Health Organization, among all countries, the United States is ranked twenty-seventh in life expectancy, eighteenth in diabetes, and first in obesity.

nate these disease processes from taking place. Instead, one can slow them down so they don't progress nearly as quick. Let me cite an example: The process of cancer is ongoing in all of us. Cancer cells regularly develop from one's normal cells when some toxin or stressor damages a healthy cell's sensitive DNA. The result is rapid cellular reproduction with the potential for out-of-control growth. This is the first of many steps of the cancer process, but it does not usually go completely unchecked because the body with a healthy, strong immunity has important cellular mechanisms that can control cancer cells from spreading. While a diagnosis of cancer might be made today, the condition probably began many years, even decades, ago. The cancer progressed because the body was exposed to far too many environmental or food toxins or did not have the capability to slow down the

tumor's runaway growth. Eventually, the mass becomes large enough to be seen on X-ray or trigger symptoms.

So how can someone alter this scenario by placing a brake on cancer's silent spread?

First, there are some well-known reasons why cancer secretly progresses. Epidemiologist John Potter, from the University of Minnesota, states that "at almost every one of the steps along the pathway leading to cancer, there are one or more compounds in vegetables or fruits that will slow up or reverse the process." *Time* magazine's January 21, 2002, cover story read, "New discoveries [from food] can help prevent everything from obesity to cancer to heart disease."

What are the factors that trigger these cellular changes to start cancer, and what are the things that could slow it down? Here are three common factors that can speed up the process of cancer:

5

- Chemicals called free radicals are produced in the body due to toxins in the environment (in particular, from air and water pollution), radiation (we're exposed daily from three forms: ultraviolet, medical x-rays, and cosmic), and aging itself when you don't eat the proper foods.
- Nitrogen compounds are generated from overcooking foods containing protein, a common source is grilling steak, but since most foods contain some protein, overheating can do the same for chicken, fish, and even vegetables.
- Chronic inflammation, a typical problem caused by imbalances of dietary fat and the body's hormones, and excess stress.

A variety of nutrients in foods will actually stop or slow the cancer-forming process. Here are some of these vital nutrients:

- Sulforaphane, lipoic acid, and alpha-tocotrienol are powerful phytonutrients that can block the damage from free radicals.
- Glutathione, the body's most potent antioxidant, can block the actions of nitrogen compounds.
- Flavanoids, gingerol, curcumin, sesamin and other nutrients in fresh, organic fruits, vegetables, and other plant foods can block the process of inflammation.
- Tangeretin, limonine, and tocotrienols can block other areas of cancer progression.

You may not have heard of these nutrients, but they're all readily available in a healthy diet that includes vegetables, fruits, seeds, and nuts, especially in their raw state. These are whole foods, not processed or precooked ones, and in many cases are found only in organically grown items. That's because the agriculture-food industry genetically removes these nutrients from many foods to increase shelf life and make them sweeter in taste.

In an ideal world, everyone should be allowed the opportunity to live to an age where one can die with dignity, not from war, disease, or chronic illnesses such as a stroke, heart attack, or debilitating tumor, but from what some consider "natural causes."

The phrase "natural causes" is quite vague, almost more a legal name rather than scientific. There are no guidelines in the book of death certificates to assist doctors or coroners with their final decisions. The result is that there is little consensus on what the name "natural causes" mean. Instead, I'll refer to "normal life span."

The human body's cells can't keep replicating forever. In fact, all animals live to about six times their skeletal maturity, except for humans. The human skeleton matures at around twenty years of age, so natural death in humans should be around 120 years.

Dying at seventy years of age or sixty or fifty of some ailment means that a life has ended prematurely. A serious illness or

6

disease took over and the body could not outlive it.

But this book tells you not only how to keep ahead of preventable sickness, but it also shows you how to remain physiologically younger than your chronological age. There's no reason why you can't walk, swim, ride a bike, or play tennis or golf well into your 80s and 90s. And if we can clean up our toxic environment and food supply, living past 100 could someday be a reality for many.

You don't have to wait for disease and sickness to exhibit symptoms before you do something about your own health. Take action now. You can't depend on the current health care system for either a quick fix or long-term remedy. The ultimate responsibility for your own health is entirely in your hands.

Health versus Fitness

Health is only part of the overall picture for aging gracefully. You also need to be fit; you need muscles for movement, to keep your bones strong and protect you from falls, to burn body fat, and avoid being overweight.

But fitness is the not the same as health. Instead, they're actually two different but mutually dependent states. This realization came to me early in private practice while I was running the 1980 New York City Marathon. My purpose, I thought, was a self-demonstration of health, but in the end, when I crossed the finish line after running 26.2 miles through New York City's five boroughs, I suddenly became aware that in my single-minded pursuit of fitness, I had neglected my health.

All went well during the marathon through the first ten miles. The excitement swept me along at a slightly quicker pace than I'd planned, yet I felt great. By fifteen miles I felt tired but was able to continue. Within the next couple of miles, however, I began to shiver. Despite drinking plenty of water, I felt dehydrated. And I was craving cotton candy. At eighteen miles, I stopped to check my feet. They were numb, and I wanted to be sure they were still there. "My hamstrings are cramping," I said out loud. I wasn't thinking rationally, and all I could remember was my goal to finish the race. Alarmed by how awful I looked, two paramedics tried to remove me from the course. But I wouldn't let them. Somehow, I painfully fought my way onward. I have very little memory of those last few miles in Central Park.

A finisher's medal was hung around my neck. I cried with joy over the ultimate success of passing my four-hour endurance test. But the next moment I discovered myself herded into the first aid tent. It looked like a war zone. There were casualties all around me. Doctors and nurses were running in and out. Sick-looking runners lying on cots groaned in pain. Ambulances came and went. I thought to myself, *Are these people really healthy? And am I?* I knew right then that running the marathon had not proven my health at all. I was fit enough to run 26.2 miles. But

7

clearly fitness was something quite different from good health.

That marathon experience was an epiphany—and affected my lifelong interest in the respective areas of fitness and health. I later came up with two definitions. They are as follows:

• Fitness: The ability to perform physical activity. You personally define the limits of your overall fitness. Perhaps your goal is only to walk a mile a day or train for a marathon or triathlon.
• Health: The ideal balance of all systems of the body—the nervous, muscular, skeletal, circulatory, digestive, lymphatic, and hormonal.

Improving fitness is associated with physical activity. Only a few generations ago, most people were naturally active, working physically to accomplish their daily chores. Today, our society has turned sedentary. We have escalators, elevators, SUVs, and television remote controls. Some people drive around a parking lot for five or ten minutes to get a parking space closer to the front entrance of a shopping mall. (I remember once seeing a driver circle the parking lot at a health club several times looking for a space close to the front door.) Others wait minutes for an elevator just to go to the second floor. People can fulfill most of their daily needs literally at the push of a button.

This radical change from a vigorous to an inactive lifestyle has taken place, genetically speaking, in a very short time frame. The human genes of today are still programmed to be hunter-gatherers—walking and running to hunt food, lifting and dragging it for long distances, gathering firewood before cooking and eating it. But most people are no longer even close to that level of activity. The human body can't adapt to such a major change without dire consequences—as a society, we literally have become severely deficient in physical activity. This deficiency has adversely affected muscle function leading to low back, knee, hip, and spinal problems; blood sugar and stress hormones leading to fatigue; diabetes; immune, and intestinal disorders; and contributes to heart disease, cancer, and brain dysfunction. And along with poor diet, it's the reason for our overfat epidemic.

Since a majority of the population has lost the need to be physically active, it must satisfy that requirement artificially—through exercise. But balancing fitness with health is equally important. While most people are sedentary, many who do work out often overtrain. But obsessively working out can lead to poor health and physical and mental breakdowns. Many elite athletes are fit but unhealthy. They get sick or chronically injured—and wonder why.

How much activity does the average person require? Less than you think, and it depends on other factors, including what one physically does throughout the day. A consistent regimen of walking for thirty minutes each day may be enough for many people. For others, forty-five minutes of some combination of easy running, biking, and swimming five times a week is effective.

When health and fitness are balanced, the result is optimal human performance. And it should relate to more than just athletics. There's performance in family, career, and relationships. Throughout my practice, I had the pleasure and excitement to actually see my patients and clients improve their performance, and thus succeed at achieving their goals. This included winning triathlons or marathons, finding career success, and being the best-possible parent. The secret to their success—whether it was harmony in the home, workplace, or receiving a first-place trophy at the Ironman—was balanced health and fitness.

How to Use This Book

The Big Book of Health and Fitness is a road map that will help guide you through the beautiful journey of life. There are many paths you can follow to succeed. You have free choice in this matter. You can avoid the illnesses that are commonly accepted as part of the aging process—and get old too fast or die too slow. While you can't control the passing of the years, you can actually control physiological aging. As such, you can look,

act, and feel younger than your age in years. How that's accomplished is the basis of this book.

This book provides vital how-to information in a balanced format of both art and science. I've also compiled much of the science through education and clinical research and the published research of thousands of other researchers and clinicians who have come to the same basic conclusions.

The art facet entails a unique understanding of both health and fitness. Having been in the trenches of patient care, I've learned what genuinely works and what's unfounded hype. I will share these extensive clinical and personal health care experiences, often citing case histories of real patients.

I have worked with patients from all walks of life, from the most healthy to the most frail, from professional world-champion endurance athletes to couch potatoes, from newborns and their moms to adolescents. Many had unique imbalances that not only caused dysfunction but also detracted from their quality of life, reducing their human performance. These problems were the result of dietary and nutritional imbalances while others stemmed from deficiencies in the aerobic system or the stress-coping mechanisms. It was clear that addressing these problems immediately and individually was important not only to improving health in the short term but also to avoiding serious disease in the long run.

Two Key Tools: Evaluation and Application

Two of the key tools this book offers are evaluation and application. First, evaluate or assess yourself. Through the process of self-evaluation, you can assess those unique imbalances. Only then can you apply the most effective therapy, whether it is a particular dietary modification, exercise routine, or other primary remedy to correct specific problems that cause imbalances in the brain and body.

What makes this evaluation process relatively easy are the questions you'll be asked to answer. These are the same questions that the most effective clinicians use to find out what's really wrong with a patient, the cause of the problem, and the best way to correct it. The assessment process is when I had spent most of my time with a patient. And the majority of vital information was obtained by obtaining answers to specific questions. Your answers will help guide you through a process of formulating a strategy to improve your health in an individualized way.

Once you make a successful evaluation or self-assessment, the appropriate remedy is the easy part. These are presented in an easy-to-apply format—such as how to balance fats to avoid chronic inflammation, the many sources of phytonutrients in healthy foods necessary to help fight cancer and stave off diabetes, how to build the aerobic muscles to burn more fat for energy, and even therapies you thought had to be done by health care professionals such as biofeedback.

The book begins by defining the main issues, terms, and concepts important in understanding how best to trail blaze your own path to better health. Since your health is deeply dependent upon the foods you eat, most of the first section extensively discusses diet and nutrition, with some of the content challenging many long-held popular beliefs, such as the need for more protein to build strong bones, why snacking is good for you, and how dietary fat is healthy.

Physical activity is basic not only to fitness but also to good health, and thus the second section of this book discusses developing or modifying physical activity that is most appropriate to your needs. It offers options and an individualized approach to improve fitness in simple and enjoyable fat-burning, weight-loss ways without the risk of injury.

Finally, the third section discusses common clinical conditions of specific body parts and of bodywide problems. These include the brain and how it can repair itself and grow new functions at any age, how the gut—the intestine—is the gateway to optimal nutrition and immune activity, how the heart and blood vessels adapt well with age if given the chance, why chronic inflammation is the first stage of most chronic diseases and how to avoid it, and how to truly regulate excess stress. This section of the book ties together all the information and wisdom of the preceding two sections in a truly holistic way.

HEALTH CARE JUST GETS SCARIER

Even though it's now being legally challenged in the federal courts, the health care legislation passed by Congress and signed into law in early 2010 was designed to keep a lid on runaway costs and provide access to affordable health care coverage for almost all Americans. The legislation's purpose was also to hold insurance companies accountable, guarantee more choice, and enhance the quality of health care. Of course, I am only summarizing the bill's intent with broad brushstrokes. The final bill that reached President Obama's desk ran just over one thousand pages.

But within eight months of the new law, health care consumer advocates' worst fears were coming true. According to a November 20, 2010, article in *The New York Times*, "There is a growing frenzy of mergers involving hospitals, clinics and doctor groups eager to share costs and savings, and cash in on the incentives." What this ultimately means for the sick, injured, and chronically ill is lower standards and diluted health care "by reducing competition, driving up costs and creating incentives for doctors and hospitals to stint on care, in order to retain their cost-saving bonuses." For example, three of the largest hospital networks in Kentucky negotiated a merger, prompted in part by the new law. And in Upstate New York, three regional health care systems have sought federal permission to combine their operations, which include hospitals, clinics, and nursing homes. This type of consolidation is happening all over the country.

With cost containment, a major financial challenge for doctors and hospitals, patient care and treatment will suffer. Judith A. Stein, director of the nonprofit Center for Medicare Advocacy, told *The Times* that "she was concerned that some [health] care organizations would try to hold down costs by 'cherry-picking healthier patients and denying care when it's needed.'"

Several weeks later after *The Times* article appeared, a U.S. federal judge struck down a key component of the health care reform law—that nearly all Americans are required have health insurance. Legal experts expect that his ruling will eventually be put to the test in the Supreme Court. Meanwhile, any real health care savings or benefits will not go into effect for several years. So for the time being anyway, there will be a continued and steady rise in insurance rates.

This certainly doesn't appear like an optimistic or hopeful scenario for the average American. The health industrial complex just keeps getting bigger, more complex, and costlier for those in need of medical services. All this is just a snapshot of the health care environment in 2011. It will continue to change back and forth, up and down, round and round as lobbyists, politicians, lawyers, and the courts have their influences. All the while, consumers—you—won't have much, if any, input. While health care will keep changing with the political landscape, it won't and can't get fixed because the overall system is broken beyond repair.

But the good news is that you have the power to address as well as remedy the real issue—how to remain healthy, fit, and active throughout your entire life. You can accomplish this by taking responsibility for your own health, choosing not to depend or rely on whatever dubious health care proposals are the current trend, and not allowing politicians and corporations to dictate your health care.

The Big Book of Health and Fitness contains the most up-to-date information that is scientifically based and clinically relevant presented in a user-friendly format, with specific actions you can take to understand and prevent common diseases. By correcting and diverting seemingly subtle problems, you can prevent disease, modify the aging process, and drastically improve the quality of your life. You have more control over your health—through food, nutrition, stress control, exercise, and other factors—than you ever imagined. The remedies for the greatest of ailments have been there in plain sight all along. By redirecting and rethinking your responsibility in health care, you can immediately begin reaping the benefits.

This book will help you determine which lifestyle factors best match your particular needs. By the end of the book you will know not only how to live most healthfully, and full of enjoyment, but also how to die most successfully.

You'll want to first read this book from beginning to end, paying close attention to the areas that pertain to you most—you'll know which ones those are because of the questions you'll answer. After you read the book, you'll already be making modifications with food, exercise, stress, and other factors. Then, you'll be able to continuously refer to particular parts of the book for a better understanding and a review of various topics. In doing so, you'll regularly fine-tune your body and brain and want to share the information with friends and family, perhaps influencing others in their personal quest for better health and fitness.

If you're ready to take more responsibility for your own self-health, please read on.

Dr. Philip Maffetone

Choose Your Food Wisely

CHAPTER 1

EATING THE RIGHT FOODS WILL IMPROVE YOUR HEALTH AND GIVE YOU MORE ENERGY

One of my patients was a forty-seven-year-old IBM executive who told me a story that I want to share with you. I will use a different name for him. John had gone to his regular doctor for an annual physical examination. Many tests were performed, including an EKG for the heart, a chest X-ray for the lungs, various blood and urine tests that included cholesterol, triglycerides, sugar, and protein, blood pressure—a complete evaluation with pages of tests and numbers. The next week when John returned for the results, the doctor said, "Good news, everything looks great, there's nothing wrong anywhere." It was just like the year before, and previous years. True, everything from blood pressure to cholesterol, clear lungs to good heartbeat was great news. But John asked the doctor, "Then why do I have these headaches, and why is my energy so low? And why does my stomach always bother me after eating?" The doctor had no answer other than to say that he had ruled out disease. Just like in previous years.

In ruling out disease, John's doctor performed a vital service. But it was only the first step in evaluating John's health and fitness. Though John appeared to be free of disease, he had symptoms that made him uncomfortable and were interfering with his quality of life. What's more, these symptoms could be pointing to bigger problems down the road. John's complaints were not imaginary, and they're quite common. They exist in that gray area between optimal health and disease. These are common examples of functional problems—clues that things have gone wrong with the body.

John's physician later helped me with my evaluation by ruling out more serious problems, but now we needed to find out what was really wrong. It's not normal to have headaches, indigestion, and low energy at any age. If John had these complaints now, how would his body be functioning in ten or fifteen years when he will want to retire and live a high quality of life in his golden years? Probably much worse.

The first thing I did during our first meeting was to ask John many questions—when did the headaches begin, when were they worse and better, where exactly did the head hurt, and others pertaining to his headaches. I did the same with energy—including when was it either low or high. I also asked about sleeping habits, exercise, stress, footwear, dental health, and many other seemingly unrelated issues that can provide vital information in determining the causes and formulating a successful treatment plan.

I also performed an extensive dietary evaluation, asking John to write everything he ate and drank for a five-day period. A computerized analysis of his food list, performed in much the same way that many research studies on diet and nutrition are conducted, was carried out.

I also took his blood pressure in the lying, sitting, and standing positions to see if it changed as it should. In addition, I evaluated the muscles in the head, neck, and shoulder areas and performed many other evaluations. I finally felt there was sufficient information to make certain recommendations.

One of the most important recommendations had to do with food. John was obtaining less than the RDA (recommended daily allowance) levels of various nutrients from his diet—including vitamin B_1 and B_6 to folic acid, magnesium, and zinc. I provided a long list of foods to include in his diet, including whole eggs, fresh and raw vegetables, and raw almonds and cashews as well as foods to avoid, which included corn, soy, and safflower oil products made with white flour and sugar, and Coke.

In addition, John would benefit from eating a larger breakfast that was healthy, such as a vegetable omelet instead of just a bagel with orange juice. And an apple in the midafternoon instead of a snack from the company's candy machine.

Because of his high level of work stress, I suggested an easy thirty-minute walk each day that would help his body counter much of the job stress while at the same time develop his run-down aerobic system to help burn more fat for energy.

I also performed some hands-on therapy that included some simple biofeedback to improve muscle function in his jaw and neck. Over the next three weeks, most of John's physical symptoms disappeared. By six weeks, his energy, as he gratefully told me, was the highest it's been since high school. The headaches were gone.

The remedy was so simple: all John had to do was alter his diet and get regular non-strenuous exercise.

SELF-EVALUATION: TAKE THIS QUICK HEALTH SURVEY

Below are just some of the questions I asked John, along with all new patients, to help guide my initial evaluation. Health surveys like this one will appear throughout this book, and can help guide you in individualizing your health. Ask yourself these questions:

- Are you often fatigued?
- Do you have frequent physical discomfort or pain?
- Do you often have intestinal distress, constipation, or diarrhea?
- Are you unhappy with your current health care provider?
- Do you feel and act your age or older than your age?
- Do you have a history of chronic illness that's not completely resolved, such as heart or circulatory problems, any types of cancer, intestinal disorders, inflammatory conditions ("itis" problems), blood sugar problems, or any undiagnosed signs or symptoms?
- Are you significantly less able to do things today than ten, twenty, or more years ago?
- Are you less healthy and happy now than earlier in your life?
- Do you often or regularly take medications (prescription or over-the-counter)?
- Do you worry more or have less passion for life compared to when you were younger?
- Do you have significant stress from work, relationships, family, or other sources?
- Do you have difficulty learning new things or remembering?
- Do you often have difficulty falling asleep or staying asleep?

A person in optimal health will not have many "yes" answers. The more "yes" answers, the more changes you'll need to turn them to "no" answers—but it won't be as difficult as you think.

Another patient named Sara had a somewhat similar situation as John's—daily problems affecting the quality of life that her doctors could not fully understand or diagnose. A high school teacher in her midforties, Sara was physically active. She would visit the gym four or five times a week and go for long walks on the weekends. She was a model of health for most of her peers. But Sara indicated that in the past three years, she was gaining weight, had difficulty sleeping through the night, waking at least twice each night unable to get back to sleep for an hour, and fatigued during the day. In the past year, she developed nearly uncontrollable craving for sweets each evening and consumed many unhealthy products.

Sara complained about these problems to her doctor, and after a variety of tests, which were all normal, it was suggested that Sara's hormones may be out of balance. The recommendation was hormone replacement therapy. "All women at your age need them," her doctor informed her. But Sara didn't take too kind to that notion, especially after all the hormone tests came back normal. Her doctor said that she had to try some kind of therapy; otherwise, her condition would just get worse. "Besides," her doctor emphasized, "you'll look younger."

Sara had too many women friends who developed unpleasant side effects after starting hormone replacement therapy and thought there must be a better way.

My history and examination of Sara included a dietary analysis, exercise evalua-tion on a treadmill, and other tests, including those for stress hormones, none of which her doctor performed. I also asked Sara to record her morning temperature before getting out of bed. As suspected from her history, the temperature was consistently low, usually around 97°F.

Based on the symptom picture, the low body temperature and high levels of stress hormones, I felt that one of Sara's problems was that her thyroid gland was not working properly. It appeared to be underactive, but not so much as to be diagnosed as hypothyroid—her blood tests for thyroid hormones were all normal.

In addition, Sara was wearing herself down by exercising too hard. This began when she first noticed a slight weight gain—working out harder and eating less, she thought, would solve the problem. But while exercising at a higher heart rate meant she would burn more calories, she now trained her body to burn more sugar and less fat. And her weight gain was not nearly as dramatic as the increased level of body fat—her clothing size had increased noticeably over a three-year period after remaining about the same for twenty-five years. Harder exercise also produced more physical stress, and the added body fat was emotionally alarming. Finally, Sara had added soccer coaching to her already-busy work and social schedule. An evaluation of her cortisol hormone confirmed that she was in a high stress state.

To keep her weight from increasing, Sara decided to reduce her midday meal to almost nothing, just a small plain salad, keeping calories to a minimum. But within a couple of months, she could not control her evening hunger. She was now eating more food at dinner and snacking on unhealthy items throughout the evening.

I recommended a number of lifestyle changes. She needed to eat more food and, in particular, consume smaller amounts of healthy items more frequently, primarily during the day. Her diet was also significantly low in certain omega-3 fats, called EPA, which are important for thyroid function, and she was given a specific dietary supplement containing these fats. Part of my list of recommended foods for snacking included fresh fruit, almonds, and cheese, along with some recipes for healthy desserts.

I also asked Sara to wear a heart rate monitor during exercise so her workouts would be more aerobic and thus burn more body fat—not just while exercise but during the other twenty-three hours of the day. (See chapter 14 on using a heart rate monitor.)

About a month later, Sara's friends began asking her if she was losing weight—they could see it in her face, they claimed. After encouraging her to not weigh herself, explaining that scale weight measured mostly water and was not a good indication of body fat, she could not provide an answer. But her friends were right—as she was following the recommendations strictly, her clothes started fitting noticeably looser, and she was getting thinner. Her good energy returned, and after about two months, she was sleeping soundly through the night without waking. Her body temperature also rose to a normal 98.6°F.

It's important to note that, of the thousands of patients I saw through my career, the recommendations and treatments I provided were always different for each individual despite similarities in symptoms. In the cases of John and Sara, for example, both experienced fatigue—but the causes and remedies were different.

In the presence of abnormal signs and symptoms, problems can exist that are not diseases. These are called functional problems and are the most common complaints heard from most people. Functional problems are

Signs and Symptoms

Throughout this book the terms "signs" and "symptoms" will often be used. Signs are more objective complains we can see, such as a bruise on the skin, a fracture seen on X-ray or a swollen eye—all signs of trauma. Or they're an objective measurement such as body temperature, a cholesterol reading, or an electrical reading of the brain. Symptoms are more subjective and more difficult to see. Fatigue and pain are two common symptoms of some problems in the body.

Signs and symptoms often appear together: the symptom of fatigue is sometimes caused by the sign of low levels of iron in the blood.

caused by many possible imbalances in the body, but many have one thing in common: they are often associated with low energy.

The most common single complaint heard by health care professionals is fatigue. The lack of energy does not just make one tired but can adversely affect many parts of the body. All the organs, glands, muscles, and especially intestines and brain require energy all the time. Without adequate energy, the body can't function as optimally as possible, contributing to functional problems. Many people are unaware that they don't have sufficient energy to be healthy—in many cases, they've gotten so used to having low energy they think it's normal. It's not. Today, low energy is a problem in younger and younger individuals—even in children who wrongly drink or eat sugary treats for quick energy, which only worsens the underlying condition.

Getting back your energy is easy. It almost always has an obvious and important relationship with the foods you eat, and it's the first step to achieving optimal health.

Getting Unlimited Physical and Mental Energy

The human body must produce large amounts of energy for all physical and mental activities. If it does not, getting tired may be the least of one's problems. The whole body may function with less efficiency. The result— one feels older because one ages faster. But normally, at all ages, the body's great built-in energy-generating mechanisms should pro-

vide one sufficient power to function quite well, and the result is that one should feel like one did in one's prime. Before discussing the details of these energy systems and what can go wrong, let's take a step back to answer an important question: where does this energy come from? The answer is both simple and complex.

Basically, energy comes from the sun. Light energy from the sun comes to earth and is converted to chemical energy in plants through the process of photosynthesis. We eat the plants, and most of us eat animals that eat plants. The chemical energy we take in from food is converted to mechanical energy that fuels all our physical and mental activities.

More directly, the energy produced by the body comes from the foods we eat. This energy is obtained from the basic macronutrients in food—carbohydrate, fat, and protein. Though many foods contain all three, there's usually a predominance of one of these in each food. Consider the following examples:

- Carbohydrates are predominant in bread, sugar, rice, pasta, fruit and fruit juice, cereal.
- Fats are dominant in oil, butter, cheese, egg yolk.
- Protein is highest in meat, fish, poultry, egg white, cheese.

The majority of energy is produced from two of these food groups—carbohydrate and fat. Only a small amount, up to 15 percent of total energy, is produced from protein (by conversion of certain protein building blocks, amino acids, into carbohydrate).

All three macronutrients are converted into energy in two steps. First, they are digested in the intestine and absorbed into the blood: as glucose from carbohydrates, fatty acids from fats, and amino acids from protein.

In the second step, after these food compounds go through the liver, the blood carries them to the cells where the molecules of glucose, fatty acids, and amino acids are further metabolized (chemically broken down). The hydrogen atom, the common building block of all three, is released as a result of further actions. This atom contains one electron that is highly charged with energy. This electron is finally converted to a substance called ATP (adenosine triphosphate), which is the form of energy used by the body.

Dietary carbohydrates, fats, and proteins each have different amounts of hydrogen molecules and, therefore, varying amounts of potential energy when we consume them. Fats have by far the most hydrogen, one reason we can get much more energy from the fats in food. Fats can actually provide more than twice the potential energy you get from either carbohydrates or proteins.

Where does all this energy-generating activity take place? Mostly it occurs in two types of muscles:

- The body's long-term energy comes from the aerobic system, with its aerobic fibers (a type of cell) contained in virtually all the muscles.

- The body's short-term energy comes from the anaerobic system, with its anaerobic fibers contain in all the muscles.

All throughout the body, aerobic muscles primarily use fat as fuel to produce energy. In particular, when the aerobic muscles are functioning optimally, an individual can derive a lot of energy from fat. In fact, the majority of one's energy at any given time can come from fat, and the energy supply is virtually endless—the average lean person has enough stored fat to endure a one-thousand-mile trek!

While the body continually generates energy from both sugar and fat, the more one derives from fat, the better is one's overall health and human performance. By improving one's fat-burning metabolism, which will be discussed in greater detail in chapter 4, the positive end result is having more physical and mental energy. Moreover, the body will store less fat, and it will be able to maintain a more stable blood sugar level because there won't be a craving for sugar for energy.

When the body doesn't produce adequate amounts of energy from fat, it instead relies too heavily on sugar. The consequence is the common symptom of fatigue. It comes in physical and mental forms, or in a combination of both. Some people say they just can't perform as they did when they were younger. But age is no excuse for a lack of energy. Physical fatigue may strike at a particular time of the day, or it may make one feel exhausted from the time one awakens.

Mental fatigue is also common, making it difficult to think clearly or make decisions. This can affect anyone from students and executives to children and adults at all ages.

To avoid both physical and mental fatigue, while accessing unlimited energy from one's fat-burning system, two things must occur. First, you need to provide that system with the proper fuel in the form of healthy food. Second, you need to develop the body's powerful aerobic system and maintain it regularly with physical activity.

Both fat and sugar are almost always being burned for energy at all times. It's a question of how much of each one uses. Let's say that you are currently getting half of your energy from fat and half from sugar. When you improve your aerobic system and fat-burning capabilities, you may be able to obtain 70 percent of your energy from fat and 30 percent from sugar. In fact, those individuals who burn higher amounts of fat not only have more energy but also less aches and pains, better mental focus, increased muscle function, and overall improved health.

But many people only get 10 percent of their energy from fat, forcing a full 90 percent to come from sugar. That's an inefficient and unhealthy way to obtain energy. This is the typical situation in people who are fatigued and attempt to obtain more energy from sugar because they can't get much from fat. And when fat is not used for energy, the excess is stored in the body.

Measuring Fat and Sugar Burning

This mix of fuels used for energy can be easily measured in a person and is something I have done during my years in practice and during other research. So when I say you can improve your fat-burning capability, it is because I have seen and recorded these changes in actual patients. These measurements are taken using a gas analyzer, which measures the amount of oxygen a person inhales and the amount of carbon dioxide exhaled. The ratio of carbon dioxide to oxygen gives the percentage of fat and sugar that is used for energy. This is referred to as the respiratory quotient or RQ (sometimes called respiratory exchange ratio or RER). I usually don't recommend getting tested because for most people, when fat burning is poor, there are plenty of signs and symptoms of this deficiency. These include the obvious—increased fat storage. Others include fatigue, blood sugar problems, hormone imbalance, poor circulation, and even common physical injuries. Best of all, as fat burning improves, the body is able to correct many of its own problems.

UNDERSTANDING FUNCTION AND DYSFUNCTION

The symptom of fatigue is an example of one that's more commonly not associated with disease. However, fatigue, like many other signs and symptoms, is indicative of something in our body is not working properly; and if left unchecked, these problems can not only worsen quality of life, lead to unnecessary medication, (which could produce harmful side effects,) and may even be the earliest indication of a disease process. In the majority of cases, food not only contributes significantly to the problems but is also a remedy.

The seemingly innocent signs and symptoms like low energy or recurring headaches are functional problems. They are often and erroneously associated with the process of aging. While they may be common in people as they get older, they're not normal. These functional problems are also referred to as functional illness.

There are often no particular names for various early stages of disease development. But there may be subtle clues in the form of signs and symptoms, often vague in nature, and they could cause uncomfortable problems to the people who have them and ultimately cause illness. These are known as functional problems, or functional illness, and are associated with some specific dysfunction in the body.

Functional problems are sometimes referred to as predisease, preclinical, or in the case of cancer, premalignant. Functional illness is that gray area between optimal health and disease. Altogether, the signs and symptoms of function illness are the most complained about in health care. They are also the most self-medicated for by those who have them, although drugs don't correct the problem; it only masks the symptoms.

Fatigue, headache, indigestion, back pain, allergies, weight gain, and dozens of other complaints are not normal and seldom caused by aging. But these ailments are so common that people have accepted them as part of growing old. Through the years, pharmaceutical companies have cleverly filled the shelves of grocery stores and pharmacies—and now their websites—with products made to medicate and cloak these functional signs and symptoms. A pill for every illness or problem might be the motto of the giant pharmaceutical industry. But numbing the symptom with a drug does not make it go away, won't correct the cause, and worse yet, it can turn off the body's attempt to let it know that there's something wrong.

Primary versus Secondary Problems

An important distinction to make when there is more than one functional problem is cause and effect. Typically, when two functional signs or symptoms exist, usually one is primary and the other secondary. In the example of Sara, she developed intense cravings for sweets in the evening. That's a secondary symptom of a blood sugar problem and related to her more primary problem of inadequate eating of healthy food during the day. Primary problems are often the most quiet and typically being asymptomatic, meaning they don't produce symptoms. Rather than recommending Sara to eat more food in the evening to satisfy her cravings, I determined what the primary problem was—insufficient food intake during the day—and addressed it by recommending more healthy food consumption throughout the day.

Those with chronic problems often accumulate many different signs and symptoms. One problem leads to another and then another. Over the years, people are caught in the web of functional problems and don't know where to turn—doctors often see these patients as candidates for psychological therapy or even drugs to relax them, sometimes labeling them as hypochondriacs.

I call this common complex web of functional signs and symptoms the domino effect. It's like lining up a series of dominoes near each other. All one needs to do is knock down the first one and many others will fall. What caused the last one—the common complaint—to fall? Obviously it wasn't the one before it, or the one before that, but the first one—the primary problem. The body works the same way. Let's use the example of a nutritional problem. Many people have low levels of calcium in their bodies, which can cause bone fractures and muscle dysfunction. Just taking a calcium supplement or drinking milk is not the answer because, often, calcium absorption from the intestines may be poor, so your blood—and therefore bones and muscles—never gets adequate amounts of this nutrient. But more primary to malabsorption is low levels of vitamin D. Since foods don't provide adequate amounts of D, the cause may be due to inadequate sun exposure, our best source of this nutrient. Vitamin D not only helps the intestines better absorb calcium from the diet but it also helps metabolize calcium so the bones and muscles get more of their share.

In many cases, the primary dysfunction, the initial problem that causes the rest, is unnoticed. It may be weeks, months, or years, as the dominos fall, that more obvious signs and symptoms begin to appear. In the end, you get a headache, fatigue, or depression—and in many cases, disease. When you try to treat the last domino with some medication, the cause of the problem isn't addressed—and remains.

Being able to differentiate between primary and secondary problems is important for all of us—especially health care professionals who can be more objective in their evaluations. Unfortunately, with today's health care deficiencies, time is one thing many patients don't get.

The classic example of this scenario is treatment of a diseased organ. A heart bypass operation or removing a cancerous growth might temporarily alleviate the problem. But what about addressing the root cause of the problem? If it's not found, how long will it take before another major problem arises, if it hasn't already?

As you become more intuitive about your health and as you better understand how food affects you, it will be easier to understand your body's signs and symptoms—it's as if your body is calling out to get your attention for assistance. This is an important part of taking responsibility for your own health.

Fueling our body and brain with proper food provides energy to help balance our health and fitness and increase human performance. This comes in the form of food—each bite one takes should be associated with building up the body, at every age, rather than tearing it down.

Choose Your Food Wisely

Food is the foundation of everything you do. Without the right fats for the aerobic system, energy will be limited. Without the thousands of nutrients from fresh vegetables and fruits, the immune system can't stop the process of illness and disease. And without the balance of macronutrients—the proper amounts of carbohydrates, fats, and proteins your particular body needs—the brain can't continue to thrive.

In order to achieve optimal human performance, wise decisions about the foods you eat are essential. The best foods help the body produce nearly unlimited energy, increase fat burning to avoid weight gain, and achieve optimal brain function at all ages.

You need these important nutrients every day. That's because the body is constantly making new cells and, in fact, always replacing itself, so it's actually making new parts all the time. The body has around a trillion cells. Some have a normal life span of only a few months, such as red blood cells. Others last much longer, such as bone cells. So different areas of the body renew themselves more often than others. Some cells last our whole life—brain cells are not always replaced but still rely on many vitamins, minerals, fats, and proteins to maintain optimal function. The building blocks that are used to produce and maintain this new body come from the foods one eats. So in a real sense, you really are what you eat.

Just as each of us has a different set of fingerprints, the specific requirements for carbohydrates, fats, and proteins, along with the right amounts of vitamins, minerals, and fiber, can vary from person to person. To build and maintain optimal health, you must supply your body with the right mix of fuels and nutrients that matches your individual needs. This is much easier than you think. Or used to be.

All animals on earth know how to eat. However, most humans have lost their instinctive ability to make wise food choices and instead look elsewhere—diet books, TV shows, magazine, and newspaper articles—for advice. Unfortunately, we are inundated with messages about how and what to eat—usually from the most unreliable sources, the same companies that sell them. Much of this information is misleading and actually promotes eating unhealthy foods. In fact, even the U.S. government is involved in this disinformation campaign.

In *The New York Times*, a recent headline read, "While Warning about Fat, U.S. Pushes Sales of Cheese." With dwindling sales, fast-food chain Domino's Pizza needed marketing help. They got it from an organization called Dairy Management, with the result of a new line of pizzas with 40 percent more cheese. After a $12-million marketing campaign, sales soared. But the healthy change for Domino's gave the junk food much more dairy—containing the worse kind of saturated fat that contributes to chronic inflammation, a stepping-stone to illness such as cancer and heart disease, not to mention a significant addition of calories. The problem? Dairy Management is a marketing creation of the U.S. Department of Agriculture (USDA), the very government agency promoting a federal antiobesity drive that discourages overconsumption of fast food and saturated fat. And Dairy Management is looking for ways to get more dairy into the American diet. The largest source of saturated fat is cheese.

Only a few weeks earlier in the fall of 2010, at the National Restaurant Association's annual meeting, First Lady Michelle Obama asked everyone to help fight obesity, specifically mentioning the increased consumption of cheeseburgers and macaroni and cheese. But along the way, as the *New York Times* reported, confidential agreements approved by agriculture secretaries in both the Bush and Obama administrations, Dairy Management has helped expand cheese-laden choices on the menus of restaurants, including Taco Bell, whose popular steak quesadilla averages eight times more cheese than all other food items on the menu.

The U.S. government, along with the dairy industry, finances Dairy Management—with an annual budget of nearly $140 million. The *New York Times*'s investigation reported that "the organization's activities, revealed through interviews and records, provide a stark example of inherent conflicts in the Agriculture Department's historical roles as both marketer of agriculture products and America's nutrition police." And that "in one instance, Dairy Management spent millions of dollars on research to support a national advertising campaign promoting the notion that people could lose weight by consuming more dairy products, records and interviews show. The campaign went on for four years, ending in 2007, even though other researchers—one paid by Dairy Management itself—found no such weight-loss benefits."

It's not just the dairy lobby that's at fault here, or the USDA. The problem is much more systemic. One reason for the widespread presence of heavily biased information is how the editorial process works—many critical articles and interviews never get published or aired because the information clashes with advertisers who also sponsor "scientific studies"—often with the public not suspecting there's a conflict of interest.

There is an endless stream of money devoted to selling unhealthy food. Large corporations spend billions of dollars telling us what we should eat. The effect is Pavlovian. How many times have you seen a food or beverage commercial on TV and suddenly had an intense craving for whatever was being advertised? And how often did you feel the need to buy a certain product because a talk show "health expert" said that it can improve your health? The answer to both questions is often this: that's because of the seductive power of media.

The brainwashing starts at an unbelievably early age. According to a November 2010 study by Yale University's Rudd Center for Food Policy, children as young as two years old are seeing more fast-food ads than ever before, and restaurants provide largely unhealthy defaults for the side dishes and drinks that come with kids' meals.

The reports authors looked at the marketing efforts and menus of twelve of America's largest fast-food chains. They examined the calories from fat and sugar in more than three thousand kids' meal combinations. The study revealed that the fast-food industry spent more than $4.2 billion on marketing and advertising in 2009, focusing extensively on television, the Web social media sites, and mobile applications. Preschoolers in 2009 saw 21 percent more ads for McDonald's, 9 percent more ads for Burger King, and 56 percent more ads for Subway than they did in 2007.

McDonald's has thirteen different websites, including those targeted toward children. Each month, 365,000 kids ages two to eleven and 294,000 teens ages twelve to seventeen visit those sites. Even parents are affected by the Golden Arches's marketing blitz: 30 percent of parents surveyed wrongly thought chicken nuggets—which are laden with refined carbohydrate and fat—were healthful or somewhat healthful choices for their kids.

Finally, the report discovered that most fast-food restaurants that do offer healthful alternatives for kids—sliced apples instead of fries, for example—usually don't present them up front by the cash register and continue to serve fries as the default option ("Do you want fries with that?") unless the customer specifically asks for the apples.

Likewise, we cannot rely on the government to provide meaningful guidelines for minimal nutritional requirements. We saw this with its pushing milk and cheese consumption. Over the years, the USDA has also come up with many different dietary recommendations—I often referred to these as pyramid schemes—with carbohydrates forming the base of its food pyramid. Fruits and vegetables are the base of my pyramid. Carbohydrate foods (which includes many fruits) would be nearer to the middle of my pyramid. And what's more, it would not include refined items such as most bread and pasta or processed cereal. Instead, my slimmer carbohydrate layer would be made up of fruits, legumes, and limited amounts of 100 percent whole grains. Proteins and healthy fats would share a layer in my pyramid; in fact, many nutritional experts are now beginning to realize that many people, including those over age fifty, do not meet protein requirements.

While these are often associated with updates in scientific information, special interest groups and lobbyists such as the sugar, wheat, and corn industry heavily influence these recommendations.

In 2011, the plate replaced the pyramid. After spending millions in research, the USDA introduced its new colorful icon, named "My Plate," in the hopes of simplifying the basics of healthy nutrition for the American public. The plate image is divided into TV dinnerlike quadrants, with four portions of nearly equal size: vegetables, fruits, protein, and grains; there's also a fifth or side serving of "dairy." While the round symbol is an improvement over past pyramids, it's still vague and imprecise because it omits critical details such as eating good fats or the need to avoid large amounts of processed grains and sugar. Nor is there any recommendation how large each of the servings should be, or even the size of the plate.

The truth is that each person should have his or her individualized nutritional game plan. There is no "one plate fits all." But you can build your own healthy-eating foundation or model by adopting these easy-to-follow recommendations:

- The first is to only eat real food—not processed or artificial, but foods provided by nature. For most people, fast junk food is the largest component of their diet. It includes refined carbohydrates—cereal, bread, bagels, rolls, and pasta—including sugar and sugar-containing foods.
- Another key feature of a healthy food plan is balancing fats by eating sufficient amounts of healthy ones such as omega-3 fats in fish and monounsaturated oils in almonds, avocados, and olive oil and avoiding all unhealthy ones such as trans fat and corn, peanut, safflower, and other vegetable oils. Low fat can mean low energy and poor health.
- Consume sufficient amounts of high-quality protein, with animal sources being the most efficient.
- Eat sufficient amounts of fresh vegetables and fruits—the source of thousands of little-known nutrients.
- Drink adequate amounts of pure water, something many people fail to achieve.

By choosing your foods wisely, you'll learn to avoid the unhealthy, destructive items and consume only healthy choices that help your body build the best new cells every day. Having this kind of power will change your life. You just need to know how to best harness this knowledge.

CHAPTER 2

CARBOHYDRATE INTOLERANCE AND THE TWO-WEEK TEST
Learning How to Move Past Low Energy, Fatigue, and Weight Gain

I rarely talk about "classic cases" because each of us has unique needs. But an exception is in order, at least in the general presentation of the following scenario. One of my former patients named Susan had a long list of signs and symptoms. At age fifty-two, she felt twenty years older than her chronological age. She was a postal worker with a great sense of humor, which kept her plugging along from day to day. She told me that first time things didn't feel right was about ten years earlier when she began to experience weakness and shakiness if she didn't get to lunch on time. Then these feelings started occurring just before a delayed dinner. Each year after that, it seemed that a new complaint such as swelling in her hands would pop up. Susan also realized that, while shopping for new clothes, she was now larger in the waist and hips. At her annual physical, her doctor noticed that her blood pressure was too high. Her blood tests were normal except for high levels of fats in the blood called triglycerides. Susan was given medication to reduce blood pressure, but no other recommendations other than to return for a checkup in six months.

Six months later, Susan returned to the doctor's office for a blood test. Now she complained of being extremely tired after lunch, becoming so sleepy she was almost unable to perform her work. She considered retirement. Following dinner, she could not do any mental or physical activity, only watch TV with the result of falling asleep within a half hour. She told the doctor that her mild intestinal bloating was becoming more of a problem.

But the doctor didn't seem to be concerned about those symptoms. He said that she seemed more depressed than usual, which she confirmed. Then he explained that her blood fats, triglycerides, were alarmingly high. And her blood pressure was also not being well controlled by the medication. After getting a change in blood pressure medication and new prescriptions for high triglycerides and an antidepressant, Susan reluctantly made another appointment. But when she returned home, she decided to seek out another health care practitioner who could find the causes of her problems. She also did not fill the new prescriptions and decided to stop taking her blood pressure medication.

Susan visited my clinic a few months later, referred by a neighbor who was also a patient. I read the survey forms Susan filled out, looked through her diet diary, and asked more questions about her family history and other lifestyle habits. Virtually all her signs and symptoms appeared to come from high levels of the hormone insulin—which helps convert the sugar absorbed from carbohydrate foods to energy, but also stores some as body fat—and was later confirmed in a blood test. The high insulin appeared to be caused by eating too much refined carbohydrates—the main foods in her diet. To test this notion, I asked her to eliminate all white flour products, such as bagels, pasta, rolls and bread, and sugar and sugar-containing foods, including the daily container of yogurt she ate for lunch, (which contained seven teaspoons of sugar,) the two bottles of Gatorade, and a bowl of low-fat ice cream after dinner. She would be allowed to eat all other foods and was instructed to eat enough so as not to get hungry. Susan called the clinic every two to three days with questions about what to eat and not eat as she was serious about getting better.

Susan's next visit two weeks later was remarkable. Her clothes were becoming looser, and she lost eight pounds. She was full of energy; she was no longer sleepy even after meals. Her feelings of depression and intestinal bloating were gone. I measured her blood pressure, and it significantly decreased.

A blood test from this visit later showed normal insulin and triglycerides.

Extraordinary results? Yes for Susan. But from my own perspective, I had gotten used to seeing these life-changing results following a change in diet. Years earlier I had become acutely aware of the damage done by refined carbohydrates—I studied the delicate blood sugar mechanisms in textbooks, and once in private practice, I learned how to help patients fix their carbohydrate dysfunction—with all its signs and symptoms.

Food and nutrition is such a vast topic with many important components that it would appear difficult to find a starting point. But beginning with a discussion of carbohydrate-rich foods makes sense because its overconsumption is one of the primary causes of ill health, including functional problems, disease, and being overly fat.

If we could magically make white flour and sugar disappear from our food supply—including all the products made from them—the nation's health would improve drastically and almost overnight. And there would be countless stories like the one of Susan. While this won't happen soon enough in our society because there's too much money involved in their existence, it can happen for you—but only if this is a primary problem undermining your health and fitness. I'm not saying all carbohydrates are unhealthy; it's the processed ones that tens of millions of people are unable to tolerate.

Food history in the United States tells an interesting but sad story. In the early 1900s, companies began refining healthy, natural foods at a more rapid rate than ever before. More processing of food meant a longer shelf life, less spoilage, and higher profits. This change coincided with a huge transformation in the retail environment. No longer were shopping markets comprised of many single-food sellers—the butcher, the bread vendor, the fresh-produce stand, and the honey farmer. These small family businesses were being eliminated in favor of products from big corporations that were mass-produced and processed as well as packaged foods that would become staples in the American diet. After World War II, the transformation quickened, as small markets were being replaced by new supermarkets—a one-stop store where shoppers could get everything they needed without going to separate retailers.

Instead of bread turning stale after one day, it would appear fresh for many days and even weeks. That's because the part of the wheat most vulnerable to spoilage is the oil contained in the germ of the wheat berry, and along with the bran, these parts were removed in manufacturing. Unfortunately, these same parts are where most of the nutrition is found. Bread also had to be sweeter in taste. Adding more sugar helped accomplish this task.

Now the so-called pure white items became common household ingredients—

buckets of pure white flour and white sugar would be in almost every kitchen in the United States by the 1950s. Almost overnight, America's food supply exchanged quality for quantity. These ingredients became a staple—not just cookies, cakes, and candies but whole meals like cereal, pancakes, and pasta. Cooking was made easy for housewives—boxes of white flour and sugar, which sometimes only required the addition of water, produced "homemade" items for breakfast, lunch, and dinner, along with desserts and snacks.

An epidemic of chronic illness—in particular, cancer and heart disease—began to emerge from this new American diet. Alarmed by this trend, longtime radio nutritionist Dr. Carlton Fredericks and writer Adele Davis began pointing out the dangers of unhealthy eating. The most dangerous culprits were white flour and sugar. Most people ridiculed their ideas.

Twenty years later, the majority of Americans would be overly fat; the obesity epidemic was ready to explode.

The trend in carbohydrate overconsumption continues today, propelled by companies selling products made from the same refined carbohydrates and sugar, just repackaged, renamed, and even remarketed as healthy. At one time it was just called sugar, technically referred to as sucrose. Now, there are alternative names created by the industry as a means to trick consumers into thinking it's not the same old sugar: raw sugar, cane sugar, dextrose (corn sugar), high-fructose corn syrup, maltose, glucose, and more. Most of these names have been formulated by marketing people to counter the negative image of sugar that's been building in recent decades. Cane juice, raw sugar, and now corn sugar will be substituted for high-fructose corn syrup, which has been getting too much bad press.

The bottom line, sweet for the sugar industry but sour for our health, is that sucrose (made from refined sugar cane and sugar beets) and high-fructose corn syrup are the two most common refined sugars consumed today. In the last twenty years years, annual sugar consumption has risen from 25 to 135 pounds per person. In 1900, it was 5 pounds annually—as much as some people consume today in one week! Or consider this: a twelve-ounce can of Coke or Pepsi contains 40 grams of sugar, or about nine teaspoons of the white stuff. Both are America's favorite soft drink beverages supported by lavish advertising and marketing campaigns that extend all the way to school classroom.

And the government is right there showing its support, with the United States Department of Agriculture (USDA) telling Americans to eat more sugar. The first USDA dietary recommendations were made in the early 1900s—sugar was one of the five food groups (along with meat/milk, cereal, vegetables/fruits, fatty foods). It was a guide called

Food for Young Children released in 1916 and would soon be followed by others. Through the years, generations of people followed the USDA recommendations, which became simplified as food pyramids in the 1980s. The result was that people ate a diet that contained more sugar and other refined carbohydrates because the foundation of these recommendations were carbohydrate foods. In addition, government officials continued to be heavily influenced by the U.S. sugar industry. This was shown in the 2006 election; with sugar prices a potential target for reform in 2007, the U.S. sugar industry, which donated $2.7 million to U.S. House and Senate incumbents, staved off any change. The process continued when, in 2011, the USDA replaced the pyramid with the "My Plate" icon suggesting similar, but a slightly improved (with the addition of fruits and vegetables), food plan.

For more than 99 percent of our existence on earth, humans consumed diets that were relatively low in carbohydrates—with zero-refined forms—but higher in natural fat, protein, and vegetables. More importantly, significant amounts of plant foods were also consumed, especially vegetables, fruits, nuts, and seeds.

Looking further back in human history, we see two other dramatic changes that influenced our dietary habits. This first one was about five thousand years ago. It was a revolution for humans, the transition from the prehistoric to an organized society. This is sometimes called the first Agricultural Revolution, or Neolithic Revolution, beginning, perhaps, in the eastern Mediterranean Sea and Mesopotamia where civilization began. Humans made the transition from hunting animals and gathering wild plant foods to domesticating livestock and farming. It also included growing foods, especially barley, the primary starch in the region.

But it was the Industrial Revolution, especially in the United States during the second half of the 1800s, with its machinery to process carbohydrate crops, which brought highly refined unhealthy food in great supply to the kitchen table. For the first time in their history, humans began consuming large amounts of adulterated food, most notably highly processed wheat and sugar.

Here's an example of what the new machinery could do: easy-to-grow and cheap wheat become the major crop, which was processed to increase shelf life and make it easier to use in cooking. As I mentioned earlier, this was accomplished by removing the healthiest portions of the plant—the germ and bran, the most nutritious parts—leaving only the starch, the least nutritious part. Today, most people have never tasted or even seen whole unrefined wheat berries—instead they are quite familiar with the pure white fine powdery flour which, when consumed, acts like pure sugar.

The production of sugar increased dramatically as a result of new machinery, and by the nineteenth century, sugar was transformed from a food for the rich to a staple throughout the world that millions of people could afford. Today, annual sugar production worldwide is over 270 billion pounds. Sugar's marketing success is exemplified in the newest epidemic: obese babies. This is due to the latest highly processed baby cereals and fruit juices, which are actually worse than eating pure sugar.

CEREAL KILLERS: GETTING KIDS HOOKED ON SUGAR

Saturday-morning children cartoon shows have long been a golden meal ticket for the breakfast cereal industry. Here was a young, captive, and impressionable market ready to be exploited for maximum economic gain. Television commercials targeted to kiddies often feature cartoon mascots. For example, Huckleberry Hound, that fun-loving Hanna-Barbera blue cartoon dog from the early '60s, promoted Kellogg's Frosted Sugar Stars because he "loved these sugar-toasted oats."

Another popular mascot for Kellogg's was Sugar Pops Pete, a gun-twirling prairie pup who was sheriff in a Western town. He ruled from 1959 to 1967 with an iron paw, going up against bad guys like Billy the Kidder while singing the following jingle: "Oh, the Pops are sweeter and the taste is new. They're shot with sugar, through and through!" In the early '80s, Pete was replaced by Poppy, a female porcupine who carted around a suitcase with a full breakfast setting. Why the luggage? It was in response to a new food industry standard that mandated cereal be made "part of a complete breakfast."

Sugar Corn Pops was originally called Corn Pops when it debuted in 1951 and was the sponsor of *The Adventures of Wild Bill Hickok* radio show. Kellogg's described the brand as "crunchy sweetened popped-up corn cereal." Its actual ingredients included milled corn, sugar, soluble corn fiber, molasses, salt, and partially hydrogenated vegetable oil. Because it paid to have sugar in the name, the cereal switched to Sugar Corn Pops, yet it later reverted to Corn Pops in the '70s when a health-conscious public persuaded cereal companies to drop "sugar" from their brand's name. (Many "new" cereals were now marketed as containing "$\frac{1}{3}$ less sugar." What about the remaining two-thirds?) In January 2006, the name of Corn Pops was shortened to just Pops, but after several months of poor sales, it was changed back to Corn Pops. In 2009, a new animated mascot for Corn Pops was created—the Sweet Toothasaur.

Shoppers will find the following product description in large type on the cereal box's front panel: "Crispy, Glazed, Crunchy Sweet."

Why not simply call sugar-fortified cereal "breakfast candy"?

With annual sales of over $13 billion, Kellogg's of Battle Creek, Michigan, is the world's leading manufacturer of cereal (it also makes cookies, crackers, toaster pastries, cereal bars, fruit-flavored snacks, frozen waffles, and vegetarian foods). Other cartoon-mascot sugar-fortified cereals in its portfolio include Frosted Flakes, Froot Loops, Cocoa Krispies, and Frosted Krispies.

But why stop with cartoon figures? Why not hook up with Hollywood? Kellogg's created a movie tie-in brand called Pirates of Caribbean. This sugar-enriched cereal featured a large photo of actor Johnny Depp, a.k.a. Captain Jack, on the front panel.

In 2010, Kellogg's voluntarily recalled twenty-eight million boxes of Apple Jacks, Corn Pops, Froot Loops, and Honey Smacks due to an odd soapy or metallic smell and flavor coming from the packager's liners. The company had received about two dozen complaints from consumers, including those who reported nausea and vomiting. The liners were made with the chemical 2-methylnaphthalene, which is a component of crude oil and is chemically related to naphthalene, an ingredient found in mothballs and toilet deodorant blocks that the Environmental Protection Agency considers a cancer-forming agent.

Even though the cereal had been withdrawn from store shelves, its replacement still contained that other silent killer: sugar.

Carbohydrates and Insulin

To better understand the harmful effects of sugar and refined carbohydrates, let's consider the basic physiology of how the body reacts to the consumption of these foods.

Common carbohydrate foods—including breads and other items made with flour such as rolls, muffins, pancakes, waffles, cereals, and pasta—are among the highest in refined carbohydrates. Even products that list "whole wheat" contain mostly, or all, refined flour.

Other carbohydrates include the many forms of sugar people use at home and work, in recipes, coffee and tea, and on cereal. Hidden sugars found in many foods, from ketchup and cocoa to processed meat and fish and virtually all desserts, are also significant sources of carbohydrate. One of the main problems associated with eating these foods has to do with insulin.

Insulin, which is a hormone made by the pancreas, is responsible for converting the blood sugar into immediate energy or storage as body fat for later use. Just the mere taste of sugar on the tongue stimulates the release of insulin. Once swallowed, sugar and other carbohydrates foods are digested and absorbed into the blood as glucose (blood sugar). This stimulates the release of insulin as well, with more sugar causing higher productions of insulin.

With insulin responsible for converting the increase in blood sugar into immediate energy or fat storage, a carbohydrate meal undergoes three key actions:

- About 50 percent of the carbohydrate you eat is quickly used for energy in the body's cells. This is how the sugar industry promotes its product—as an energy food.
- Up to 10 percent of the carbohydrate you eat is stored as a reserved form of sugar called glycogen. This occurs in the muscles, where glycogen is later turned back into glucose for energy use, and in the liver, where it helps maintain proper blood sugar levels between meals and during nighttime sleep.
- About 40 percent or more of the carbohydrate you eat is converted to fat and stored. This is the reason why so many people have excess body fat—a significant amount of the carbohydrate foods consumed, particularly refined flour items and sugar, even if it's nonfat, are converted to stored body fat.

It should be noted that small amounts of insulin may also be produced if one consumes a protein-only meal, and in some people, a high-protein meal can stimulate significant amounts of insulin. But usually, it's carbohydrates that trigger the insulin mechanism.

The more carbohydrates consumed, the more insulin produced. Some individuals are even more vulnerable, including people with higher-than-normal body fat content, those with a family history of diabetes, sedentary people, and those consuming large amounts of carbohydrates over a lengthy period. In these cases, carbohydrate consumption can lead to a whole range of problems, from functional problems such as fatigue and intestinal bloating to diseases like diabetes.

The functional problems are not well defined and difficult to assess; that is why many health care professionals dismiss them. The more advanced illnesses and diseases have different names depending on the point in time they occur—an early-stage condition may be referred to as insulin resistance, and a few years later it may be diagnosed as hyperinsulinemia, and a several years after that, type 2 diabetes. But these problems are just different names on a spectrum I term "carbohydrate intolerance."

Carbohydrate Intolerance

With generations of people overconsuming sugar and other refined carbohydrates, many now have carbohydrate

35

intolerance—or CI—the most well-hidden epidemic.

The full spectrum of CI begins as a hidden problem; it can progress to a functional disorder producing symptoms like fatigue that negatively affects quality of life and can gradually result in serious illness such as diabetes or heart disease. An individual may find himself or herself at any point along this spectrum. To check how your body handles carbohydrates, the following survey will be useful. Perhaps you are carbohydrate intolerant and don't even realize it.

While best viewed as a series of a single escalating progression of the same problem, carbohydrate intolerance (CI) has distinct stages:

- In the early stages, the symptoms can be elusive, often associated with difficult-to-diagnose blood sugar problems, fatigue, intestinal bloating, and loss of concentration.
- In the middle stages, the worsening condition may be referred to as carbohydrate-lipid metabolism disturbance or hyperinsulinism and cause more serious conditions such as hypertension, elevations of LDL and lowering of HDL cholesterol, elevated triglycerides, and increases in body fat.
- In the long term, carbohydrate intolerance manifests itself as more serious problems, including obesity and various diseases such as diabetes, cancer, and heart disease. These end-stage conditions are part of a set of diseases now well recognized and referred to as syndrome X, or the metabolic syndrome.

Carbohydrate Intolerance Health Survey—Some Common Signs and Symptoms

- Poor concentration or sleepiness after meals
- Increased intestinal gas or bloating after meals
- Frequently hungry
- Increasing abdominal fat or facial fat (especially cheeks)
- Frequently fatigued or low energy
- Insomnia or sleep apnea
- Waist size increasing with age
- Fingers swollen/feeling "tight" after exercise
- Personal or family history: diabetes, kidney or gall stones, gout, high blood pressure, high cholesterol/ low HDL, high triglycerides, heart disease, stroke, breast cancer
- Low meat, fish, or egg intake
- Frequent cravings for sweets or caffeine
- Polycystic ovary (ovarian cysts) for women

Children and CI

Carbohydrate intolerance also exists in young people—even newborns as the mother's blood sugar and associated carbohydrate and insulin metabolism are shared with the fetus. Children of mothers with CI are at much higher risk for disease later in life. For example, those with CI have an estimated tenfold greater risk for developing diabetes. Some children, who ultimately become diabetic, display symptoms of carbohydrate intolerance for twenty or thirty years before the onset of the disease.

In addition to children and even newborns, other groups of people are vulnerable to CI, including those who are physically inactive, under stress, taking estrogen, dark skinned, and those with a family history of diabetes and other diseases of the metabolic syndrome. Aging is also frequently accompanied by increased carbohydrate intolerance.

Taking the Carbohydrate Intolerance survey is only the first step in reclaiming your optimal health. The next step is taking the Two-Week Test, which will help you determine just how sensitive your body is to carbohydrates.

Carbohydrate Intolerance Health Survey for Children

- Low or high birth weight (5½ pounds or less, 9 pounds or more)
- Taller than average for age
- Increased weight or body fat
- Parent or grandparent is diabetic (adult onset)
- Sleep problems
- Mother: increased stress during pregnancy
- Increased aggression or anger
- Attention-deficit hyperactive disorder (ADHD)
- Overeating sweets or carbohydrates upsets
- Physical activity low
- Family history: high blood pressure, high cholesterol or triglycerides, heart disease or stroke, breast cancer
- Constant craving for sweets

The Two-Week Test

The Two-Week Test will tell you if you are carbohydrate intolerant and, if so, how to remedy it. Yet I must emphasize that this is only a test and not a permanent diet, and it will only last two weeks—you will not be eating like this forever. And most importantly, this is not a diet or should be pursued beyond this fourteen-day period. Nor should you experience hunger during the Two Week Test—you can eat as much of the noncarbohydrate foods as you want and as often as you need.

Many thousands of people have used my Two-Week Test to get healthy, fit, and significantly improve their energy levels. Others have found it to be the best way to start burning body fat. Still others have reduced or

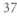

eliminated medications they once required. Of all the clinical tools I developed and used for assessment and therapy through my career, the consistent results from the Two-Week Test surprised me the most—at how a person can go from one extreme of poor health to vibrant health in such a short time. It's simply a matter of removing a major stress factor—refined carbohydrates and excess insulin—in a person's life and allowing the body to function the way it was originally meant.

HOW I DEVELOPED THE TWO-WEEK TEST

I developed the Two-Week Test in the mid-1980s. After spending almost seven years trying to wean carbohydrate-intolerant patients off white flour and sugar, it was exhausting work—almost like dealing with drug addicts. My goal was to lower carbohydrate intake to find the level that would eliminate signs and symptoms of excess insulin. The process went too slowly. One evening I was reading *The Merck Manual*, the most popular medical reference book used by health care professionals, to look up basic facts about assessment and treatment procedures. There was a single sentence, almost an aside, about elevations of insulin and how reducing carbohydrates might be necessary in some patients with hyperinsulinemia. Then I recalled a 1971 study from the *New England Journal of Medicine*. It was tucked away with copies of other studies in a folder called "Blood Sugar and Insulin" in my filing cabinet. As I paged through the study called "Effect of Diet Composition on the Hyperinsulinemia of Obesity," the proverbial pieces to the puzzle starting falling into place. Then I recalled another study. I searched the file hoping to find it. There it was, from Columbia University's Department of Medicine and published in the *Journal of Clinical Investigation* in 1976 ("Composition of Weight Lost during Short-term Weight Reduction")—it showed that ten days of restricted carbohydrate foods resulted in not only the loss of weight but significant reduction of body fat.

This information was not really new to me; it was the reason I was weaning patients' off insulin-provoking foods. But for some reason, the short excerpt and the other two studies brought everything into clearer focus. I asked myself, "If weaning patients off their unhealthy carbohydrate addiction was so difficult, why not go cold turkey so they could experience the immediate benefits?" They would actually feel better quickly because insulin levels would drop right away, and within the first few days, they would begin to experience life without harmful levels of this hormone rather than by slowly reducing those foods, which could take weeks or months to attain the same effect.

At first, this new test period I devised lasted ten days—the same period of time used in one of the studies I had reviewed. But the first few patients I used this new approach on needed more time off carbohydrates to fully appreciate the positive effects, especially with regard to burning body fats. I added four more days to the trial or testing period. Two weeks worked much better.

To be sure patients understood this was not a diet, I referred to it as a test. It eventually became known in my office as the Two-Week Test.

The Two-Week Test was unique. Not because it helped me better understand the patient's sensitivity to carbohydrate foods. But more importantly, rather than conducting a blood or urine test that provided numbers that most patients could not easily understand or translate to real-life changes, this new approach required individuals to take an active role the process of self-evaluation. During the testing period, he or she would actually feel what it was like to have normal insulin levels, optimal blood sugar, and in many cases be finally free of signs and symptoms associated with CI—all within a short time frame. This was a far superior method of educating the patient.

For those individuals who were not carbohydrate intolerant and didn't feel any different during the test, it ruled out CI as a common health problem. But patients who were overweight, had blood sugar problems, and simply could not escape the damage of eating refined carbohydrates, they now knew what it would take to quickly change their health.

It is not the purpose of the Two-Week Test to restrict calories or fat. It merely restricts many carbohydrate foods. And there's no need to weigh food. Just eat what you're allowed and avoid what's restricted for a period of two weeks. Nor is its purpose to avoid all dietary carbohydrates or go into ketosis (an extreme metabolic state of fat burning when little or no glucose is available for energy) like with some diet programs whose long-term success is questionable; in fact, once someone goes off one of these diets, weight gain is typical.

Before the Test

Before you start the Two-Week Test, jot down any health problems that you might have, such as insomnia or fatigue. This may take a few days since you might not recall

39

them all at once. This aspect is important because after the test, you will review these complaints to see which ones have improved and which have not.

Next, weigh yourself before starting the test. This is about the only instance I recommend using the scale for body weight—it's not a measure of body fat, but in this case it's a good pre- and postevaluation. During the test you may lose some excess water your body is holding, which will show on the scale, but you'll also go into a high fat-burning state and start losing body fat (which won't show on the scale). I've seen some people lose only a few pounds during the test, and some twenty or more pounds. This is not a weight-loss regime, and the main purpose of weighing yourself is to have another sign of how your body is working, especially after the test.

Before you start the test, make sure you have enough of the foods you'll be eating during the test—these are listed below. Go shopping and stock up on these items. This requires a little planning, so make a list of the foods you want to eat and the meals and snacks you want to make available. In addition, go through your cabinets and refrigerator and get rid of any sweets, foods containing them, and all breads and products made from refined flour. Otherwise, you'll be tempted. Many people are addicted to sugar and other carbohydrates, and you may crave these foods for the first few days without them.

Planning what to eat and how often is important. Schedule the test during a two-week period that you are relatively unlikely to have distractions—the holidays or times when social engagements are planned can make it too easy to stray from the plan. Don't worry about cholesterol, fat or calories, or the amount of food you're eating. This is only a test, not the way you'll be eating all the time.

Most importantly, eat breakfast within an hour of waking.

Following the test for less than two weeks probably will not give you a valid result. So, if after five days, for example, you eat a bowl of pasta or a box of cookies, you will need to start the test over.

Foods to Eat During the Test

You may eat as much of these foods as you like during the Two-Week Test:

- Eggs (whites and yolk), unprocessed (real) cheeses, heavy (whipping) cream, sour cream.
- Unprocessed meats including beef, turkey, chicken, lamb, fish, and shellfish
- Tomato, V8 or other vegetable juices
- Water—drink it throughout the day in between meals
- Cooked or raw vegetables such as squash, leaf lettuce and spinach, carrots, broccoli and kale, but no potatoes or corn
- Nuts, seeds, nut butters
- Oils, vinegar, mayonnaise, salsa, mustard, and spices
- Sea salt, unless you are sodium sensitive
- All coffee and tea (if you normally drink it)

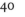

Be sure to read the ingredients for all foods as some form of sugar or carbohydrate may be added. These include peanut butter, mayonnaise, sour cream, and even sliced meats.

Foods to Avoid During the Test

You may not eat any of the following foods during the Two-Week Test:

- Bread, rolls, pasta, pancakes, cereal, muffins, chips, crackers, rice cakes, and similar carbohydrate foods
- Sweets such as cake, cookies, ice cream, candy, gum, breath mints
- Products that contain hidden sugars, common in ketchup and other prepared foods (read the labels)
- Fruits and fruit juice
- Processed meats and fish such as cold cuts and smoked products, which often contain sugar
- All types of potatoes, corn, rice, and beans
- Milk, half-and-half, and yogurt
- So-called healthy snacks, including all energy bars and sports drinks
- All soda, including "enhanced" mineral water and diet drinks

A Note on Alcohol

If you normally drink small to moderate amounts of alcohol, some forms are allowed during the test:

- Alcohol allowed: dry wines and pure distilled spirits (gin, vodka, whiskey, etc.), and those mixed with plain carbonated water, including seltzer, tomato juice, or V8.
- Alcohol not allowed: sweet wines, all beer, champagne, alcohol containing sugar (rum, liqueurs, etc.), and those mixed with sweet ingredients such as tonic, soda, or other sugary liquids. If in doubt, avoid it.

Below are some other suggestions for eating, food preparation, and dining out, which may be helpful during the Two-Week Test. You may find these suggestions useful after completing the test as well.

Meal Ideas

Eggs
- Omelets, with any combination of vegetables, meats, and cheeses
- Scrambled with guacamole, sour cream, and salsa
- Scrambled with a scoop of ricotta cheese and tomato sauce
- Boiled or poached with spinach or asparagus and hollandaise or cheese sauce; with bacon or other meats
- Soufflés

Salads
- Chef—leaf lettuce, meats, cheeses, eggs
- Spinach—with bacon, eggs, anchovies
- Caesar—Romaine lettuce, eggs, Parmesan cheese, anchovies
- Any salad with chicken, tuna, shrimp, or other meat or cheese

Salad Dressings

- Extra virgin olive oil and vinegar (balsamic, wine, apple cider), plain or with sea salt and spices
- Creamy—made with heavy cream, mayonnaise, garlic, and spices

Fish and Meats

- Pot roast cooked with onions, carrots, and celery
- Roasted chicken stuffed with a bulb of anise, celery, and carrots
- Chili-type dish made with fresh, chopped meat and a variety of vegetables such as diced eggplant, onions, celery, peppers, zucchini, tomatoes, and spices (no beans)
- Steak and eggs
- Any meat with a vegetable and a mixed salad
- Chicken parmigiana (not breaded or deep-fried) with a mixed salad
- Fish (not breaded or deep-fried) with any variety of sauces and vegetables
- Tuna melt on a bed of broccoli or asparagus

Sauces

- Plain melted butter.
- A quick cream sauce can be made by simmering heavy cream with mustard or curry powder and cayenne pepper or any flavor of choice. It's delicious over eggs, poultry, and vegetables.
- Italian-style tomato sauce helps makes a quick parmigiana out of any fish, meat, or vegetables. Put this over spaghetti squash for a pastalike dish. Or make lasagna with sliced grilled eggplant or zucchini instead of pasta.

Snacks

- Hard-boiled eggs
- Rolled slices of fresh meat and/or cheese wrapped in lettuce
- Vegetable juices
- Raw almonds, cashews, pecans
- Celery stuffed with nut butter or cream cheese
- Guacamole with vegetable sticks for dipping
- Leftovers from a previous meal

Dining Out

- Let the waiter know you do not want any bread or bread sticks to avoid temptation.
- Ask for an extra vegetable instead of rice or potato.
- Chinese: steamed meat, fish, or vegetables (no rice or sweet sauce).
- Continental: steak, roast, duck, fish, or seafood.
- French: Coquille Saint-Jacques, boeuf a la Bourguignonne.
- Italian: Veal parmigiana (not breaded or deep-fried), seafood marinara.

Avoid all fried food as it usually has breading or is coated in flour.

After Taking the Test

Reevaluate your original list of complaints after the Two-Week Test. Is your energy better? Are you sleeping better? Feeling less depressed? If you feel better now than you did two weeks ago, or if you lost weight, you probably have some degree of CI and you're unable to eat as much carbohydrate as you did before the test. Some people who have a high degree of CI will feel dramatically better than they did before the test, especially if there was a large weight loss. Some people say they feel like a new person after taking this test. Others say after a few days of the test, they feel young again.

Any weight loss during the test is not due to reduced calories, as many people eat more calories than usual during this two-week period. It's due to the increased fat burning resulting from reduced insulin. While there may be some water loss, especially if you are sodium sensitive, there is real fat loss.

If your blood pressure has been high, and especially if you are on medication, ask your health care professional to check it several times during the test, and especially right after the test. Sometimes blood pressure drops significantly and your medication may need to be adjusted, or eliminated, which should only be done by your health care professional. For many people, as insulin levels are reduced to normal, high blood pressure lowers too.

If nothing improved during the test—and it was done exactly as described above—then you may not be carbohydrate intolerant. But if the Two-Week Test improved your signs and symptoms, the next step is to determine how many carbohydrates your body can tolerate, without a return of these problems. This is done by adding a single-serving size of natural unprocessed carbohydrates to every other meal or snack. The purpose is to determine if any of these carbohydrates cause the return of any of the original signs or symptoms, including weight gain. At this stage, having just completed the test, your body and brain will be more aware of even slight reactions to carbohydrate foods—basically, you'll be more intuitive to how your body responds to food. This is done in the following manner over the next one to two weeks:

- Begin adding single-serving amounts of natural, unprocessed carbohydrates at every other meal or snack. This may be plain yogurt sweetened with a little honey for breakfast or an apple after lunch or dinner.
- For a snack, try tea with honey.
- Avoid all refined carbohydrates such as sugar and refined flour products (like white bread, cereals, rolls, or pasta).
- Other suggestions include brown rice, sweet potatoes, yams, lentils, and beans.

Most bread, crackers, cereals, and other grains are processed and should be avoided—even those stating "whole grain" or "100 percent whole wheat." Read the ingredients carefully. If you can find real-food whole grain products, they can be used. These include sprouted breads, whole oats (they take thirty to forty-five minutes to cook), and other dense products made with just ground wheat, rye, or other grains. If in doubt, avoid them during this one- to two-week period.

I want to emphasize again not to add carbohydrates in back-to-back meals or snacks because insulin production is partly influenced by your previous meal.

With the addition of carbohydrates, be aware of any symptoms you had previously that were eliminated by the test, especially for symptoms that develop immediately after eating, such as intestinal bloating, sleepiness, or feelings of depression.

Most importantly, if any signs or symptoms that disappeared during or following the Two-Week Test have now returned, you've probably exceeded your carbohydrate limit. For example, if your hunger or cravings were greatly improved at the end of the test and now they've returned, you probably added too many carbohydrates. If you lost eight pounds during the test and gained back five pounds after adding some carbohydrates for a week or two, you've probably eaten too many of them. Likewise, if blood pressure rises significantly after it was reduced, it may be due to excess carbohydrate intake. If any of these situations occur, reduce the carbohydrates by half; otherwise, experiment to see which particular foods cause symptoms and which don't. Some people return to the Two-Week Test and begin the process again.

In some cases, people can tolerate simple carbohydrates, such as fresh fruits, plain yogurt, and honey, but not complex carbohydrates such as sweet potato, whole grains, beans, or other starches. This may be due to the difficulty in digesting starches in some people with CI. In other situations, some individuals can't tolerate any wheat products due to a sensitivity or even allergy to gluten (discussed in the next chapter. During this posttest period, these dietary factors are often easy to determine.

After a one- to two-week period following the Two-Week Test, by experimenting with natural carbohydrates, you'll have an excellent idea about your body's level of tolerance. You'll better know which foods to avoid, which ones you can eat, and those that must be limited. You'll become acutely aware of how your body feels when you eat too many carbohydrates.

From time to time, you may feel the need to go through a Two-Week Test period again to check yourself, or to quickly get back on track after careless eating, such as during the holidays, vacations, or periods of stress.

Many people find the loss of grains in the diet leaves the digestive tract sluggish and a little constipated. After years of eating lots of carbohydrates, your intestine gets used to that type of bulk. If you become constipated during the Two-Week Test, or afterward when a lower amount of carbohydrate in the diet is maintained, it could be due to a number of reasons:

- First, you may not be eating enough fiber (this topic is discussed in more detail in chapter 7). Bread, pasta, and cereals are significant sources of fiber for many people.

- Psyllium is a high-fiber herb that is an effective promoter of intestinal function. Adding plain unsweetened psyllium to a glass of water, tomato juice, or healthy smoothie can keep your system running smoothly—start with one teaspoon a day for a few days to make sure it's tolerated and then use up to about one tablespoon a day. Another way to add psyllium to your diet is to use it in place of flour for thickening sauces or in place of bread crumbs to coat meats and vegetables. If you require a fiber supplement, be sure to use the ones that do not contain sugar, so read the labels. There are some sugar-free psyllium products on the market, and you should not have trouble finding one.

- Dehydration may be another reason for constipation at this time. If you don't drink enough water, you could be predisposed to constipation. During the Two-Week Test, you'll need more water—up to two to three quarts or more per day—which is really a normal amount for a person of average weight.

- After the test, vegetables, legumes such as lentils, and fruits are also great sources of fiber. So if you become constipated, it may simply be that you need to eat more vegetables and fruits as tolerated.

- In addition, adequate intake of natural fats, discussed later in this book, can also be helpful in preventing constipation.

Occasionally, some people get tired during or after the Two-Week Test. Most commonly it's from not eating enough food and/or not eating often enough. The most common problem is not eating breakfast. And many people should not go more than three to four hours without eating something healthy.

Maintaining Your Food Balance

Once you successfully finish the Two-Week Test and add back the right amount of tolerable carbohydrate foods, you should have an excellent idea of your carbohydrate limits—the amount of carbohydrate you can eat without producing abnormal signs or symptoms. This is best accomplished by asking yourself about mental and physical energy, sleepiness and bloating after meals, or any of the problems you had previous to taking the Two-Week Test. You may want to keep a diary so you can be more objective in your self-assessment. In time, you won't need to focus as much on this issue as your intuition will take over, and you'll automatically know your limits.

Once you find your level of carbohydrate tolerance, you're on your way to balancing your whole diet. Yet another important aspect of carbohydrate foods to be more aware of is which of the many choices available in supermarkets, farmer's markets, and elsewhere are truly healthy and which to avoid. While there's nothing radical about

Case History

Bob was determined to renew his health in a natural way. He was overweight and always exhausted, and his blood pressure, cholesterol, and triglycerides were too high. He started the Two-Week Test and initially felt quite good. But within a few days, he began getting tired and irritable. After I spent talking with Bob for just a few minutes, it was clear that he was doing several things wrong. Because the test caused him to spend more time in bathrooms, he did not drink much water during the day. In addition, since he thought about how many calories he was eating, he became calorie conscious and ate less. To make matters worse, he thought that yogurt was in the cheese group and was eating two or three containers of fruit yogurt each day. When I told Bob that the yogurt had six to seven teaspoons of sugar in each single-serving container and to forget about the calories for now and plan his water intake better, he started his test again. After the first week, he was feeling great and even better by week 2. Within a month, his energy remained high, and a couple of months after that, a visit to his regular doctor showed his blood pressure and blood fats were back to normal, and he had lost fourteen pounds.

the notion that refined carbohydrates are unhealthy, there are many radical diet plans that make it seem like all carbohydrates are deadly. They're not. Finding your level of tolerance is what's most important, and then eat only healthy carbohydrates—this is among the topics of the next chapter.

To summarize, here are the basics of the Two-Week Test:

- Write a list of all your signs and symptoms.
- Weigh yourself.
- Plan your meals and snacks—buy sufficient foods allowed on the test and get rid of those not allowed so you're not tempted.
- Eat as much as you need and as often to never get hungry.
- Always eat breakfast.
- After the test, reevaluate your signs and symptoms, including weight.
- Begin adding natural, unprocessed carbohydrates to every other meal or snack and evaluate whether this causes any of your previous signs or symptoms (or weight) to return.

CHAPTER 3

CARBOHYDRATE FOODS
The Good, the Bad, and the Really Harmful

Not all carbohydrates are created equal. A candy bar is full of carbs—the bad kind that leads to blood sugar problems, brain chemistry changes, and weight gain. A serving of fresh fruits or lentils is also full of carbs—the good kind that will give you sustained energy and curb your appetite.

As I pointed out in the previous chapter, refined carbohydrates—the most common ones being white flour and sugar—are harmful for most if not all people. In addition, the increased consumption of refined carbohydrate foods in the diet replaces many other healthy items—vegetables, fruits, eggs, fish, and meat. These items contain more nutrients to help build optimal health and fitness daily.

Another problem is that by regularly consuming sugar and other refined carbohydrates, you can sensitize your taste buds for more preference to sweetness than other tastes such as bitterness. Most vegetables have a slight bitter, nonsweet taste, and those who have become accustomed to the sweet tastes of sugary foods find mild bitterness unpleasant—the result being they end up disliking most vegetables such as leaf lettuce, broccoli, and squash. Even less sweet fruits such as blueberries, plums, and certain varieties of peaches are considered not taste-worthy when one's taste buds are always seeking sweetness.

Sugar Addiction: Why Is It So Hard to Kick?

What is it about sugar that makes it so difficult for many people to wean themselves from it by performing the Two-Week Test? Does the dependency have to do with a person's sweet tooth? Is the addiction to sweets an acquired habit? And why are some individuals able to live quite happily without sweets as part of their regular diet?

Through the years, I discovered that many of my former patients were initially unable to even consider the test because giving up sugar and sugar-containing foods, as well as refined carbohydrates, was much too difficult to contemplate. Even the lure and promise of optimal health, including weight loss, more energy, and better mental focus, was insufficient. They rather remained in the rut of their own choosing.

So why is sugar so addicting?

Many people with a sugar dependency argue that foods don't taste the same without being sweetened. Since sugar is such a widely used ingredient found in many processed products, from so-called healthy breads to cereals (even added to "bland" brands like Wheaties and Cheerios) and energy bars to even staples like tomato sauce, finding out which foods don't contain sugar or high-fructose corn syrup is often a nutritional challenge.

Scientific research of sugar's chemical effect on the body has shown that it triggers the brain's pleasure and reward centers—emotional areas responsible for the release of "feel good" neurotransmitters called dopamine. These are the same brain areas stimulated by cocaine, nicotine, opiates (such as heroin and morphine), and alcohol. This addiction is not an imaginary thing in the minds of millions of sugar junkies—it's associated with real physiological changes in the brain. Since the brain's pleasure areas are also close to the pain centers, withdrawal from sugar is often described by many people as being painful—not unlike experiencing romantic pain, the loss of a loved one, or eliminating nicotine or caffeine.

Psychoactive compounds present in cocoa and chocolate, salsolinol being the main one, might be why chocolate can also so be addicting. But the high levels of added sugar contained in most chocolate products are probably more addictive than the chocolate alone.

Sugar may also be a primary factor while other addictions are secondary. In this case, treating the sugar problem—getting a person off the white stuff—might be the first step in eliminating other harmful substances such as alcohol, nicotine, caffeine, or harder drugs like heroin and cocaine. Other modalities such as hypnosis, acupuncture, behavior modification, and psychotherapy can be useful. In my clinical experience, when helping patients who were addicted to drugs—from alcohol to amphetamines and caffeine to cocaine—the most successful cases with a positive outcome were initiated by first eliminating sugar and other refined carbohydrates.

If you are sugar-dependent, ask yourself this: "After a big meal of pasta, bread, soft drink, and dessert, does my behavior change?" Do you become sleepy, moody, or have a loss of concentration? When you avoid sugar altogether, do you experience cravings? Do you tend to eat sugary foods even though you know you shouldn't and feel you should better control yourself? Are sweets a comfort food for you? These questions about sugar addiction are similar to indications of drug addiction and the reason researchers and clinicians see an overlap between sweets and drugs. The sugar-bingeing cycle is perpetuated when sugar is unavailable, which is then followed by the urge to abuse the drug (sugar) again.

Let's look at some behavioral aspects of sugar addiction. Which of these statements applies to you when it comes to eating sugar-containing foods and other refined carbohydrates?

1. Eating until feeling uncomfortably full.
2. Eating large amounts when not physically hungry.
3. Eating much more rapidly than normal.
4. Often eat alone because you're embarrassed by how much you're consuming.
5. Feeling guilty, depressed, or disgusted after overeating.

6. Marked distress or anxiety regarding binge eating.

Binge-eating episodes are associated with three or more of these factors. These questions might provide criteria for a clinical diagnosis of binge eating with sugar. The most recent edition of *Diagnostic and Statistical Manual of Mental Disorders* (a thick book published by the American Psychiatric Association that provides descriptions and characteristic symptoms of different mental illnesses) defines "binge eating" as a series of recurrent binge episodes in which each one is defined as eating a larger amount of food than normal during any two-hour period. Without any exaggeration, I've been told this identical eating history by thousands of patients throughout my career—people who were not, in my opinion, mentally ill, but were binge eaters—and for the most part, because they simply couldn't wean themselves from sugary or highly processed foods.

In the study on addiction ("Sugar and Fat Bingeing Have Notable Differences in Addictive-like Behavior"), published in the *Journal of Nutrition* (2009), Nicole Avena and her colleagues at Princeton University's Department of Psychology state the following: "Individuals with a preference for bingeing on sweet foods tend to binge more frequently." In addressing an obvious question—why don't people binge on foods such as broccoli?—the authors write, "There must be some property

49

of palatable 'dessert' and 'snack' foods rich in sugar and/or fat that promotes binge eating. Sugars and fats are well known to have different effects on physiology and brain chemistry, which may be related to their different effects on behavior."

Baclofen is a medication known to reduce the intake of certain drugs of abuse. It's been used to treat those addicted to morphine, heroin, cocaine, and alcohol. Since sugar has behavioral and brain chemical similarities to drug abuse, it is the reason some researchers say sugar can be addicting. The same Princeton research team sought to determine whether Baclofen would have an effect on binge eating. Specifically, would Baclofen reduce sugar bingeing? It didn't. (However, they also tested to see if the drug reduced binge eating of fats which can also be a powerful addiction—it did.)

Maybe they are in denial, but many people have trouble accepting the notion that sugar is so addicting. It's not perceived in the same way as tobacco or alcohol. In fact, "more scientific studies are needed to study if sugar is indeed addicting" is the argument often voiced by the sugar industry and its well-paid lobbyists who also exert influence in the media and government. (To this day, the tobacco industry continues to argue that "more studies are needed" to determine whether cigarette smoking or secondhand smoke is truly harmful.)

But because sugar is strongly addictive, this knowledge is put to generous use by the same companies that put the sweet stuff in our food and drinks. They carefully place sugar-laden foods in easy-to-access locations, such as at the checkout counter; many are also placed at eye level for children to see while sitting in the shopping cart.

Halloween is the start of the so-called holiday season. It's not just in North America, but the nutritional horrors of Halloween candy-bingeing are experienced in most of Europe, China, Japan, and elsewhere. For candy manufacturers, it's their biggest moneymaking holiday. New York City's Economy Candy Store alone sells six thousand pounds of sugary treats for Halloween. Surveys show that thirty-six million children in the United States between the ages of five and thirteen collect candy. Of course, millions more children—and adults—of all ages gobble down pounds of sweets for days and weeks after Halloween, finishing just in time for the next holiday feeding frenzy. Thanksgiving, Christmas, New Year's, and right up to the Super Bowl parties are devastating from a health perspective. Just within the span of two months, many people have gained weight, lost health, got the flu, and must visit their doctor for help.

The Glycemic Index

The glycemic index (GI) is a list of carbohydrate foods rated by how much your blood sugar increases after eating them. The GI can refer to a single food or a whole meal. Changes in blood sugar and insulin can vary

A SUGAR-FREE SOCIETY?

If society placed sugar and other highly refined carbohydrates in the same heavily taxed and regulated category as cigarettes or booze or, better yet as illicit drugs like cocaine, crystal meth, or heroin, there would be a loud and angry revolt by a jittery public. State, city, and even federal government agencies would ban these foods due to the astronomical cost of health care associated with their addiction. Companies that produced cereals, candies, cookies, ice cream, soda, fruit juice, and sugar itself would be sued, much like the tobacco class-action lawsuits of recent history. One can easily imagine secret after-school chocolate-cookie-chip deals, black-market sugar fetching several hundred dollars per pound or only available by prescription, and the successful flourishing of sugar-addiction clinics where the treatment of choice would be artificial sweeteners such as saccharin, aspartame, and alcohol sugars. Drug cartels would shift their resources to establishing sugar cartels that would take over the supply chain by creating a network of well-guarded sugarcane plantations. In the major cities, clandestine sugar beet grow houses would keep local law enforcement officials busy.

But sugar is too much a part of our daily existence for it ever to become banned. Remove it from our lives and society would come crashing down. If we were to extrapolate the past twenty-year rise of per capita sugar consumption, which increased by 500 percent, and looked ahead two decades, the average supersized, overweight American will be eating over six hundred pounds of sugar each year. Another way to view this alarming number is by imagining your garage filled with sixty ten-pound bags of raw sugar.

With some countries such as England, Taiwan, and South Korea banning sugar-fortified food commercials on children's television shows, restricting or banning soda in schools, and with restaurants being required to post calories in menus, the nutritional battle lines have already begun to form.

Science is catching up, too, with studies showing what's already obvious—banning fast-food advertisements in the United States could reduce the number of overweight children by 18 percent, say the researchers from the National Bureau of Economic Research (NBER), a nonprofit research organization dedicated to studying the science and empirics of economics in the American economy. The study was published by the *Journal of Law and Economics* (2008) and performed by NBER economists Shin-Yi Chou of Lehigh University and other researchers.

But let's not wait for the government or science to get us to act first. Just like with other addictions, we are ultimately the responsible party. Each of us holds the power to control or eliminate (depending on one's definition) sugar addiction despite the ongoing propaganda from big corporations who continue to market their life-threatening foods to an unsuspecting, trusting, and overweight public.

greatly from person to person. But generally, both rise more rapidly with more refined carbohydrate intake.

The glycemic index (GI) is not new. The index was first used by H. Otto and his colleagues in 1973 and published in a German scientific journal. Briefly, it said carbohydrate foods elicit a glycemic response by the body—varying elevations in blood sugar that depended upon the type of food. In 1981, the first list of these foods—the glycemic index—was published. Since then, the use of the GI has grown steadily, and today it is commonly employed in research and medicine and among large numbers of health- and weight-conscious individuals as indicated by the many low glycemic-type best-selling books over the past two decades. Along the way, many foods, which had to be tested on humans one by one, were added to the list, and now there are almost 2,500 different food items.

In general, fruits, dairy products, and legumes have a lower GI; breads, breakfast cereals, rice, and products made from grains usually are high GI, but some are available in low-GI versions.

To determine the GI of a carbohydrate, researchers give subjects a single food following an overnight fast; it was then measured the changes in blood sugar. The GI is expressed as a percentage of the blood sugar changes to two reference foods—either glucose or white bread, which both have a GI of 100—but of the same carbohydrate content. Below is a sample of some foods from the glycemic index:

As you can see, some foods, such as cornflakes, have a reaction in the body that's

FOOD	GI (RELATIVE TO WHITE BREAD = 100)
Donut	107
Pancakes	114
Muffin (plain)	66
Scones	131
Fruit punch	95
Gatorade	111
Cornflakes	133

significantly greater (33 percent more) than plain white bread. So a bowl of cornflakes for breakfast would be much worse, from a standpoint of rising blood sugar and insulin, than eating two or three pieces of white bread.

Foods with a GI of 55 and below are considered low glycemic, and those above, higher glycemic. In the middle areas of this general scale are moderate glycemic foods.

High-GI foods, which produce the greatest glucose response, include bagels, breads, potatoes, sweets, and other foods that contain refined flour and sugar. Many processed cereals, especially those containing the sugar maltose, which has a high GI, produce an even higher glycemic response. Even foods you may think are good for you can trigger high amounts of insulin, including fruit juice and bananas. The biggest problems in most diets may be wheat products, potatoes, fruit juice, and sugar or sugar-containing products.

Carbohydrates with a lower GI include some fruits, such as grapefruits and cherries, and lentils. Noncarbohydrate foods, proteins, and fats usually don't cause a glycemic problem, although in some people, even meals high in protein and/or fat can trigger an abnormal insulin response. In these situations, eating smaller and more frequent low-glycemic meals often solves the problem, as discussed in a later chapter about healthy snacking. Most vegetables contain only small amounts of carbohydrates (except high-starch ones like potatoes and corn).

Carrots were at one time believed to be a high-glycemic food, but studies have shown the glycemic effect of this root vegetable to be relatively low.

Studies show that the GI may be important in the treatment and prevention of many chronic diseases, including diabetes, some cancers, heart disease, and in weight control.

The development of the GI marked a major paradigm shift from most previous studies on this subject because it considered the body's response to food instead of the number of grams or calories of carbohydrates. The concept that people can respond differently to foods containing the same amount of carbohydrates was not new—it's been part of the holistic philosophy for centuries. But to mainstream medicine, this was a breakthrough. I have used and referenced the GI in my writings for years.

Three Factors That Influence GI

The glycemic index of a food—and the whole meal it is part of—is also influenced by other ingredients:

- The natural fiber contained in foods can moderate the GI. Refined carbohydrates usually have reduced amounts of fiber, one reason they have a higher GI. Without fiber to slow digestion, absorption of glucose is more rapid, just like pure sugar. So eating a cookie or piece of cake, typically made from white flour, will cause more of an increase in blood sugar and insulin compared to eating a piece of fruit or whole grain crackers with the same amount of carbohydrate and calories but with a higher fiber content.

- The fat content of a food also affects its GI—fat lowers the glycemic index. Lower amounts of fat also result in quicker digestion and more rapid absorption of sugar. A meal containing some fats, such as olive oil or butter, slows digestion and absorption, resulting in a lower in GI.
- Like fiber and fat, the protein content of a food or meal also affects its GI. As protein levels rise, in general, the GI lowers.

The GI is not a list of healthy versus unhealthy food. In fact, most of the foods on the list contain refined carbohydrates and are unhealthy. Many people have learned that to lower a food's GI they could add fiber, fat, or protein because these ingredients slow glucose absorption. For example, a French baguette has a high GI of 95, but add butter and it's lowered to 68. That's interpreted as, "Hey, I'm eating healthy." No, it's still junk food. You'll still convert 40 percent or more of that carbohydrate into body fat!

The GI has two other drawbacks. The first is that its accuracy is now being questioned. Foods grown and prepared in different location can vary, including ripeness of fruit, physical forms of foods (for example, whole or ground), processing of foods, and how the food is prepared. My own research shows that an important factor not considered in the calculation of the more than 2,500 foods on the GI is the effect of a food's sweetness during the testing process. Stimulation of sweetness by the taste buds in the mouth can cause immediate changes in blood sugar and insulin before the food being tested is digested and absorbed. As different people chew their food for varying lengths of time, and each can have very different taste sensation, this can affect the final outcome; these factors have not been considered in the research.

Another problem is that people misread the GI numbers. Bananas are a good example. The average GI for five different bananas studied is 51. While many people would think that's acceptable, this is the same number as ice cream and almost the same (52) as sweet corn, two foods a health-conscious person would avoid. And consider the range of GI for different bananas, which are different varieties and from different geographical regions: from a low of 30 to a high of 75! Clearly some bananas—the small "baby" bananas—have a much lower glycemic index while the common large ones are much higher.

Without considering the overall picture, the GI has become just another fad diet for legions of overweight people to pursue. Society has gone from being calorie-fixated to GI-obsessed, seeking out those foods that are low glycemic, or that can be made low-glycemic by adding fat or fiber, thinking they're healthier—but that is simply not always true. Because sugar addiction remains the real, underlying, primary problem.

Cardiovascular Disease and Sugar

For decades, most "authorities" blamed the dramatic rise in heart disease, stroke, and other cardiovascular problems on dietary fats—with cholesterol singled out as the main villain. This thinking or antifat approach was an easy sell to the public, who accepted low- and no-cholesterol recommendations despite almost-zero evidence that it ever contributed to illness or disease. Millions of people suddenly avoided eggs, and the chicken-laying industry was nearly wiped out in favor of highly refined carbohydrate foods: breakfast cereals, instant pancake mixes, and frozen waffles—virtually all of which contain added sugars. Sure, a few prominent voices objected to the new anti-egg hysteria, but multimillion-dollar ad campaigns engineered by the large processed-food companies made sure that "everyone knows eating eggs raises your cholesterol"—but in reality, they don't.

The fact is, refined carbohydrates and sugar can cause the same problems that were once blamed on dietary cholesterol: triglyceride and cholesterol blood test numbers that increased the risk of heart disease. While an entire chapter is devoted to this subject in section III, here are some important factors about sugar and refined carbohydrates that can significantly increase the risk of heart disease:

- *Triglycerides.* Abnormally high levels of triglycerides in the blood—which raise the risk of heart disease—are usually the result of a diet high in refined carbohydrates. The increased triglycerides are due to the conversion of dietary carbohydrates by insulin into fat—triglycerides. In my experience, a blood test that measures fasting triglycerides levels over 100 mg/dl (milligrams per deciliter) might be an indication of carbohydrate intolerance—even though 100 is in the so-called normal range (where 150 or 200 is considered the upper limit of normal). Instead of medication to lower triglycerides, the most popular therapy, treating the cause of the problem—eliminating refined carbohydrates—will usually normalize triglycerides quickly, often during the Two-Week Test.

- *Cholesterol.* The now-well-known blood cholesterol picture associated with an increased risk of heart disease includes low levels of the "good" HDL cholesterol and high levels of the bad LDL (these two types of cholesterol are discussed in greater detail in chapter 24). A diet of refined carbohydrates can produce just this type of cholesterol imbalance. A study by Jean Welsh and her colleagues from Emory University published in the *Journal of the American Medical Association* in April 2010 showed that added sugars used in many packaged foods are a common cause of high LDL cholesterol and reduced HDL. (Research has not shown that eating eggs or other cholesterol in the diet causes the same problem—in fact, consuming egg yolks can reduce your risk because they can raise your good cholesterol.)

- *High blood pressure.* Most people with hypertension, which raises the risk of heart disease, have CI. There is often a direct relationship between insulin levels and blood pressure—as average insulin levels elevate, so does blood pressure. In addition, sodium sensitivity is a common secondary problem in some individuals—consuming too much sodium causes water retention along with elevated blood pressure. By significantly reducing or eliminating refined carbohydrates, blood pressure usually normalizes, and often sodium sensitivity as well. As with high triglycerides, this can occur during the period of the Two-Week Test (changes in blood cholesterol usually take longer, depending on the person).

Carbohydrate Foods: The Good and the Bad

Once the Two-Week Test has helped you determine the amount and type of healthy carbohydrates your body can tolerate, it's likely that some of these types of foods will remain a stable part of your diet. When choosing carbohydrate foods, it's important to emphasize that not all carbs are created equal. It's not a level playing field. Some carbohydrates are more natural than others; in general, the more highly processed the carbohydrate food is, the worse it is for you. Highly processed carbohy-

drates generally have a higher glycemic index than those that are processed less or not processed at all. Most commercially processed bread, bagels, rolls, cereals, and other grain products, and those containing sugar, are so highly processed with virtually no nutritional value they can only harm your body and brain, impairing physical energy and mental clarity. This does not mean you can't enjoy eating great gourmet meals, including certain desserts, such as cheesecake, brownies, and fudge. They can be delicious and nutritious when made with healthy ingredients without sugar and white flour.

So what carbohydrates should you eat? Here's a healthy start:

- *Fruit.* At the top of the list of healthy carbohydrates is fruit. In addition to containing vitamins and minerals, fruit also contains important phytonutrients, which include thousands of plant nutrients important for health and disease prevention (some include beta-carotene, tocotrienols, and gingerol). At the low or good end of the glycemic index are cherries, plums, grapefruits, apricots, melons, berries, and peaches. Apples, pears, baby bananas have a more moderate glycemic index, with grapes, oranges, and large bananas scoring higher. Pineapple, watermelon, and dried fruits are among the highest-glycemic fruits and should be eaten sparingly, if at all. Most people who are CI can tolerate some amount of fresh fruits, although sometimes they can only eat from the low glycemic group.

- *Legumes.* These are defined here to include lentils, peas, and beans—they are usually tolerated by many people, but often in small amounts. Lentils have much less starch, and beans have the most. These foods are thought by many to be high in protein but instead contain much more carbohydrate. For instance, a serving of red beans typically may have six grams of protein and 16 grams of carbohydrate, with five of these carbohydrate grams as fiber. Because of the presence of both protein and fiber, the glycemic index of red beans and other legumes remains relatively low for a carbohydrate food. Overall, because of their composition, most beans, including lentils, have a moderate glycemic effect and are a good alternative to refined-carbohydrate foods.

- *Vegetables.* This large group of plant foods contains varying amounts of carbohydrates, but mostly in very small amounts. Some vegetables, however, contain moderate to high amounts of carbohydrates and therefore warrant discussion here. Among them are corn and potatoes, which should be eaten sparingly, if at all. In fact, a baked potato is full of carbohydrate—about 37 grams as much as a single serving of cooked pasta—and a higher glycemic index than even some cakes and candy. "New" potatoes—those very small red varieties—have a much lower glycemic

index than all others. The reason potatoes and corn are such high-glycemic foods is because they have been genetically modified to be larger and taste sweeter than a few generations ago.

- *Whole grains.* "Whole grains" has no legal or regulated definition, so manufacturers often use it to fool you into thinking a product is not processed, when most are. Whole grains are best purchased in their natural form whole and uncut, rolled, or otherwise processed. These include oat groats, wheat and rye kernels, quinoa, buckwheat, and millet. You often won't find them in most grocery stores and may have to obtain them from a health-food store. While many people with CI don't regularly tolerate these foods, those that can may use them to replace the refined versions:

1. Whole oat groats can replace the common processed oatmeal cereals and quick-cooking oats. Whole oats take about forty minutes to cook.

2. Long-grain brown is a good choice to replace white rice and all instant rice.

3. Products labeled WILD RICE are not really rice—they're a seed from a reedy grass. It's fairly low in carbohydrate and an even better choice as a rice replacement.

4. There are a number of breads on the market made from whole, sprouted grains, and most have a lower gly-

cemic index. Read the labels because many also contain "wheat flour" (which might be white flour) and even sugar.

5. Other possible foods include amaranth, quinoa, and buckwheat. These should be purchased whole, not ground or cut.

Wheat: The Shaft of Life

Next to sugar, wheat may be the most unhealthy food staple of the Western diet, contributing significantly to ill health and disease. We all know how bad sugar is for health due to its high-glycemic nature—but wheat and wheat products can actually be worse due to an even higher glycemic index, so eating that single piece of whole wheat bread is not unlike eating a spoonful or two of white table sugar. And much of this wheat turns to stored body fat. That "fat-free bagel" you were thinking of having for breakfast? Think again. It will just turn to stored body fat.

Wheat is another politically linked success story, just like the tobacco, sugar, and dairy industries whose well-connected lobbyists spend millions on politicians and governmental officials. The goal is driven by corporate profits, not whether the feeding of America unhealthy food and drinks is a public safety issue. And considering the health risks, wheat's place on any food pyramid or "My Plate" is a scheme that serves those who are addicted and the companies that sell it.

Wheat is a common cause of intestinal problems, allergy and asthma, and skin problems; it prevents absorption of various nutrients, contributes to weight gain, even severe obesity—and occasionally causes death.

The reason for wheat's failure as a healthy food staple is twofold; the protein component of wheat, called gluten, is highly allergic in many people, including infants who are unfortunately given this as their first solid food. Many people are adversely affected by gluten without realizing it, with a slow, silent buildup of chronic illness. Gluten is what makes bread rise, so most baked goods and packaged foods are full of it.

The second reason wheat is unhealthy is that almost all wheat products are high glycemic—from bread, bagels, and muffins to cereals, and additives to many packaged foods to wheat flour itself, a key ingredient in almost all cookbook recipes.

Gone are the days when people would buy real whole wheat berries, grind them, and make flour or sprout them for use in food products. While the berries still contain gluten, they're not high glycemic. But almost all wheat used today is highly processed, losing its most nutritious components of the germ, essential oils, and bran.

The list of specific conditions associated with wheat keeps growing—from autoimmune diseases, such as arthritis, type 1 diabetes, lupus, multiple sclerosis, and chronic inflammation to infertility and skin disorder (such as eczema, acne, and psoriasis), and even cancer.

Wheat allergy is among the common allergies in children and adults, along with milk, soy, peanuts, and corn. The most practical way to assess this is to note how you feel after ingesting a wheat-based product or meal. The most common symptom is intestinal bloating, but signs and symptoms are associated with skin, breathing, and edema, and may be immediate or delayed. If you're sensitive to wheat, significantly reducing or eliminating it from your diet is the most effective remedy.

Here are some other ways that wheat affects the body:

- In the intestines, wheat can bind vital minerals from food and prevent their absorption. These include calcium, magnesium, iron, zinc, and copper.
- Wheat can reduce digestive enzymes, especially those from the pancreas, rendering proteins and fats less digestible. This could cause whole proteins to be absorbed, triggering allergies. And by not digesting fat, essential fatty acids may not be absorbed, contributing to inflammation and hormonal balance.

- Combining exercise and wheat can trigger allergic reactions in some people, although it's not common. This occurs when a person eats some form of wheat and exercises within a given time period. This is followed by some allergic reaction, showing itself as a skin rash or hives, and occasionally more severe problems including anaphylaxis and even death. This may also include breathing difficulty. It is sometimes difficult to diagnose because of the need for both triggers (wheat and exercise) around the same time period. It's conceivable that some of the deaths reported in athletes during competitions are due to this problem.
- Wheat can sometimes cause mental or emotional symptoms, including depression, mood swings, attention problems in children, and anxiety. Long-term illness associated with wheat allergy includes dementia due to cerebral (brain) atrophy.
- Osteoporosis may be strongly associated with wheat allergy.

If you're in doubt about what wheat may be doing to your health, consider strictly avoiding it for a couple of weeks or a month. You just may become a healthier new person.

WHAT ARE WE WAITING FOR? THE CELIAC HEALTH CRISIS IS ALREADY HERE

My longtime friend and pediatric specialist Coralee Thompson, MD, who was my co-author for the book *Healthy Brains, Healthy Children,* has seen firsthand the implications of celiac or wheat-related illnesses, especially among children with severe learning or neurological disorders. She contributed the following essay for *The Big Book of Health and Fitness*:

When 50 million people worldwide are afflicted by a serious illness, isn't it time for a public health movement to occur? It's long overdue. One in about a hundred adults and children has a disease whose incidence has been worsening for several decades without being addressed by mainstream medicine. And about a third of the population carries one or two of the genes that trigger this disease. It's a problem that can destroy one's life—not unlike cancer and heart disease—and can kill you.

The condition? Celiac disease, also called gluten-sensitive enteropathy or—simply put—wheat intolerance (although it's more than just wheat). It's all the same problem on a spectrum of severity—some are devastated by it, some die of it, and others are just plain sick with seemingly elusive and difficult to diagnose problems. It could manifest as vague intestinal discomfort, or be painful, and often become serious with malabsorption of nutrients, arthritis, or liver disease.

The incidence is common: there are four times as many Americans with celiac disease as the number of people who have heart attacks. While many people have died from celiac, most are just miserably ill, with others living a low quality of life. Unfortunately, most health care professionals are still not informing their patients of the problem, or its very simple treatment.

What's the easiest and most effective treatment? Eliminate all gluten from your diet. This includes all types of wheat and other gluten-containing grains such as durum, semolina, spelt, kamut, rye, barley, and triticale. You will not miss out on anything very nutritious by avoiding these gluten foods. However, by substituting fresh vegetables, fruits, and other healthy items, you'll obtain much more nutrition.

A recent article published in the *Journal of Family Practice* may help spread the word to health care professionals and patients about celiac disease and its pandemic nature. (A "pandemic" refers to a more serious global problem while an "epidemic" is usually more regional in its spread.) The article discusses many of the scientifically documented aspects of the disease and the clinical features doctors should be more aware of. While other conservative medical journals are starting to publish more studies, as well as reviews and commentaries of this common ailment, it's still too often presented as some rare condition that is difficult to treat when, in fact, it's a common problem with a simple remedy.

Unfortunately, unlike bird or swine flu, celiac disease is not sexy enough for our 24/7 media-driven society to sensationalize or highlight even though it's worse than the flu. In fact, there is very little media coverage of celiac, no Jerry Lewis telethons, no charity fun runs or walks, and no major marketing campaigns to educate children or adults. Nor have we gotten past the decades-old indifference and in some cases mockery by the powers that be in medicine and government who more than ignored the problem. Lobbyists have long fought to protect the agribusiness companies that make and sell gluten products from initiating educational campaigns by the government, schools, and medical societies.

Despite being first described by the Greek physician Aretaeus more than two thousand years ago, most doctors today still ignore gluten sensitivity in their patients. But small numbers of sufferers and a handful of health care professionals who knew the disease was real have been speaking out for many years, despite the ongoing ridicule, often being treated as fanatics with claims that celiac isn't real in most patients who have it. I can't stress this enough: it's not an imaginary disease concocted by hypochondriacs.

Part of the problem has been that no drug or medical procedure can successfully treat celiac; however, a variety of prescription and over-the-counter drugs continue to be marketed to millions of patients to treat the signs and symptoms of the disease—from intestinal complaints of pain and discomfort, to fatigue, depression, dermatitis, headaches, and immune distress. Perhaps this was also a part of the pharmaceutical companies' campaign to maintain a silence as to its existence—if millions of people no longer needed to take drugs to treat secondary symptoms, these pill-dispensing companies would stand to lose billions of dollars.

Those carrying the gene for celiac disease—probably about a third of the world—can easily express the condition. Eating enough wheat can trigger the celiac gene to express itself, resulting in the illness. And this is just what's been happening. Since 1950, the incidence of celiac disease has increased by almost 500 percent. It's not just more recognition and diagnosis of the condition but also a worsening of the pandemic. While the experts are still calling this explosion a "medical mystery," it seems clearly evident that this condition is yet another example of environmental pressure—namely, diet stress—on existing vulnerable genes. In particular, it's people stuffing down bagels, bread, pasta, cereal, muffins, and many other foods containing gluten. It's giving babies and young children wheat as their first and primary foods instead of vegetables, fruits, and meats, and using crackers and cookies as a reward.

SIGNS AND SYMPTOMS

When celiac disease manifests, the body produces antibodies (literally meaning "against the body") resulting in an autoimmune process that particularly affects the tiny fingerlike structures of the small intestine called villi. These villi are responsible for the absorption of nutrients from the food we eat. When these antibodies destroy the villi, numerous problems occur, resulting in malabsorption of nutrients from the diet. Vitamin K and iron are examples of nutrients that just pass through the gut unabsorbed.

Celiac disease can also cause physical problems such as exhaustion, dermatitis (skin conditions), bone (osteoporosis) and muscle problems, adrenal dysfunction, and mental stress including depression can also occur. And it can manifest as a disease process including type I diabetes, thyroid and pancreatic problems, gall bladder and liver disease, lupus, chronic hepatitis, and even cancer. In addition, Down and Turner syndromes, rheumatoid arthritis, fibromyalgia, alopecia areata, scleroderma, and Sjorgen's are other associated problems.

Assessment and Treatment

If you suspect celiac disease, a simple blood test for these antibodies may reveal the condition:

- Endomysial antibody
- Tissue transglutaminase antibody
- Antigliadin antibody
- Total serum IgA

The ability to evaluate these antibodies has made diagnosing celiac disease much easier and cost effective. Not long ago, intestinal biopsy—which required surgery—was the gold standard for a celiac disease diagnosis.

Another easier and effective way to assess the problem yourself can be accomplished by simply performing a dietary evaluation: eliminate all gluten and see how you feel—avoid all types of wheat and other gluten containing grains, as I mentioned above (durum, semolina, spelt, kamut, rye, barley and triticale). It's important to read the ingredients on all packaged foods. And it's not unusual for a food without wheat to be processed in a manufacturing plant where wheat is used for other food, only to be contaminated by the "wheat-free" food item. Moreover, wheat and other offending items are often hidden ingredients in some food items. Avoid foods and ingredients as instant coffee, beer and malt products, soy sauce, food coloring and flavoring, sugar, so-called instant foods, canned items, and even dietary supplements and prescription and over-the-counter drugs.

Rather than be bogged down by the hundreds of packaged foods that may contain gluten, avoid them all and simply eat real and unprocessed food. By purchasing fresh vegetables and fruits, whole meats, eggs, real cheese, raw whole nuts and seeds, and other natural choices, you can make safe, healthy, and tastier meals without the risk of consuming wheat. And you'll save money.

A small food industry has evolved, taking advantage of those who are gluten intolerant. Unfortunately, many of the processed food items are unhealthy: highly processed, high in sugar, packaged convenience foods. Those seeking real health should avoid these as well.

Is such a simple treatment for such a potentially debilitating disorder that easy? Yes. I could fill a separate book with successful case histories of adults and children who, by eliminating gluten, have dramatically improved their health. More scientific research is not needed. No drug or medical therapy will be found to cure the problem. There's no newly developed surgical procedure that's useful. No company will profit from therapy for celiac disease. In other words, too many businesses won't benefit from celiac treatment, and that is another reason why it's not as well-known or discussed as other medical conditions.

The remedy for celiac disease is extremely simple—and it's your choice. Avoid all wheat and all foods containing gluten.

What about Sweeteners?

Sweeteners are carbohydrates, or sugars, in their purest form. They range from highly processed and higher-glycemic products such as table sugar (sucrose) and maltodextrin to the lower glycemic sources such as honey and agave. As with other carbohydrate foods, the least processed and more natural sugars are best for use as sweeteners.

Most sweeteners are complex carbohydrates, making them more difficult to digest. Worse, they are high glycemic. These should always be avoided. They include all maltose sugars (maltodextrin, malt sugar, maple sugar, and syrup), corn sugars and syrups (high-fructose corn syrup), all cane sugar (white or brown), rice syrups, and molasses.

Perhaps the best sweetener to use is honey. It's a simple carbohydrate that doesn't require digestion, unprocessed, and low in glycemic index. But I recommend honey only in moderation and not to exceed your carbohydrate limit.

Honey has been used for centuries as both a sweetener and a remedy, and it remains today as the most natural sweetener available. Honey contains a variety of vitamins, minerals, and amino acids, including antioxidants. In addition, honey has anti-inflammatory and antimicrobial effects. Scientific studies have substantiated honey's therapeutic value and even its ability to improve endurance in athletes.

Honey is also perhaps the only carbohydrate food that does not promote tooth decay through acidity. In general, proteins and fats raise salivary pH, making it more alkaline, while carbohydrate foods lower pH, making it more acidic. Honey is the sweet exception—a carbohydrate that may raise pH levels. In addition, honey has an overall beneficial effect on oral health due to its antibacterial effect and ability to reduce dextran, a sticky, sugary substance that helps bacteria adhere to the teeth.

Like fruit, honey is primarily a blend of fructose and glucose, with different types of having ratios of each. Those that crystallize the fastest are the ones with the highest glucose content, and thus the higher glycemic index. Since fructose has the lowest glycemic index of all sugars, honey with higher fructose content will have the lowest glycemic index. Sage and tupelo honey, for example, are known for their high-fructose content while clover honey has a medium-fructose content, and alfalfa honey is higher in glucose.

When shopping for honey, look for a number of attributes. Dark honey may be the most therapeutic and have the most nutrients. Buckwheat honey is said to contain the highest amounts of antioxidants. Raw, unfiltered honey retains more beneficial qualities. Heat, light, and filtering remove some of the beneficial properties of honey.

Agave is exceptionally high in fructose. Although it has a low glycemic index, it lacks the therapeutic benefits that honey contains.

Due to its high fructose content, some individuals don't tolerate it. Intestinal distress is the most common symptom, and to those with high-triglyceride levels, high-fructose intake may worsen the condition.

What about Artificial Sweeteners?

I recommend avoiding artificial sweeteners in virtually all situations because I believe fake sugars can have an adverse effect on your health. Some say the research is still not clear on this issue, but I say why wait when there's enough information about its harmful effect. Their use is linked to various health problems from headaches to indigestion.

Artificial sweeteners are used in many food items: diet soda, chewing gum, ice cream, iced tea mixes, and many other products. If you want to avoid them, you must read the labels.

While substances such as saccharin are not recommended for children or pregnant women, and aspartame has been related to an increased incidence of migraine headaches and allergic reactions, another fact has been

---

CHRONIC CARBOHYDRATE INTOLERANCE: THE METABOLIC SYNDROME

There is a complex of related diseases that include biggest killers of today: heart disease, cancer, stroke, and diabetes. These diseases kill more people in the United States each year than those died in all our wars combined. Together, these conditions are referred to as the metabolic syndrome (or syndrome X). The specific disorders include the following:

- Diabetes (type 2)
- Hypertension
- Obesity
- Polycystic ovary
- Stroke
- Breast cancer
- Coronary heart disease
- Hyperlipidemia (high blood cholesterol and triglycerides)

Unfortunately, once some of these diseases develop, they are more difficult to treat conservatively, and more extreme care may be needed. However, even these conditions can improve with the right dietary control, which includes solving the problem of excess carbohydrate intake.

---

ignored: the use of artificial sweeteners is most often accompanied by increased consumption of food. In other words, if you use artificial sweeteners, studies show you often end up eating more food, usually sweets. What's worse is that you may store more fat as well. Researchers are unclear why this happens, but certain factors seem to be implicated. It may be a learned process by the body. The tasting of sweet substances may cause the body to store, rather than burn, fat. Or it may be related to the dehydration that accompanies consumption of artificial sweeteners. This may trigger the brain to increase the appetite and food intake as a means of restoring water balance. Eating low-calorie substances will lower the body's metabolism. This will not only cause the body to store more fat but also activate the need to eat more food.

Some people argue that artificial sweeteners reduce calories. You may be fooled into believing that you are buying a more-healthful, low-calorie food when you choose a product made with fake sugar. But you're avoiding only fifteen calories per teaspoon when using an artificial sweetener. This is not a significant caloric factor.

In recent years, alcohol sugars have become popular as a source of low-calorie sugar. They include xylitol, mannitol, and sorbitol, with new ones being developed—but they all have a common feature, ending in the letters *ol*. One of the newest alcohol sugars is erythritol—and it's certified organic!

They are a hydrogenated form of a carbohydrate. Xylitol is the most commonly used alcohol sugar and is made from glucose.

Alcohol sugars don't break down very well in our intestines and so don't get absorbed to stimulate insulin like regular sugar.

A key to overall self-health care is properly understanding how carbohydrates affect you—which ones you can easily tolerate and which ones must be avoided. In general, all refined carbohydrates should be eliminated and then replace them with fresh fruits, legumes; and if your body can handle beans and whole grains, add them to your diet. Plus, there's no need to give up all snacks and desserts. By using small amounts of honey as a sweetener, a variety of healthy, great-tasting items can be made, as you will see in the recipe section of this book. Wisely choosing your carbohydrate foods will provide you with many health and fitness benefits, from a leaner, more active physical body to better mental focus and stamina.

CHAPTER 4

IGNORE THE BIG FAT LIE
Why Having the Right Balance of Fats in Your Diet Will Significantly Improve Your Health

For decades, "fats" have been considered a four-letter word. But nothing can be farther from the truth. In fact, fats are one of the most beneficial substances in the diet and are often the missing ingredients in developing and maintaining optimal health and fitness. Fats play a key role in controlling inflammation and pain, hormone balance, and energy production.

An ongoing, well-financed misinformation campaign against fat has misled the public into creating an epidemic of fat phobia—all while the obesity rates have increased. Manufacturers took natural fats out of foods and replaced them with refined carbohydrates, including sugar. Billions of dollars are spent promoting and selling the low-fat and fat-free message. It's a message that is unhealthy and false.

Even worse is the manufacturing and marketing of low- or nonfat-packaged foods or meals. These products are highly processed and often require chemical additives to remove the natural fats and oils. One problem is that when fats are removed from a food, the taste deteriorates. Consider low-fat yogurt. Manufacturers reduce the tasty fat component but must add something back to make the product more palatable. This usually is sugar. No-fat products are often more sweetened. Many low- and nonfat yogurts have 20 to 30 grams of sugar added!

Low- and nonfat foods with all this added sugar also adds body fat. With the altered food product now at higher glycemic threshold, 40 percent or more of that added sugar will only turn to stored body fat after eating it. Yet consuming a more natural product, such as plain whole milk yogurt, is much less fattening.

In addition, as noted earlier, removing many fats from foods reduces your intake of essential fats and fat-soluble nutrients, especially vitamin A. And there's the satiety factor—low- and nonfat items do not provide the fullness one obtains from a natural, healthy meal. The result may be that you eat more food because you don't yet feel full. All this contributes to ill health and adds extra body fat.

So you need to ignore the hype, misinformation, and ongoing public relations campaign regarding fat as something evil. Instead, the real role of fat is underappreciated and ignored, usually at the expense of a person's health and well-being.

To find out why fat should be an important part of your menu, let's first look at whether you have a dietary fat imbalance. Just as too much fat is dangerous, so is too little.

The health survey below can help you determine your risk for dietary fat imbalance:

HEALTH SURVEY

- Does aspirin (or other NSAIDs) improve any symptoms?
- Do you have chronic inflammation ("itis" conditions such as arthritis, bursitis, tendonitis)?
- Do you have a history or increased risk of heart disease, stroke, or high blood pressure?
- Do you eat restaurant, takeout or fast food more than once or twice weekly?
- Are you carbohydrate intolerant?
- Do you follow a low-fat diet?
- Do you often have feelings of depression?
- Do you have a history of tumors or cancers?
- Do you have reduced mental acuity?
- Do you have diabetes or history of diabetes?
- Are you over age fifty?
- Do you have increased blood fats—triglycerides and cholesterol?

As with previous health surveys, if you answered any of these as "yes," it may indicate an imbalance of fats in your diet, with more "yes" answers increasing the risk.

68

Just What Is Fat?

The term "fat" also includes oil. As one of the three main macronutrients in our diets (the other two being carbohydrates and proteins), fats are found in concentrated forms such as vegetable oils, butter, egg yolk, meats and fish, and dairy, along with nuts and seeds. Smaller amounts of fat are contained in most other natural foods including broccoli, spinach, squash, and most vegetables, lentils, and all beans.

Virtually all natural fats are healthy—but the key to optimal health and fitness is consuming them in balance. In general, eating too much of one type of fat, such as too much saturated fat from dairy products or too much omega-6 fat from vegetable oil, is an example of a fat imbalance that can adversely affect health. Balancing fats is as important as controlling carbohydrates.

In addition, eating "bad" fat—those that are artificial and highly processed, such as trans fat and those used in fried foods, can cause serious health problems. Foods such as chips, french fries and fried chicken, packaged snack foods, and restaurant items usually contain bad fat.

Natural fats have been a staple for humans throughout evolution. In fact, we would not be here today if not for dietary fat's nutritional value. Certain dietary fats consumed in balanced proportions can actually help prevent many diseases. For instance, we now know that dietary fats are central to controlling inflammation, which is the first stage of chronic disease such as cancer and heart disease. Other common illnesses, some of which are predisease conditions, can also result from fat imbalance: cataracts, arthritis, physical injuries, osteoporosis, ulcers, allergies, and asthma.

To better understand the role of fat in one's diet, let's look at body fat, which is important for optimal health and fitness. But too much or too little is a problem. Stored body fat is increased and decreased several ways as shown in the chart below.

There's no "normal" level of body fat as everyone has a unique physical body with

---

INCREASING FAT STORAGE

- Forty percent or more of the carbohydrates (including sugar) you eat turns to fat and are stored.
- Most fat consumed goes into storage right away (smaller amounts are used for energy).
- Overeating protein foods can also be stored as fat.

DECREASING FAT STORAGE

- Physical activity burns stored body fat (especially easy aerobic exercise).
- Eating a meal, or even a snack, can stimulate body-fat burning (a process called thermogenesis) and occurs more effectively after consuming foods containing fats.

varying needs. Below are some of the benefits of stored body fat. Listed here are some of the benefits of stored body fat:

- *Energy.* The aerobic system depends on both stored body fat and the fats circulating in the blood as the fuel for muscles, which power us through the day. Fat produces energy and prevents excessive dependency upon sugar, especially blood sugar. Fat provides more than twice as much potential energy as carbohydrates do, nine calories per gram as opposed to only four calories. Your body is capable of obtaining much of its energy from fat, up to 80 or 90 percent, if your fat-burning mechanism is working efficiently. The body even uses fat as a source of energy for heart-muscle function. These fats—called phospholipids—normally are contained in the heart muscle and generate energy to make it work more efficiently.

- *Hormones.* The hormonal system is responsible for controlling virtually all healthy functions of the body. But for this system to function properly, the body must produce proper amounts of the appropriate hormones. These are produced in various glands and depend on fat for proper production—the thymus gland regulates immunity and the body's defense systems; the thyroid regulates temperature, weight, and other metabolic functions; the kidney's hormones help regulate blood pressure, circulation, and filtering of blood. Cholesterol is one of the

fats used for the production of hormones such as progesterone and cortisone. Even if body fat is too low, problems can arise: the combination of low-fat diets and reduced body fat can cause some female athletes to experience disruptions in their menstrual cycle, and in older women, menopausal symptoms; in men, low levels of testosterone can weaken bones.

- *Eicosanoids.* Hormonelike substances called eicosanoids are necessary for such normal cellular function as regulating inflammation, hydration, circulation, and free radical activity. Produced from dietary fats, eicosanoids are especially important for their role in controlling pain and inflammation. Many people who have inflammatory conditions, such as arthritis, colitis, tendonitis—conditions whose names end in "itis"—probably have an imbalance of dietary fats. But in many more people, chronic inflammation goes on silently. Eicosanoids are also important for regulating blood pressure and hydration, preventing constipation or diarrhea, and can trigger menstrual cramps, blood clots, and tumor growth.

- *Insulation.* The body's ability to store fat permits humans to live in most climates, especially in areas of extreme heat or cold. In warmer areas of the world, stored fat provides protection from the heat. In colder lands, increased fat stored beneath the skin prevents too much heat from leaving the body. An example of fat's effectiveness as an insulator is in the Eskimo's ability to withstand great cold and survive in good health. Eskimos eat a high-fat diet and, despite this, have a very low incidence of heart disease and other ailments.

In warmer climates, fat prevents too much water from leaving the body, which can result in dehydration that causes dry, scaly skin. Some evaporation is normal, of course, but fats under the skin regulate evaporation and can prevent as much as ten to twenty times more water from leaving the body.

- *The brain.* About 60 percent of the non-water part of a healthy brain is fat. During our own development, the incorporation of fat into the brain—in particular the essential fatty acids including A, B, and most especially C fats—enabled us to better create, learn, remember, and grow our brains at a much faster rate. This is especially important not only for all children from birth but all adults as well.

The covering of neurons—the specialized brain cells that communicate with each other—have a high monounsaturated (oleic) fat content, the same type of fat found in olive oil, almonds, and avocados. Overall, C fats (EPA and DHA) are the most common fat in the brain.

Many brain disorders, including cognitive dysfunction such as Alzheimer's disease, can be prevented with the right fats, and these conditions can also be treated with fats such as fish oil.

- *Healthy skin and hair.* Fat has protective qualities that also give skin the soft, smooth, and unwrinkled appearance that many people try to achieve through expensive skin conditioners. The healthy look of skin—and hair—comes from the fat inside our bodies. Fats, particularly cholesterol, serve as an insulating barrier within the skin. Without this protection, chemical pollutants can more easily enter the body through the skin. Hair loss starts with an imbalance of dietary fats that triggers inflammation in the scalp.

- *Pregnancy and lactation.* The effective functioning of fat-dependant hormones improves fertility for both would-be parents. Once conception does take place, fats continue playing a key role in the health of mother and child. The uterus keeps the newly conceived embryo thriving by providing nutrition until the placenta can begin to function, usually a period of a week or more. Adequate progesterone, a hormone produced from fats, is primary for the embryo to survive the first critical week, preventing miscarriage (spontaneous abortion). The placenta itself must also develop and produce hormones for the fetus—accomplished in large part from the rising production of estrogens and progesterone as the pregnancy continues.

Following birth, breast-feeding helps protect the baby against allergies, asthma, and intestinal problems through its high-fat content, particularly cholesterol. The baby is highly dependent upon the fat in the milk for survival, especially during the first few days. During this time, the fatty colostrum content of breast milk is of vital nutritional importance.

- *Digestion.* Fats play a primary role in digestion. Bile from the gall bladder is triggered by fat in the diet, which is the first step in the digestion and absorption of essential fats and fat-soluble vitamins (A, D, E, and K). Most dietary fats are digested—broken into smaller particles—in the small intestine. The pancreas, liver, gall bladder, and large intestine are also involved in the digestive process. Any of these organs not working properly could have an adverse impact on fat metabolism in general, but the liver, which makes bile, and the pancreas, producing the fat digestive enzyme lipase, are particularly important. Without sufficient fat in the diet, the start of the digestive process—the gall bladder secreting bile—would not be effective.

Fat helps regulate the rate of stomach emptying, helping protein digestion, and satisfies physical hunger by increasing satiety—the signal given to the brain that you're full. With a low-fat meal, the brain keeps sending the same message: eat more! Because you never really feel full, overeating follows (the reason some people actually gain weight on a low-fat diet).

Fats also slow the absorption of sugar from the small intestines, which keeps blood sugar and insulin from rising too high and too quickly (recall that fat in the meal lowers its glycemic index). Additionally, fats protect the inner lining of the stomach and intestines from irritating substances in the diet, such as alcohol and black pepper.

- *Body support and protection.* Stored fat offers physical support and protection to vital body parts, including the organs and glands. Fat acts as a natural built-in shock absorber, cushioning the wear and tear of everyday life, and helps prevent organs from sinking with age due to the downward pull of gravity.

By controlling free radical production, fats can physically protect our cells against the harmful effects of X-ray exposure. In addition to medical X-rays, we are constantly exposed to X-rays from the atmosphere—cosmic radiation penetrates most objects, including airplanes. The average person gets more cosmic radiation exposure during an airline flight from New York to Los Angeles than from a lifetime of medical X-rays.

- *Vitamin and mineral regulation.* Most people know that vitamin D is produced by exposure of the skin to the sun. Sunlight chemically changes cholesterol in the skin through the process of irradiation to vitamin D_3, which is then absorbed into the blood. Without the vitamin D, cal-

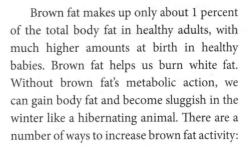

cium and phosphorous would not be well absorbed, and deficiencies of both could occur. But without cholesterol, the entire process would not occur.

Vitamins A, E, and K also rely on dietary fat for proper absorption and utilization—a low-fat diet could be cause a deficiency in these vitamins. Certain fats circulating in the blood, called prostaglandins, help carry calcium into the bones and muscles. Without these fats, calcium levels in bones and muscles can be reduced resulting in the risk for stress fractures, osteoporosis, and muscle dysfunction. Unused calcium may be stored, sometimes in the kidneys, increasing the risk of stones, or in the muscles, tendons, or joint spaces as calcium deposits.

Two Types of Body Fat

Our body fat is as important as the fat we eat. The human body possesses two distinct types of body fat, referred to as brown and white. Both are metabolically active, living parts of us. Total body fat content ranges from 5 percent in male athletes to more than 50 percent of total body weight in obese individuals. Much of the fat we consume and the fat produced from eating carbohydrates turns to white fat. It's also our stored form of energy, used during physical activity (unless we're not active enough, then we don't burn it, and it remains in storage). Other attributes of white fat are protection of body parts as noted above.

Brown fat makes up only about 1 percent of the total body fat in healthy adults, with much higher amounts at birth in healthy babies. Brown fat helps us burn white fat. Without brown fat's metabolic action, we can gain body fat and become sluggish in the winter like a hibernating animal. There are a number of ways to increase brown fat activity:

- Food frequency can affect brown fat to either increase or decrease fat burning. Eating several times a day—five to six smaller healthy meals instead of one, two, or three larger ones—can trigger thermogenesis, an important postmeal metabolic boost to increase fat burning. However, if caloric intake is too low, brown fat can slow the burning of white fat. This can happen on a low-calorie diet and when meals are skipped.
- The body's brown fat is stimulated by certain dietary fats. These include omega-3 fats, especially from fish oil and olive oil. While supplements of fish oil may be the only way to obtain adequate amounts of EPA, some supplements can be harmful—conjugated linoleic acid (CLA) can actually reduce brown fat activity.
- Caffeine—contained in tea, coffee, and chocolate—can increase brown fat activity. But too much caffeine can trigger stress, reducing fat burning and promoting fat storage.
- Refined carbohydrates, including sugar, and other high glycemic items can reduce fat burning.

In addition to foods, stimulating brown fat can be accomplished with various lifestyle routines:

- *Skin temperature.* If we get too hot during the day or overdress during exercise, brown-fat activity can lead to less burning of white fat. This is why wearing extra clothes or "rubber sweat suits" during exercise, a common weight-loss myth, can be dangerous.
- Likewise, soaking in a sauna, hot tub, or steam room regularly after exercise may offset some of the fat-burning benefits of physical activity. While these activities increase sweating, resulting in some water-weight loss, the sacrifice is reducing brown fat activity. Hot tubs and saunas do come with health benefits, but to avoid the reductions in fat burning take a minute or two to cool the body in a cold shower or tub afterward.

Brown fat is stimulated by cold. Most of our brown fat is found under the skin around the shoulders and underarms, between the ribs and at the nape of the neck. Cooling these areas can help increase fat burning. (These are also the specific areas to keep from overheating during exercise.)

Low body temperature is associated with reduced fat-burning. Poor thyroid function is often associated with body temperatures below the normal 98.6°F.

- Physical activity increases fat-burning too. The best kind being the easy-aerobic type, such as walking, which trains the body to burn more body fat all day and night. This issue is discussed in detail in section II.

Unfortunately, most research on brown fat comes from the pharmaceutical industry, which is looking for new drugs to stimulate brown fat. But as noted above, we already know enough healthy habits to stimulate brown fat so we can burn more white fat.

Balancing Your Dietary Fats

Now that you have a general understanding of healthy body fat, I want to outline how to balance your consumption of certain fats in your diet. In general, this is accomplished in three steps. The first two are simple—when using dietary fats and oils:

For cooking, use only olive oil, butter or ghee ("drawn" or purified butter), coconut oil or lard.

Avoid all vegetable oil (such as soy, safflower, corn, and peanut) and trans fat (from margarine and other processed fats and oils).

The third step is to consume omega-6 and omega-3 fats in a ratio of about 2:1. Most people consume much more omega-6 fats and have a ratio of 5, 10, or 20 to 1. This is the crucial part of balancing fats and needs much more explanation.

The issue of balancing fat consumption is quite involved. Volumes have been written on the subject, and many scientists have devoted their entire careers to this topic. But I have simplified the explanations to help you achieve this important task.

There are three common forms of fats in our diet—the differences are due to their chemical makeup. As such, they have varying characteristics for use in cooking and function quite differently in the body. These three forms of fats are referred to as mono-unsaturated, polyunsaturated, and saturated.

Monounsaturated—the Mono Fat

Mono fat is associated with improved health and disease prevention and should make up the bulk of fat in your diet. Mono fat—also referred to as oleic or omega-9—helps reduce the risk of cancer, heart disease, and obesity. The Mediterranean diet, with its lower incidence of ill health, is relatively high in mono fat. An example of how this fat can prevent disease is by its influence on cholesterol: it can raise good HDL and lower bad LDL cholesterol, greatly improving cardiovascular health. In addition, mono fats can help control inflammation, reduce the harmful effects of too much saturated fat, and its presence in foods is associated with phytonutrients—important plant compounds discussed in chapter 7.

Mono fat is also very stable with a naturally long shelf life. As discussed later, polyunsaturated fat is unstable and easily oxidizes and can form dangerous oxygen free radicals from exposure to air, light, and heat. Not so for mono fat. Due to its chemical structure, it's virtually immune to oxidation, making it safe for cooking and storing without refrigeration. This is one reason why olive oil, made up mostly of mono fats, has been used as a food ingredient and in cooking for centuries in many cultures.

Mono fat is found in many foods and oils. Avocados, almonds, and macadamia nuts contain higher amounts. Olive oil is very high in monounsaturated fat and is the best oil for use on salads and in recipes.

Polyunsaturated Fat

Many foods naturally contain polyunsaturated fat. They have become a staple in the American diet. Two essential fatty acids—so named because we must consume these vitaminlike nutrients as we can't make them in our bodies—are found in "poly" fats: they are termed "omega-6" and "omega-3." There are varying amounts of each in different types of poly oils, and most importantly, they play a vital role in regulating inflammation and pain.

While a small amount is necessary for health, high amounts of omega-6 poly fats are potentially dangerous. They're found in vegetable oils often used in cooking and salads and high in packaged foods. Those with the highest amounts of omega-6 fats are contained in safflower, peanut, corn, canola, and soy oil. They're even found in infant formulas and dietary supplements.

Polyunsaturated fat is easily oxidized to chemical free radicals, making it a potentially dangerous oil. Oxidation occurs when this type of fat is heated or exposed to light and air. When we consume oxidized fat, this free-radical stress can damage cells anywhere in the body, speed the aging process, turn LDL

THE MIGHTY OLIVE AND WHY IT MAKES ONE OF THE BEST COOKING OILS

History tells us that olives were native to the Mediterranean region over five thousand years ago. The olive tree may be the oldest cultivated plant. In addition to its use as food, the oil from olives became a staple for the people in the region, and eventually the world.

The best olive oil to use is the least processed and most nutritious—organic extravirgin olive oil. My favorites are from Italy, Spain, and Greece. The "first-press" oil is obtained from the whole fruit without heat or chemicals. The highly nutritious phytonutrients, especially a group of compounds called phenols, are abundant in this oil, which gives it a light bitter taste and dark green color. Much lower amounts of phenols are present in other grades of olive oil not labeled as EXTRAVIRGIN.

Most countries that produce olive oil adhere to the International Olive Oil Council (IOOC) standards when it comes to classifying their products. While the IOOC has a United Nations charter to develop criteria for olive oil quality and purity standards, the United States has not adopted them. The USDA, which allows lower quality olive oil to be sold, still uses a 1948 classification system (although this is expected to someday change).

An important IOCC criterion for olive oil is that it cannot be diluted with non-olive oils, and must conform to sensory and analytical standards. The oils must be obtained directly from the olive fruit without the use of solvents or other chemicals.

The highest quality olive oil is labeled as ORGANIC and EXTRAVIRGIN OLIVE OIL. Only about 10 percent of the oil produced is extravirgin (I have no data on how much of this is certified organic). This oil can vary widely in taste, color, and appearance, much like fine red wines. Choose a brand that meets your taste.

Other products labeled as OLIVE OIL or PURE OLIVE OIL are not extravirgin and of lower quality. Those labeled as LIGHT or EXTRALIGHT are examples of marketing gimmicks, are very low quality, and should be avoided.

---

cholesterol "bad," and significantly increase the need for antioxidant nutrients. The fat content of most people's diet is very high in omega-6 fats from vegetable oils.

One way to make poly fat work toward optimal health, rather than contributing to functional problems and disease, is to balance the consumption of omega-6 and omega-3 fats. To accomplish this, avoid all vegetable oils and processed food because they are generally high in poly fat; instead, use extravirgin olive. Before discussing this issue in more detail, let's discuss saturated fat because it's part of the balancing act.

Saturated Fat

Of all the dietary fats, the saturated form is always considered the worst. But saturated fat is important for energy and hormone production, cellular functioning, and optimal brain function.

Saturated fat, like the poly form, is made up of many different fatty acids of varying attributes. Here are some:

- Palmitic acid is found in high amounts in dairy fat—in milk, cheese, cream, yogurt, and butter. It can raise cholesterol. Palm-kernel oil is also high in palmitic acid, but palm fruit oil is not and actually can lower LDL cholesterol. Some of the dietary carbohydrate that converts to fat become palmitic acid. High blood levels of palmitic acid may predict type 2 diabetes, heart disease, stroke, and carbohydrate intolerance. But it's not the presence of palmitic acid that's the problem—when all fats are balanced, palmitic acid does not seem to be such a health problem.
- Arachidonic acid—AA—is another fatty acid that gives saturated fat a bad name. Small amounts of AA are essential for health, especially for the brain, the fetus,

newborns, and growing children. But too much AA is very unhealthy. These fats are found in dairy, egg yolks, meats, and shell-fish. But these foods are not nearly the problem compared to the high amounts of omega-6 fat in the diet, commonly found in vegetable oil, because this fat can be converted in the body to AA. The result can be chronic inflammation, bone loss, and increased pain. As discussed below, AA plays a key role in balancing fats.

- Stearic acid is another fatty acid found in saturated fat. It has various health benefits on the immune system. Foods containing higher amounts include cocoa butter and grass-fed (but not corn-fed) beef. And stearic acid can be converted to healthy mono fat.
- Lauric acid is a fatty acid that plays an important role in energy production, and it has antiviral and antibacterial actions, especially in the intestine (and the stomach in particular, against *Helibacter pylori*). Coconut oil, high in saturated fat, has high levels of lauric acid (and contains very little polyunsaturated fat), making it an ideal fat for cooking.

In animal foods, which contain relatively high amounts of saturated fat, the most important factor that determines the level of healthy fatty acids is the food consumed by the animal. As noted above, grass-fed beef contains a much healthier content of fatty acids compared to corn-fed beef. For the same reason, wild animals usually contain healthier fatty acid profiles than animals that are fed grain in confinement. In plants, the soil plays a certain role in determining fatty acid content, with natural fertilizers a healthier choice over chemical types.

Mono, poly, and saturated fats are found in most foods. A few foods contain predominantly one type of fat or another, but most contain a combination of all three fats. Many people are surprised to learn, for instance, that the fat in an average steak is about half monounsaturated and half saturated, with a small amount of polyunsaturated.

The ABCs of Fats: Optimal Balance

While it might first appear to be an excessively complicated subject, balancing your dietary fats is as easy as learning the ABCs. I developed this model in the mid-1980s, as a way to teach health care professionals about the subject of fat balance, for patients to implement the ideas, and in my own published articles on the subject.

There are three fatty acids that require balance for optimal health. I mentioned them above—they are omega-6, AA (arachidonic acid), and omega-3. I'll refer to these three as A, B, and C fats, respectively.

Approximate Percentage of Mono, Poly, and Saturated Fats/Oils in Some Foods			
Oil	Mono	Poly	Saturated
Olive oil	77	9	14
Canola oil	62	32	6
Peanut oil	49	33	18
Corn oil	25	62	13
Soybean oil	24	61	15
Safflower oil	13	77	10
Coconut	6	2	92
Egg yolks	48	16	36
Steak	49	4	47
Cheese	30	3	67
Butter	30	4	66
Almonds	68	22	10
Cashews	62	18	21
Peanuts	50	32	18
Sesame	40	42	14

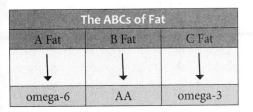

The ABCs of Fat		
A Fat	B Fat	C Fat
↓	↓	↓
omega-6	AA	omega-3

In the body, the A, B, and C fats influence inflammation: the A and C fats are anti-inflammatory in their function; the B fats trigger inflammation.

Actually, inflammation is only one of the concerns. Without sufficient anti-inflammatory chemicals (from A and C fats), one could develop chronic inflammation—this is the first step to other functional problems and disease, including cancer, heart disease, Alzheimer's, diabetes, and any of the "it is" problems prevalent in our society—from arthritis and tendonitis to colitis and sinusitis. In addition, too many B fats can cause bone loss, muscle imbalance, allergy and asthma, and menstrual problems. And B fats can also increase pain.

The A and C fats can counter all these problems, preventing disease, ill health, and reducing pain.

This is a key factor in optimal health and fitness: the balance of A, B, and C fats in the diet. But before explaining the details on how to do it, allow me to go a bit deeper in this explanation—it's very important.

In the body, the A, B, and C fats are converted to three respective groups of hormonelike substances called eicosanoids (pronounced i-cos-an-oids). I'll call these

groups 1, 2, and 3. Basically, A fats make group 1 eisosanoids, B fats group 2, and C fats group 3.

Eicosanoid balance is so powerful—so influential to overall health—that billions of dollars are spent by pharmaceutical companies to research and develop new drugs that attempt to balance the eicosanoids. But you can do it cheaply by eating the right foods! And while drugs that attempt to balance fats have some short-term success, they come with significant unhealthy, and sometimes deadly, side effects. Aspirin and other NSAIDS are the best example—while reducing the inflammatory chemicals made by the B fats (and group 1 eicosanoids), one side effect is that the natural anti-inflammatory eicosanoids are also impaired. But balancing fats by eating right only has healthy—and nearly miraculous—benefits.

The ABCs of Fats		
A Fats	B Fats	C Fats
↓	↓	↓
Group 1 eicosanoids	Group 2 eicosanoids	Group 3 eicosanoids

The term "eicosanoid" refers to a group of different compounds with names such as "prostaglandins," "leukotrienes," and "thromboxanes." They're involved in complex reactions from moment to moment in all cells throughout the body. For now, just remember that balanced eicosanoids, from balanced fats, regulate certain bodily functions that are central to optimal health and fitness, elimination of functional problems, and disease prevention. With this in mind, understanding how to balance the A, B, and C fats, and the 1, 2, and 3 groups of eicosanoids is vital. First let's discuss the foods that contain the A, B, and C fats.

A fats are most prevalent in vegetable oils: safflower, soy, corn, peanut, and canola. These omega-6 fats contain an important fatty acid called linoleic acid that I'll call LA for short. LA is an essential fatty acid because the body can't make them and we must eat foods containing them. When we do, LA is converted to other fats, including GLA (gamma-linolenic acid), with the end result being the series 1 eicosanoids with anti-inflammatory effects. In addition to vegetable oils, common dietary supplements of omega-6 products include black currant seed, borage, and primrose oils that contain high amounts of GLA. While the group 1 eicosanoids from A fats can produce powerful health effects, there is one potential problem. Conversion of A fats to group 1 can be impaired resulting in many A fats being converted to B fats.

A variety of factors can cause this to happen: reduced levels of nutrients (niacin, vitamin B_6, magnesium, protein), consumption of trans fats, and excess stress. This can more easily occur as we age. The remedy? Eat the best diet possible to ensure you obtain all the nutrients, avoid bad fats and moderate stress (a topic discussed in chapter 19).

When this happens, the aging factor will be minimized.

The B fats are sometimes considered bad because of the effects they can have in the body. But these effects are only bad when in excess—in other words, not balanced with A and C fats. As noted, B fats promote inflammation and pain. But these so-called problems can actually be important for health at the right time—inflammation is a vital first stage of the healing process, and the body uses pain to help us become more aware of a problem so we can remedy it. Another important function of AA is that it's very important for the repair and growth of the brain. This is especially vital in the fetus, newborns, and developing children; but as adults, we continually should be repairing and growing the brain as well. B fats are highest in dairy products such as butter, cream, and cheese, and in lesser amounts in the fat of meats, egg yolks, and shellfish. However, for most people, the largest source of AA is from A fats.

The C fats, omega-3, and are found mostly in ocean fish, with lesser amounts in beans, flaxseed, walnuts, and wild and grass-fed animals. These fats contain ALA (alpha-linolenic acid), an essential fatty acid that is converted in the body to EPA (eicosapentaenoic acid), with the final production of group 3 eicosanoids. This conversion can be impaired by the same problems that impair the conversion of A fats to group 1 eicosanoids—poor nutrition, trans fat, stress, and aging. Ocean fish already contain EPA and are very useful as a dietary supplement for people who require more omega-3 to balance fats. Flaxseed oil does not contain EPA, and while the body may convert some of it to EPA, it's very inefficient. EPA also exists in conjunction with another important fatty acid, DHA, which is especially important for the fetus through childhood.

It's relatively easy to balance A, B, and C fats. It can be accomplished first by eating approximately equal amounts of foods in the A, B, and C categories. It does not necessarily have to be at each meal, but in the course of a day or week, balance is of prime importance.

By eating a balance of A, B, and C fats, you'll consume polyunsaturated (A and C) and saturated (B) fats in the optimal ratio of 2:1. In the typical Western diet, many people consume ratios of 5, 10, or even 20:1! It's no wonder there's an epidemic of chronic inflammation, pain, and disease. (If you don't eat meat or dairy, consume approximately an equal ratio of A and C fats; in this case, some of the A fats will convert to B fats.)

Sugar Contributes to Fat Imbalance

Fat imbalances typically occur from some combination of eating too much A or B fats, and too little C fats, by a lack of certain nutrients, stress, and aging. But a significant cause of imbalance is from refined carbohydrates including sugar. Recall that insulin can be produced in higher amounts when these carbohydrates are consumed.

This causes more A fats to convert to B fats—enough said!

Two foods can help prevent too much A fat from converting to B fats. These are as follows:

- EPA found in raw ocean fish or in fish-oil supplements. Fish should be cooked very lightly as EPA is an unstable poly fat.
- Raw sesame oil, which contains the phytonutrient sesamin. Heated sesame oil will not accomplish this task (and is a very unhealthy food as the sesamin becomes sasamol, a potential cancer-causing agent).

If all this sounds too complicated, it's not. Here's how one my patients, Mary, succeeded in making the appropriate dietary changes to balance her fats and change her life. Mary had chronic health problem ever since around the beginning of high school. At first, with vague symptoms of intestinal distress, the family doctor found nothing from an initial examination and concluded there was no reason to perform other tests—he thought she would outgrow the discomfort. By college, Mary had bouts of being severely run down with exhaustion, periods of acute intestinal pain, and muscle dysfunction that caused weakness and numbness. As an active athlete in high school, she was unable to work out in college because it made all her symptoms worse. Eventually, an extensive evaluation was made as her condition worsened. But no definitive diagnosis could be made. One specialist after another gave an opinion—

and a name for a particular condition—from Crohn's disease and ileitis (two common intestinal conditions) to rheumatoid arthritis and Lyme disease.

Mary visited my clinic four years after finishing college, having tried many diets, drugs, and dietary supplements without success. I retrieved as many copies of her past evaluations from her family doctor that included blood and urine tests, reports by radiologists, neurologists and gastroenterologists, and a psychologist. The only revealing factor in the more-than-fifty pages of reports was a test that showed a moderate amount of inflammation—a C reactive protein test was moderately high—the reason so many doctors wanted to pin the name of some inflammatory condition on her.

In my dietary analysis, I was able to evaluate the balance of her A, B, and C fats—she consumed very high amount of A fats, using safflower oil for all her cooking and daily salads; ate small amounts of B fats, mostly a few eggs a week with one or two meals containing some type of meat; and she ate no fish or other sources of C fats. Her balance of fats was quite bad—excessive amount of A fats, moderate B fats, and little if any C fats. But from her recollection, Mary's diet was much worse growing up. This part of her history made sense considering when her problems began (during high school).

Here is a synopsis of the dietary recommendations I gave to Mary:

- Eliminate all vegetable oils—replace them with extra virgin olive.
- Eliminate all packaged foods, which often contain vegetable oils.
- For cooking, use only coconut or olive oil, or lard.
- Reduce restaurant and takeout food—limit it only to healthy, whole food items such as salads with olive oil, eggs, and meats that are lightly cooked without vegetable oil (butter, coconut oil, or lard was okay).
- Reduce all refined carbohydrates, including foods containing them.
- Avoid all trans fats such as margarine and similar items and foods that contain them.
- Limit all dairy to one serving three times weekly. This included butter, cheese, milk, cream, and yogurt.
- Increase fresh vegetables to ten servings per day.
- Increase protein intake—two times daily have one serving of eggs or any type of meats (unprocessed).
- Use raw sesame seed oil—one tablespoon each day on a salad.
- Take four capsules of fish oil containing EPA each day (daily dose of EPA = 1,200 mg).

The goal for Mary was to balance her dietary fats. Since she did not like eating fish, I told her to get EPA from a fish oil supplement as noted above. I saw Mary about a month later, and she was happy to report about a 50 percent improvement in her symptoms. I explained this would have come mostly from getting more nutrients in her diet—especially vitamins, minerals, and proteins to help the balance of fats—and from reducing refined carbohydrates, both of which would help improve fat balance. Significant changes in the body's fat metabolism would take another month—the bad fats in the body literally can take that long to be replaced by good ones. By the second month, Mary continued improving quite well, and by month 3, 90 percent of the complaints had disappeared. She claimed to hardly remember feeling this well. After about six months, Mary had no complaints. Butter and other dairy were allowed back into the diet in moderate amounts. The fish oil dietary supplement was reduced by half but would be maintained indefinitely as Mary did not consume any fish or beans.

How Much Fat Should We Eat?

Equipped with the knowledge of how important balanced fats are for the body, you are now in a position to dramatically improve your health and fitness by making some important dietary changes. This includes reduction of foods that contribute to group 1 eicosanoids, such as vegetable oils, and increasing omega-3 fats such as fish and fish oils. But how much total fat should be in a healthy diet? That amount depends on the individual and his or her particular needs.

You must first get over the idea that the less fat the better, or a diet that's 10 percent or 20 percent fat is ideal. Actually, a low-fat diet can be very unhealthy. Studies even show that people following a very low-fat diet can increase their risks for heart disease. This is due to the fact that their intake of essential fatty acids could be too low. On the other hand, there are populations whose intake of fat exceeds 40 percent, including people living in the Mediterranean region, and healthy Americans who on average are healthier than people who eat a lower-fat diet. In addition, the American Heart Association, the World Health Organization (WHO), the U.S Surgeon General, the USDA, and many other professional health organizations have recommended a diet that's 30 percent fat, not one that's 20 percent or even 10 percent.

Over the years, I have found that most people are healthier with at least 30 percent fat in their diet. Some may need more—35 or even 40 percent. But rather than follow these or any other grams, calories or percentages, experiment and find what works best for you. First, focus on finding your optimal level of healthy carbohydrates. Then balance your fats. As you go through this process, the amount of fat you consume will naturally fit your particular needs.

CHAPTER 5

CHRONIC INFLAMMATION
What You Can Safely Do to Eliminate It

Consider that the first stage of many functional problems, and most of the chronic diseases, both of which can easily ruin a person's quality of life if not end life itself, is chronic inflammation. And more than anyone else, you control whether this first stage proceeds or is halted. It's another way you make the choice between functional illness that progresses to chronic disease or optimal health. As I pointed out in the previous chapter, balancing healthy fats should be your prime focus. Almost everyone would agree—not just me but also your health care professional, scientists, and anyone familiar with the biochemical aspects of fats and eicosanoids.

Why do we seldom hear or read anything about this simple yet effective method of preventing disease and living a vibrant life? The big food and drug companies don't have an incentive to do so. There's much more money in selling over-the-counter and prescription drugs than educating people to balance their fats. (It's the same scenario with refined carbohydrates, which is also a main contributor to chronic inflammation.) Nor can we expect the government to inform the public about how balancing dietary fats can control if not reduce chronic inflammation.

For many people, the presence of inflammation is obvious. Perhaps you have an active inflammatory condition—some form of arthritis, a nagging injury such as low back pain, bursitis, or Achilles tendonitis—or your doctor informs you that the intestinal complaints you have are due to chronic inflammation.

But not all chronic inflammation is readily apparent or visible because the signs and symptoms may be masked. The following health survey will help guide you in determining your potential for inflammation.

Check the items that pertain to you:

- Do you eat restaurant, takeout, or prepared food daily?
- Do you consume milk, cream, butter, or cheese daily?
- Do you consume corn, soy, safflower, or peanut oils regularly?
- Do you consume margarine or products that contain trans fat (hydrogenated or partially hydrogenated oils) regularly?
- Is your diet low in fresh salmon, sardines, and other cold-water fish?
- Do you have a history of atherosclerosis, stroke, heart disease, or cancer?
- Do you have a history of "itis" conditions such as arthritis, colitis, tendinitis, etc.?
- Do you have allergies, asthma, osteoporosis, or recurring infections?

- Do you have chronic fatigue?
- Do you have increased body fat?
- Do you perform weekly anaerobic exercise, such as weightlifting, hard training, or athletic competition?
- Do you perform regular repetitive activity (jogging, cycling, walking, typing, etc.)?

Even if you check only one or two of the above items, it indicates an increased chance of having chronic inflammation.

In addition, another indication that your fats may be out of balance and your risk of inflammation is high has to do with how aspirin or other NSAIDS affect you. These drugs often provide many people with symptomatic relief of pain—but not everyone. If you do get relief from these drugs, it may indicate your fats are not balanced and chronic inflammation exists. That's because the primary action of these drugs is to artificially balance fats for you.

While the media usually won't publish stories about balancing dietary fats, they often write about studies that show certain anti-inflammatory drugs can reduce the risk of heart disease or cancer. But drugs such as aspirin can be a double-edged sword—helping a part of you while hurting another. Consider these examples:

Patients with heart disease are often prescribed daily aspirin after a heart attack. The reason for this is that aspirin "thins" the blood; it reduces the aggregation of platelets contained in blood vessels. Studies show this

85

can lower the risk of a heart attack or stroke by 22 percent compared to those not taking aspirin. However, studies also clearly show that many patients taking aspirin can have a fourfold increased risk of having a second heart attack.

In the case of asthma, a condition associated with chronically inflamed airways, taking aspirin (and other NSAIDS) may not help. In fact, studies show that up to 70 percent of these patients may not tolerate aspirin. Moreover, aspirin can actually cause asthma in some people. Studies show that aspirin-induced asthma is due to an alteration in the balance of fats.

The use of aspirin in preventing colorectal cancer has been highlighted by the media for years. But a recent study by Alaa Rostom, MD, and colleagues from the University of Ottawa in Canada showed that while some studies demonstrate reduced risk of cancer, others do not. So the results are not conclusive.

An overlooked factor in aspirin use in relation to preventing disease is cost effectiveness. This has to do with the drug's side effects. Studies show that the use of aspirin in colon cancer, for example, is not cost effective. This is due to the high expense from complications of the drug's side effects. These side effects include internal bleeding and ulcers.

Two Faces of Inflammation

Inflammation is typically thought of as swelling, pain, or discomfort, perhaps in one's joints, sinuses, or intestines. But for many people, chronic inflammation occurs without symptoms but can still trigger function illness and disease. A full spectrum of disorders are associated with chronic inflammation—from severe functional problems such as fatigue, hormonal imbalance, and reduced immunity, to serious conditions such as osteoporosis, heart disease, and cancer.

There are two forms of inflammation—acute and chronic. Acute inflammation is a normal healthy action, helping to heal more than just that little cut on one's finger. Without it, you would not recover from a day at the office, your easy walk, or even the minor bumps and bruises you acquire by being physically active. But acute inflammation can also be triggered much more significantly by various traumas such as a bad fall, overdoing it at the gym with the weight machines, infections, toxins in food and air, synthetic hormones (prescription and food contamination), and excess stress (due to the production of the hormone cortisol).

Acute inflammation is the first step in the healing or repair process after some physical or chemical injury, or stress, no matter how minor. Two other steps then follow: (1) The next is that it prevents the spread of damaged cells from these sites of injury that could cause secondary problems—a local infection can be contained due to the inflammatory response, instead of causing a bodywide infection. And (2) inflammation rids the body of damaged and dead cells that remain following an injury. Normally, the inflammatory cycle is almost like an "on-off" switch. It's turned on by inflammatory chemicals when it is needed for healing and repair. Then it's turned off by anti-inflammatory chemicals when the process is no longer needed. However, if the anti-inflammatory chemicals are not present in sufficient quantity, if the inflammatory chemicals are excessive, or there is an ongoing injury or stress that keeps stimulating inflammatory chemicals, the switch stays in the "on position." The outcome is chronic inflammation.

Chronic Inflammation

When inflammation continues to proceed into the chronic state, many health problems can start developing. This may be the beginning of those all-too-familiar "itis" conditions such as tendinitis, colitis, sinusitis, and arthritis. Chronic inflammation is also a precursor to ulceration, and it could ultimately lead to disease.

A simple blood test can confirm the presence of inflammation. The C-reactive protein (CRP) test is the most accurate screen for inflammation and can detect very low levels. This test can also predict future risk of coronary heart disease and stroke even in otherwise healthy individuals. The best suggestion is to have a CRP performed regularly when other blood tests are ordered. If the result is not normal, retest every six months until it's normal while you're balancing your fats. CRP levels should be lower than 1 mg/L, which is the lowest risk of developing cardiovascular disease (between 1 and 3 mg/L, a person has an average risk, and CRP's higher than 3 mg/L are associated with at high risk).

Other blood tests include the erythrocyte sedimentation rate (ESR). This common blood test for inflammation can be performed when blood is taken for other tests, or with a finger prick. A complete blood count measures white blood cells and may also indicate inflammation. Compare your results to the reference ranges given by the lab.

More on Diet and Inflammation

As I detailed in the previous chapter, balancing fats is a key to controlling inflammation. Here again is a quick summary:

- Balance A, B, and C fats in your diet.
- Maintain a healthy diet to ensure you get the nutrients necessary to maintain a balance of fats: vitamins B_6, E, C, and niacin and the minerals magnesium and zinc, along with adequate protein.
- Avoid specific foods and lifestyle factors that disturb the balance of fats. These include trans fat, refined carbohydrates, including sugar, and excess stress, including overexercise.

Specific foods can fight inflammation because they contain phytonutrients that help drive the A and C fats to group 1 and 3 eicosanoids that reduce inflammation. Here are the most common anti-inflammatory foods:

- *Ginger and turmeric.* Both spices are used in many types of foods. While fresh turmeric is more difficult to find in stores, fresh ginger is widely available. Ginger can be used in salads or added to salad dressing, made into a tea, pickled, or is added to many dishes for its pungent flavor. Developing a habit of using ginger regularly in your meals can be helpful in controlling inflammation. Turmeric is actually in the ginger family and probably on your spice shelf. It's commonly used as a natural coloring agent and is a major ingredient in curry powder.
- *Citrus peel.* Many people drink or eat citrus fruit but discard the best part—the peel. They are throwing out some of the most important nutritional factors. The oil in citrus peel contains limonene, a powerful phytonutrient. When eating the fruit, eat some of the skin, or at least the white parts. This is more enjoyable when the fruit is tree-ripened, which makes for a much sweeter skin.
- *Onion.* Foods in the onion family—including shallots, chive, and garlic—can also help reduce inflammation. In American culture, garlic and onions are often avoided due to the odor after eating them. But both have great therapeutic benefits and should be part of your daily diet, even if it's just in your evening meal.

Functional Illness

Chronic inflammation that's allowed to continue unchecked can lead to a full spectrum of functional problems, such as fatigue, hormonal imbalance, and reduced immunity. Fatigue is probably one of the most common consequence of chronic inflammation. Other problems associated with chronic inflammation include the following:

- *Lowered immunity.* This can result in frequent, recurring infections, including colds and flu, and yeast and fungal infections such as candida. Asthma and allergies may also develop due to the combination of low immunity and chronic inflammation.
- *Hormonal imbalance.* This can include many aspects of the hormonal system, especially the adrenal stress hormones, reducing your ability to cope with stress. Sex hormones—estrogen, progesterone, and testosterone—can also be adversely affected, resulting in diminished sex drive, reproductive function, and muscle and bone health. Reduced thyroid function can also result due to inhibition of thyroid-stimulating hormone.
- *Nervous system imbalance.* This includes increased activity of the sympathetic nervous system potentially leading to increased tension, rising blood pressure, disturbed blood sugar, and anxiety or depression.
- *Digestive distress.* Among the problems that can result are poor digestion, gas formation, heartburn, and various inflammatory conditions such as colitis (colon), gastritis (stomach), and ileitis (small intestine). Poor absorption of nutrients can be another result, creating

an entire series of potential problems throughout the body that mimic nutritional deficiency.

- *Chronic pain.* Inflammation produces pain-stimulating chemicals throughout the body. This also results in a reduced pain threshold.
- Physical injuries—especially those with "itis"—are often caused and or maintained by chronic inflammation. They include bursitis (inflammation of the bursa material that surrounds the joints), tendonitis (inflammation of a tendon which connects a muscle to a bone), arthritis (inflammation of a joint), and myositis (inflammation of a muscle).
- *Cataracts.* Another common condition that develops with age is cataracts, and inflammation plays a major role in the development of this eye disease. Chronic inflammation has been shown to predispose healthy individuals to future risk of age-related cataracts.
- *Gingivitis and periodontal disease.* These oral conditions are also associated with inflammation and may be a silent cause of chronic bodywide inflammation.
- Excessive menstrual pain is associated with chronic inflammation caused by excessive group 2 eicoanoids from too many B fats.
- *Hair loss.* This common problem in both men and women can be associated with inflammation in the scalp, specifically the hair follicles.

Chronic Diseases

In the long term, chronic inflammation can lead to more serious diseases. Here are some of them:

WHEN EATING FISH ISN'T ENOUGH—TAKE DIETARY SUPPLEMENTS

One remedy that can significantly help control inflammation and balance fats is fish oil supplements, which provide a concentrated form of C fats. Fish oil supplements contain high amounts of EPA, and in combination with reducing vegetable oils, it can help make fat balance a reality. EPA also helps prevent some of the A fats from converting to B fats. In addition, raw sesame seed oil helps prevent this process too. Be sure to buy small amounts of raw sesame oil, don't cook it, and keep it refrigerated because it's a relatively unstable polyunsaturated oil. However, don't refrigerate fish oil capsules (or any gel caps) as the cold temperatures can cause them to leak, allowing oxygen in—at the risk of rancidity and lower potency.

In addition to EPA, fish oil often contains DHA (docosohexanoic acid), which is another important C fat that's especially important for children's developing brains. In the body, DHA can convert to EPA, and vice versa.

- *Cardiovascular disease.* This includes heart disease, atherosclerosis, and stroke.
- *Ulcers.* As chronic inflammation progresses, ulceration is a common next step. In particular, this occurs in the intestinal tract. A condition such as ulcerative colitis is a combination of ulcers and inflammation. Stomach and duodenal ulcers are also associated with inflammation.

Inflammatory lung diseases include cystic fibrosis, chronic obstructive pulmonary disease, pulmonary fibrosis, and lung cancer.

Growth of a tumor is directly associated with chronic inflammation because of the excess amount of group 2 eicosanoids from B fats. Many types of cancer are the end result—including those in the pancreas, liver, brain, and skin.

ANTI-INFLAMMATORY DRUGS—HOW THEY WORK

Millions of people take various types of nonsteroidal anti-inflammatory drugs—NSAIDs—every day. They're hoping to alleviate chronic aches and pains. Anti-inflammatory drugs work as follows: In the conversion of A, B, and C fats to eicosanoids, an important enzyme called cyclooxygenase, or COX, is required. There are actually two COX enzymes, and many people are familiar with the term "COX-2 inhibitors." These are drugs that attempt to inhibit these enzymes. Aspirin and all other NSAIDs, including ibuprofen, Advil, Motrin, Nuprin, and Naprosyn, temporarily block the COX enzyme so much less of the inflammatory series 2 eicosanoids are formed. While this reduces the inflammation, these drugs can also eliminate groups 1 and 3, along with their beneficial properties. This may result in an improvement of symptoms, but it also turns off the important anti-inflammatory mechanism. In addition, the cause of the problem—fat imbalance—goes untreated.

While symptoms are often reduced or relieved, these drugs have side effects by causing chemical stress to occur throughout the whole body. Here are some of side effects of NSAIDS:

- They cause intestinal problems, including bleeding, in almost everyone taking them (even if it's not noticeable). This can cause anemia and fatigue.
- They can cause muscle dysfunction, contributing to physical aches and pains, and injuries.
- They can reduce the body's ability to repair joint and bone stress.
- They can cause kidney damage, especially when you're dehydrated.
- They can disturb sleep.

- They may not necessarily reduce all inflammation.
- They cause immune system stress.
- They can increase the risk of atrial fibrillation or heart flutter.

Instead, controlling pain and inflammation is best accomplished by eating adequate amounts of healthy fats and maintaining their proper balance. In addition to controlling inflammation and pain, eicosanoids have many other important functions. Impairing these actions can result from taking NSAIDS as well. Both groups 1 and 3 decrease blood clotting and dilate blood vessels, which lowers blood pressure and increases circulation. Group 2 eicosanoids, however, do almost the opposite, increasing blood clotting, constricting blood vessels, and increasing blood pressure. But these activities can be healthy when balanced—without the constricting of blood vessels and the raising of blood pressure, blood circulation would be poor and not enough oxygen, vitamins, and minerals would be circulated throughout the body. Or without blood clotting, you could bleed to death from a small cut. Balance is key, and NSAIDS cause an imbalance.

Too many group 2 eicosanoids can be deadly: they constrict blood vessels too much and can lead to blood clots. They can also trigger tumor growth, atherosclerosis (fat deposits), asthma and allergy, bone loss, and even promote menstrual cramps. Balancing these actions by increasing anti-inflammatory actions is vital.

Other diseases associated with inflammation are asthma, with its chronically inflamed passageways into the lung as a main component of the condition are cancer, osteoporosis, and type 2 diabetes. Even chronic fatigue syndrome and anorexia have been found to be associated with chronic inflammation.

Chronic inflammation results in a variety of end-result signs and symptoms; from arthritis and colitis to chronic muscle and joint injuries. Along the way, the process of disease may develop—an ulcer, cancer, heart disease, cognitive brain disorders such as Alzheimer's. Quality of life is greatly diminished. Health and human performance gradually destroyed. This is an all-too-common road for many people to travel on—or be wheeled along. But you can choose another road where health and fitness continues to improve with age. We've discussed the ways to do this by avoiding unhealthy refined carbohydrates and bad fats and by consuming good carbohydrates and balance natural fats. Next up is the importance of protein foods, the topic of the next chapter.

CHAPTER 6

THE POWER OF PROTEIN
Are You Eating Enough?

Once you've determined the right amount of carbohydrates for your body and balanced your fats, proper protein intake is relatively easy to determine. For example, if you find that 40 percent of your macronutrients are carbohydrates and 30 percent fat, the remaining 30 percent as protein would probably be the optimal amount for you. As convenient and oversimplified as that may sound, that's how it turns out for most people. Find the first two pieces of the puzzle and the third falls neatly into place.

However, there's no need to determine percentages—or grams calories or any other quantity. Instead, make the appropriate changes as outlined in the earlier chapters, beginning with carbohydrates, and let it all fall into place; your intuition will become a powerful ally. Coralee Thompson, MD, simplifies protein needs even more: "At each meal eat the amount of dense protein food such as meat, fish or eggs that fits in the palm of your hand." It's that easy.

Each person needs protein every day for good health and fitness. This is true at all ages, for males and females, and whether you are walking thirty minutes a day or training for a marathon. Larger body frames and those performing a lot of physical work usually need more protein. Growing children also need relatively higher amounts of protein for development. In fact, throughout life, there is still a significant and continuous need for protein.

Protein is necessary for so many healthy bodily functions. Here are just a few examples:

- Enzymes important for balancing fats, digestion, and hundreds of other metabolic activities necessary for optimal health require protein.
- Protein is essential for maintaining neurotransmitters—the chemical messengers used by the brain, the rest of the nervous system, and gut for communication.
- Protein is a key element for building new cells, especially for muscles, bones, organs, and glands, throughout life.
- Oxygen, fats, vitamins, hormones, and other compounds are regulated and transported throughout the body with the help of protein.
- Protein is necessary to make natural antibodies for the immune system.
- Protein contains key amino acids for health. For example, cysteine is necessary for the body to make its most powerful antioxidant, glutathione, and glutamine is used to fuel the intestine for optimal function, especially for digestion and absorption of nutrients.
- Protein is important for the production of glucagon in relation to controlling insulin and blood sugar.

Studies continue to show that the protein recommendations by the USDA are too low. These recommendations have resulted in reductions in protein intake by some people with dire health consequences such as muscle loss. Even the argument that protein can harm the kidneys is losing ground as new studies show that restricting dietary protein in those with kidney problems can actually increase the risk of death. Most of this confusion about protein requirements comes from old and outdated research that only measured the protein by-product nitrogen as excreted in the urine. This failed to consider the amount of nitrogen lost in sweat since this is a critical aspect of the protein-breakdown process.

How Much Protein?

So how much protein does your body require regularly? The answer to this important question depends on some of these factors: body size (larger body frames need more), overall muscle mass (those with a large muscle mass need more protein to maintain it), and level of physical activity (more activity mean more protein needs). That is why using the USDA's protein recommendation comes up short. Its suggested daily consumption of protein is the bare minimum for an inactive person. And it's based on body weight and not lean muscle mass. This amount is 0.8 grams of dietary protein per kilogram (2.2 pounds) of body weight. Based on this, a person weighing about 70 kilograms or 150 pounds should consume 60 grams of protein per day. This can be obtained with two eggs at breakfast, a salad with fish at lunch, and a small steak at dinner.

But for most active, healthy people, this amount is insufficient. Recent studies show that protein requirements should be twice that of the USDA's dietary requirement. Based on my own clinical experience, I prefer to recommend a range of normal that includes the minimum amount of 0.8 grams to about 1.6 grams per kilogram of body weight. For most athletes and those with very physical jobs, the amount of protein may still need to be increased above this level. Those involved in jogging/running, biking, swimming, and other aerobic-type exercise usually need more protein because the normal continual process of building and repairing muscle may actually be greater than that of weight lifters.

For most active, healthy people, a normal protein intake over 1.0 grams per kilogram of body weight, usually closer to the 1.6 number, is best. The following are some examples of food servings that provide these amounts of protein:

- For a 175-pound person, the daily protein intake may be 128 grams. The protein foods that would provide this include three eggs and cheese at breakfast, a salad with a hefty serving of turkey at lunch, and salmon for dinner.
- For a 145-pound person, the requirement may be about 106 grams: two eggs for breakfast, a chef's salad for lunch, and a sirloin steak for dinner.

- And for the person weighing 125 pounds who would minimally require about 90 grams of protein: two eggs at break-

Myths about Protein

The image many people have of protein-rich foods, shakes, and supplements is that they're mostly for body builders, weight lifters, triathletes, and football players. The fact is, everyone needs daily dietary protein to remain healthy and fit. Protein is a basic nutritional requirement to help build and maintain one's bones, organs, and glands. Dietary protein is also critical because it generates health-promoting enzymes for energy, hormone balance, digestion, and immune function. And protein is important for brain function.

You need to consume protein each day to replace the millions of muscle cells you lose. Otherwise, muscle mass is reduced. By maintaining them, you not only sustain your strength and ability to be agile, but you also protect your bones and prevent injury.

At one time low muscle mass was considered a problem mostly in those over age sixty, but now it's a health issue in younger adults and even children mainly due to the overfat epidemic. Lower levels of muscle are associated carbohydrate intolerance and chronic inflammation.

94

fast, tuna salad for lunch, and lamb for dinner.

If you're 200 pounds or more, or appreciably under 125 pounds, just estimate the protein requirements based on the above numbers. For example, at 200 pounds, that's 25 percent heavier, so 25 percent more than 128 grams of protein is 160 grams.

When individuals make healthy changes in their lifestyle, the resulting protein choices often increase without the person realizing it. It can happen naturally. I saw this time and again in my private practice. Such was the case with a former patient I will call Fred. He saw great success from the Two-Week Test—elimination of his aches and pains, losing body fat, and getting off the six different medications he was taking. Fred then moved on to balancing his fats. A secondary dietary analysis showed, without him first realizing it, that his protein intake rose from his original diet survey that he took during his first office visit: a change from about 48 grams to about 65 grams a day from eggs, meat, nuts, and small amounts of cheese. At age fifty-two, Fred was never physically active, but now that he was feeling healthier, he wanted to exercise to build more fitness. He first started walking and a few months later began to alternate this with jogging. He eventually added swimming three times a week to his total workout time of seventy-five minutes each day. Needless to say, Fred was building muscles—especially in his arms, legs, and shoulders. About a year after his initial visit to my clinic, I reviewed

his diet again. Now his protein intake was up to 90 grams of protein a day. Fred felt great.

Here's another case study that demonstrates the importance of a sufficient amount of protein in one's diet. Two couples visited my clinic because they were exhausted from what they claimed were years of overwork

HEALTH SURVEY: ARE YOU PROTEIN DEFICIENT?

Do you have any of these symptoms?

- Reduced muscle strength
- Muscle imbalance (aches and pains, chronic injuries)
- Hormone imbalance
- Carbohydrate intolerance
- Chronic inflammation
- Reduced physical performance or disability
- Slow walking speed (less than about two steps per second)
- Poor balance.
- Low vitamin D (blood test below 50 nmol/L)
- Difficulty ascending stairs or getting out of a chair
- Taking antacids or drugs to reduce stomach acid

Unfortunately, these are common signs and symptoms associated with chronic protein malnutrition.

and raising a family. With the kids gone, Joan and Rob, now in their late fifties, were ready to make health and fitness a priority for the years ahead. I recommended that Joan perform the Two-Week Test while Rob did not appear to have a problem with carbohydrates. Joan's protein intake initially was very low, around 20 grams, because she avoided meat and eggs and ate a low-fat diet that consisted mostly of refined carbohydrates. Rob was a meat eater, consuming about 60 grams of protein a day, although he had low levels of many vitamins and minerals because he ate very few fruits and vegetables. Both eliminated junk food, balanced their fats, and started consuming many more vegetables and fruits. After about three months, both Joan and Rob were feeling less tired and exhausted; they were exercising regularly and eating well every day. They returned about a year later for a checkup, continuing their excellent lifestyle habits. Among other things, I performed another dietary analysis. Joan's daily protein intake had increased to about 60 grams, quite adequate for a petite woman who was moderately active. Rob's protein intake increased to over 100 grams. At six feet and now biking daily for ninety minutes, Rob was enjoying his fruits and vegetables, along with meats and eggs, more than ever. Bottom line, for Joan and Rob and everyone else, is this: don't underestimate or underconsume protein.

In fact, if you require more than 100 grams a day, that's not excessive, it's what your body needs. Eating the amount of protein your body requires is not a high-protein diet; it's getting your proper requirements! Sometimes, when unhealthy people consume normal amounts of protein, they won't feel good because something else is wrong. For example, as protein intake increases, so does your need for water, which helps eliminate the normal by-products of protein through the kidneys. That's part of the old argument that protein is a stress on the kidneys; it most certainly is if you are dehydrated.

Or if you're under significant stress and your stomach does not make sufficient amounts of natural hydrochloric acid—the first chemical stage of protein digestion—protein digestion can be a problem that could give you symptoms of intestinal distress. Addressing the cause of the problem—the stress and stomach, not the protein—is the best remedy. Or another potential protein problem may occur if you combine a steak with some bread or a potato—this is a significant stress for the stomach, and indigestion often follows.

Amino Acids: The Building Blocks of Protein

Just as carbohydrates are made up of sugars and fats are composed of fatty acids, dietary protein is made up of building blocks called amino acids. They are important for new cell formation, including bones, immune function, and hundreds of metabolic activities throughout the body. For example, the

96

amino acid tryptophan is used to make certain neurotransmitters in the brain. Or recombining many amino acids provides for the manufacture of new muscle cells. There are at least twenty amino acids necessary to human nutrition, all of which are indispensable for optimal health and human performance. While some amino acids can be manufactured in the body by other raw materials from food, others called "essential amino acids" must be taken in through the diet. While amino acids that are made in the body are sometimes referred to as "nonessential," this is misleading as all amino acids are essential. In order to obtain these vital components, the intestine must do its job. First, protein must be efficiently digested in the intestine, resulting in breakdown into amino acids. Second, these amino acids must be absorbed into the body. Once absorbed, the amino acids are used either directly, such as cysteine being used to help make the immune systems most powerful antioxidant, glutationone, or they are recombined into whole proteins such as for muscle formation.

In general, animal foods are the best sources of protein and contain all the amino acids. Overall, the highest-rated protein food is eggs, followed by beef and fish.

For those who don't eat animal products, obtaining all the amino acids is not an easy task. This can be accomplished by combining enough variety since not one plant-based food, except soybeans, contains all the amino acids (although soy is very low in the amino acid methionine). Certain combinations of plant foods, such as beans and rice or whole grains and peanut butter, can provide a complete protein. However, combining meals high in carbohydrates (such as rice, beans, grains, etc.) with protein can reduce digestibility, with the result that some protein will not digest into amino acids, and some amino acids won't get absorbed. In addition, many of these foods today are processed or contain added ingredients making them an unhealthy choice. Examples include white rice, refined wheat and other grain products, and peanut butter containing added sugar and hydrogenated fat.

LOSING MUSCLE MASS IS DUE TO NATURAL AGING, BUT AN INCREASED LOSS IS UNHEALTHY AND IS KNOWN AS SARCOPENIA

Sarcopenia comes from the Greek word meaning "poverty of flesh," and it refers to the degenerative loss of skeletal muscle mass and overall body strength associated with aging. This loss of muscle mass may be caused by different factors, with an end result of increased body fat and loss of muscle. In the past few decades, sarcopenia has emerged as a major health concern due to a reduction of physical activity

97

and increased longevity. In other words, people are becoming weaker, but they are living longer. The result is a lot more broken hips and legs from falls by an increasingly aging population; and these accidents often mark the beginning of the end for many: months, if not years, of limited mobility.

Many people complain about getting old. It's what old people do. But now people in their forties and fifties are experiencing many of the same problems as those in their sixties, seventies, and eighties. They have slowed down, feel more aches and pains, and lose strength. Their balance is lost, risking falls, and broken bones. Over time, there can be a gradual reduction in height, as well as a more evident slumped-over posture. This is typically due to sarcopenia. And it's preventable! A key cause of sarcopenia is inadequate protein intake. Just eating sufficient amounts of protein foods not only can help maintain muscle mass but stave off sarcopenia.

In the September 7, 2010, issue of the medical journal *Clinical Interventions in Ageing*, researchers Louise Burton and Deepa Sumukadas from University of Dundee in Scotland reported that "many older adults do not consume sufficient amounts of dietary protein which leads to a reduction in lean body mass and increased functional impairment." They further explained that the loss of muscle mass is a strong predictor of mortality in later life and that low muscle strength, the result of lost muscle, is associated with increased risk of death.

One's muscle mass peaks in the twenties and thirties but in one's forties begins to drop depending on how much protein is consumed and the level of physical activity. By age fifty, there is a steady decline in muscles throughout the body. But it need not be the case for everyone; you control much of these changes through lifestyle— diet as well as weight-bearing or resistance exercises that will maintain your overall muscle tone and strength.

Even young people, including children, are not building their bodies. Preethi Srikanthan and colleagues from UCLA's Department of Medicine wrote in a May 2010 issue of the medical journal *PLOS*, "With the ongoing obesity epidemic in the U.S. and the disturbing increases in the incidence of obesity in children and young adults, our data suggest that we can expect to see sharp increases in sarcopenia and diabetes in the coming years. In this environment, interventions aimed at increasing muscle mass in younger ages and preventing loss of muscle mass in older ages may have the potential to reduce type 2 diabetes risk."

Because muscle do more than move our bodies or lift things, reduced amounts can, in controlling free radicals, place one at risk for carbohydrate intolerance and diabetes, increased blood fats (cholesterol and triglycerides), hypertension, and cardiovascular disease. As body function diminishes and ill heath rises, sarcopenia can worsen to a more advanced condition called cachexia—a metabolic syndrome with chronic inflammation at its root, with even more loss of the body's muscle. Where sarcopenia ends and cachexia begins is difficult to distinguish, but the key is preventing it by maintaining optimal protein intake, physical activity, and overall good health.

But there's more troubling news about to emerge on the sarcopenia scene. Like the medical rage in conducting bone scans in the last decade to detect brittle bones or osteoporosis, scanning the body for muscle mass will soon become the latest health care trend. These tests—with fancy technical names such as magnetic resonance imaging (MRI), dual energy X-ray absorptiometry (DXA), and bioelectric impedence analysis—all have their strengths and weaknesses as diagnostic tools. The tests often have difficulty in distinguishing muscle from water retention and muscle fat. But these exams will nonetheless be marketed to a public fearful of aging and declining muscle loss. The companies and individuals doing the testing will probably not inform you to eat more protein but simply to sell you some special dietary supplement or "new exercise" workout DVD.

Making Wise Protein Choices

For most people getting enough protein should not be a problem as there are many healthy options. These include eggs, meats, fish, and dairy foods. For those who won't eat these foods, getting enough protein can be a challenge. Soybeans and certain combinations of legumes and grains can supply all essential amino acids, but you risk not getting adequate protein and generally must eat more carbohydrate than needed. For most people obtaining sufficient protein is relatively easy, especially when choosing animal sources.

Choosing the best animal proteins means finding the best sources. This may be organic, grass-fed, free-range, kosher, and whatever other labels are used to differentiate the highest quality eggs, meats, fish, and dairy foods from those obtained from poorly treated animals. Beware of the modern food industrial complex, which mass produces beef, chicken, pork, and other animals in unhealthy (and often inhumane) ways. The result is dangerous food, typically used in the fast food industry, with higher risks of *E. coli* outbreaks and items containing harmful hormones and chemicals used in the raising of animals and production of these foods.

The human intestinal track is well adapted for digesting animal-source foods, having evolved from early history on a diet relatively high in meat and fish (with varying amounts of vegetables, fruits, and nuts). While the popular trend in recent decades has been toward the misconception that any or all meat consumption is unhealthy, there are a variety of unique features of an animal-food diet that are vital for health and fitness. Here are some of them:

- Animal foods contain high levels of all essential amino acids.
- Vitamin B_{12} is an essential nutrient found only in animal foods.
- EPA, the powerful C fat that helps control inflammation and the one preferred by the human body, is almost exclusively found in animal foods.
- Iron deficiency is a common worldwide problem and is best prevented by eating animal foods because it contains this mineral in a most bioavailable form.
- Vitamin A is found only in animal products. Plant foods—vegetables and fruits—contain only beta-carotene, which is not vitamin A; its conversion in the body to vitamin A is not always efficient in humans.
- Animal products are dense protein foods with little or no carbohydrate to interfere with digestion and absorption.

- People who consume less animal protein have greater rates of bone loss than those who eat larger amounts of animal protein.
- Creatine, the best source is meat, is an important amino acid to build muscle and prevent its loss.
- The amino acid glutamine, the main energy source for optimal intestinal function, is primary found in meat, especially those minimally cooked such as rare beef.

Here's the Beef about Meat

Yes, it can be tricky to be a meat-eater in a nation that believes in the almighty fast-food hamburger that might contain by-products from many different cattle, even from different states and countries. But it's no bull—if you want to be healthy, beef really is "what's for dinner." Also consider it part of a healthy breakfast, lunch, or snack. Three ounces of lean porterhouse contains 20 grams of protein, and just six grams of saturated fat, balanced by a healthy seven grams of heart-friendly monounsaturated fat. In addition to being an excellent source of high-quality protein, beef is also rich in B vitamins, glutamine, calcium, magnesium, iron, and zinc to name a few of its nutrients.

Organic and natural beef have not been treated with antibiotics or given growth-stimulating hormones. You can buy naturally raised meats in some grocery and health-food stores, and local sources may be even better. Look for nearby farms and ranches that sell meat from animals that have been raised on grass, not fed corn, and without the use of growth hormones, antibiotics, and other chemicals used by most stock growers. Whether you live near a farm that sells natural or organic meat or order from a ranch that can ship to you, you may wish to save money and buy a large quantity of beef so that you always have some on hand. The meat will keep well in a freezer until it's time to make another order.

When cooking beef, keep it on the rare side. Studies show that beef cooked medium, medium well, or well done is associated with higher rates of stomach cancer. This is due to the production of carcinogenic nitrogen compounds created during overcooking. Heat-sensitive nutrients, such as the amino acid glutamine, are also significantly reduced in meat cooked beyond rare.

Bacteria in beef are usually due to the food-handling process. While bacteria can reside on the surface of meat, it won't get inside unless the meat is ground. Almost all cases of food poisoning involving meat are from sources that have been ground ahead of time, which allows bad bacteria to flourish. For this reason, ground meat should be thoroughly cooked unless it's freshly ground just before eating it.

Before I bring up poultry and fish as potential sources of protein, allow me to start with the egg—an incredible and often maligned food staple. Eggs are more than incredible: they are the perfect food all wrapped up in one single cell. Yes, that's right—an egg is an individual cell containing the most complete and highest protein rating of any food. They contain all the amino acids, and two eggs contain more than twelve grams of protein, just over half in the white and the rest in the yolk. In addition, eggs also contain many essential nutrients, including significant amounts of vitamins A, D, E, B_1, B_2, B_6, and B_{12} and folic acid. Eggs also contain important minerals such as calcium, magnesium, potassium, zinc, and iron. Two other nutrients, choline and biotin, which are important for energy production and regulating stress, are contained in large amounts in eggs. Most of these nutrients are found in the yolk of the egg.

The fat in egg yolks is also nearly a perfect balance, containing mostly monounsaturated fats and about 36 percent saturated fat. And egg yolks contain both A and C fats.

Eggs have almost no carbohydrate (less than 1 gram), making them the perfect meal or snack for the millions who are carbohydrate intolerant. Ounce per ounce, eggs are also your best food buy with hardly any waste. And with so many ways of preparing them, eggs are delicious.

While most people love the taste of eggs, many are still concerned about eating them because of cholesterol. But studies now show that adding more eggs to your diet can actually decrease your cardiovascular risk. For most people, eggs can be part of a healthy food plan; I eat several whole eggs a day. I have them soft-boiled, as omelets, lightly fried in a little butter, and in smoothies.

Eggs are only as healthy as the hens that lay them, since the nutritional makeup of eggs, especially the fat, depends upon what the chickens eat. For this reason you should avoid run-of-the-mill grocery-store eggs that have been produced in chicken factories. Unfortunately this includes most eggs on the market. The healthiest eggs come from organic, free-range hens. Even better, buy eggs from a local farmer who lets chickens eat healthy, wild food and organic feed. Free-range means that the hens are allowed to roam where they can eat bugs and vegetable matter, yielding eggs with a better fat profile, with more monounsaturated fat, and more essential fatty acids. The so-called omega 3 eggs come from chickens fed with flaxseeds, not EPA. Often these hens are not free-range nor certified organic and are still housed in very crowded hen factories.

The domestic taming of chickens and other fowl for egg production dates back to before 1500 BC in China. Today, eggs come in many sizes and shell colors, not just white and brown. Depending on the type of chicken that laid them, some eggs have tints of green, blue, and red.

Eggs, of course, should always be stored in the refrigerator, unless you have your own hens and will be using the eggs within a few days. Because of their porous shell, there is slight evaporation of moisture from the inner egg through the shell, which changes its flavor and freshness. If you are not using them quickly, store your eggs in a sealed container to prevent loss of moisture. Never store eggs next to highly flavored foods, such as onions and fish, because they will easily absorb odors from these foods. Always store eggs with the large side up, which suspends the yolk effectively within the egg white.

Chefs know that room-temperature eggs are easier to work with; when boiled, they don't crack, the whites are easier to whip, and the yolks "stand up" more when fried. If you're separating eggs, however, the colder ones are easier to work with.

Speaking of boiled eggs, they should never really be boiled but kept just at a slight simmer until done. Furiously boiling them results in rubbery whites and less-tasty yolks.

One way to prevent the shells from breaking during boiling is to use a pin. Prick the shell on the large end of the egg with a pin. This allows the air pocket, found in the large end of the egg, to escape during cooking. Otherwise, if the air can't escape, the pressure builds, and it may crack the shell. The best way to cook soft- or hard-boiled eggs is to place them in cold water (one-half inch above the eggs) and bring to a boil. Take off the heat immediately. For soft-cooked eggs, remove after two to four minutes, depending on your taste, and run under cold water. For hard-cooked eggs, cover and let sit for ten to fifteen minutes then rinse in cold water, and keep refrigerated until ready to use. (An egg that is less than two days old is very difficult to peel when hard-boiled.)

Finally, before you buy eggs, make sure they are relatively fresh by looking at the date. Or you can shake them close to your ear; if you hear a sloshing sound, it means they've lost a lot of moisture over time and there's a big air space in them—avoid these. Eggs also contain a natural barrier—an invisible protective coating that keeps out bacteria. Never wash the eggs you're going to store because you will remove this natural protection.

The Poultry Flap

The poultry industry has done such a good job telling the public how healthy chicken or turkey is over meat and pork, but this is untrue. In fact, chickens are generally raised in more unhealthy environments than cattle because of lower sanitary standards. Today's chicken house is really an overpopulated filthy city, containing one hundred thousand birds or more, cooped up in tiny boxes or very crowded conditions. Because of this, most chickens are given many chemicals and drugs to counter common diseases and infections,

The best bird for the table is organically raised—they've not been treated with or fed any chemicals or drugs; instead, they are given certified-organic feeds and filtered water. This may be the safest of all poultry. Many grocery stores and health-food stores carry organic chickens and turkeys. In addition, you may be able to find birds such as these from a local farm.

The Catch to Fish

Fish can also be a great source of protein and some contain significant quantities of omega-3 C fats. However, just as with other protein foods, some fish are healthier choices over others. The best sources are wild fish, not farm-raised.

In general, avoid seafood that includes the so-called bottom feeders, those fish and other sea species that eat from the ocean's floor where the potential for consuming toxic material is highest. This is especially true for those species that feed close to shore. Flounder, sole, catfish, and crab are some examples of foods to avoid eating regularly. Oysters, clams, mussels, and scallops are also sources of potential pollutants. Clams are perhaps the worst seafood to eat, especially when raw, since they normally filter out and concentrate viruses and bacteria, heavy metals, and other chemical pollutants from the waters in which they live. If you enjoy eating seafood, here are some tips for doing so more safely and more nutritiously:

- Choose fish caught in waters farther away from polluted, industrial areas. These include most Alaskan and Canadian salmon, sardines, and herring.
- Look for cold-water fish like salmon, dark tuna, sardines, and other small fish that contain higher amounts of EPA.
- Eat smaller fish and crustaceans: trout, bass, and shrimp but avoid marlin, great white tuna, and swordfish. Smaller and

younger fish have not accumulated the toxins found in larger and older species.

- Avoid precooked fish and prepared or processed seafood such as breaded frozen fish or seafood, fish cakes, ground fish, and imitation crabmeat (popular at sushi bars).
- If you catch your own fish, ask local authorities about the limits of safety. Some regions recommend limiting how much of certain species you should eat in a year due to toxicity.

Unfortunately, the oceans, rivers, and lakes are becoming so contaminated that wild fish are containing levels of toxins that are dangerous. I recommend limiting fish to once or twice a month or less, and even less than that for children and pregnant women.

Other Meaty Matters

In addition to beef, poultry, and fish, other organic meats are also good sources of protein. They include the following:

AVOID FARM-RAISED AND GENETICALLY MODIFIED FISH

As bad as our natural lakes, rivers, and oceans are getting, the picture is worse for farm-raised seafood—this should always be avoided. These foods often include antibiotics, pesticides, steroids, hormones, and artificial pigments. Unfortunately, they are becoming popular due to availability and cost. Farm-raised salmon makes up 95 percent of the salmon on the market today. Since these fish are raised in confined, crowded, and unsanitary conditions, the threat of disease and parasites is great. To combat disease and parasites, some fish farmers add antibiotics to salmon feed and treat the salmon and their pens with pesticides. Some fish are also treated with steroids to make the fish sterile and growth hormones to speed them to market size and reduce production costs. In addition, since farm-raised salmon do not naturally eat crustaceans that naturally make the flesh pink or orange, salmon growers often feed color additives to pigment the flesh.

For the first time, genetically modified fish are coming to a market near you—the first genetically engineered salmon are a reality. One concern is that the production of these fish has not considered the impact on our health or that of the environment. More alarming is that genetically altered salmon won't be labeled as such, so consumers have no way of knowing what they're buying.

Sadly, this is only the first in what will probably be a long list of genetically manipulated animal foods coming to market.

- Pork and lamb are popular meats and can be found certified organic.
- Meats such as buffalo and elk have appeared in some specialized grocery stores. When choosing these meats, use the same guidelines as with beef and poultry—buy those that are organic or raised naturally at a local farm.
- Wild game, including big game animals, such as deer as well as small game such as rabbits and game birds, is also another great source of protein. Wild game meat is generally leaner but higher in A and C fats than domestic meats. While hunting your own meat is nearly ideal, there is a growing concern in some areas like the northeastern United States that the use of pesticides and other environmental chemicals has affected wild animals. But in general, wild game is much safer than store-bought meat.

Generally avoid ground meat of any kind unless it has been freshly ground right before deep freezing or eating it. A store or butcher should have a record of the day and time a particular batch of meat was ground.

Ground meat is a haven for bacteria and can ferment in your intestine much worse than whole meat. If you want to use ground meat, it's best to buy a large piece of meat and then grind it up just before cooking—most butchers, even those in large grocery stores, will do this for you. Even better is to buy a grinder for your own needs and purchase whole pieces of meat that you grind when you want it. It will be more nutritious, safer, and tastier.

Also beware of other meats that have already been cut and stored ahead of time, such as sliced meat, chopped meat, and stew meat. Try to buy as large a piece of meat as possible and cut it yourself.

Processed meats can also be unhealthy choices. Most sausage, lunch meats, and other prepared meats are not only ground but also may contain high amounts of sugar, artificial preservatives, and chemicals that you want to avoid. However, it is possible to find organic bacon and hams that have been cured with honey and with no harmful chemicals.

The most nutritious parts of the animal to eat are the organs and glands. In our society, the liver is the most common organ food, with stomach, brains, kidneys, and others only rarely eaten. However, when a lion kills its prey, it's the organs and glands that are first devoured. The muscle, what we refer to as the "meat," is often left for the scavengers. Unfortunately, with our polluted environment, organ meats such as the liver are becoming more dangerous since it's the liver's job to filter the blood and remove toxins from the body. If you enjoy liver and other organ and gland meats, be sure to find a very good source.

Say Cheese!

Cheese and plain yogurt are dairy products that contain quality protein without

105

many of the lactose-intolerant and other intestinal problems associated with milk. This is especially true if you can find products made from organic raw milk. These cheeses can be found in many stores, local farms and markets, and on the Internet.

Whichever type of milk they're made from, cultured products such as cheese and yogurt are good sources of complete protein with the lactose, or "milk sugar" reduced by friendly bacteria in the culturing process. To be sure that an item is fully cultured, meaning the lactose has been consumed by the natural bacteria, check the NUTRITION FACTS on the label; the carbohydrate should be very low. (Of course, you want to avoid the fruit-flavored and sweetened varieties of yogurt that are always full of sugar—sometimes with a half-dozen teaspoons or more!)

It's important to remember that dairy is also high in B fat. So you must be careful to eat cheese in a way that maintains balance with your intake of A and C fats. If you are recovering from an inflammatory-related illness, such as cancer, heart disease, and the others discussed in this book, limit or avoid dairy products. Like eggs and meats, the milk used to make cheese is partly a reflection of the diet of the animal. A grass-fed milk cow will produce a better product with a superior balance of fats than one that is grain-fed (the same with cows and other animals raised for meat).

In addition, avoid so-called American cheese, cheese spreads, and other processed cheeses. These highly processed products, which outsell natural cheese, are usually several types of unripe cheeses, ground up with added chemical stabilizers, preservatives, and emulsifiers.

The best cheese is made with raw milk, like the cheese made for centuries (the same way it's done in Europe). We use raw goat and cow milk to make raw cheese of various types. It's easy, and for about $5, we can make about $40's worth of delicious cheese.

Milk Proteins: Curds and Whey

Remember Little Miss Muffet eating her curds and whey? These are the two proteins found in milk. Whey protein is the thin liquid part of milk remaining after the curds—called casein—are removed.

Whey is the part of the milk containing most of the vitamins and minerals, including calcium, and it's a complete protein. During the making of cheese, which mostly is produced from curds, whey is often fed back to the animals for nutritional reasons. However, making whey cheese is great option—the one most people are familiar with is ricotta. When buying it, check the label and make sure whey, not curds, is the main ingredient (many cheap ricotta products are made with whole milk and not whey). Whey is also made into powders for use in baked goods and smoothies as discussed below.

The whey component of milk contains a group of natural sulfur-containing substances called biothiols that help produce a key antioxidant in your cells called gluta-thione. Because it helps the immune system, whey has been used to help prevent and treat many chronic conditions, from asthma and allergies to cancer and heart disease. It can also help improve muscle function. Most people who are allergic to cow's milk can usually consume whey without problems. Small amounts of lactose are found in whey (much less than is found in liquid milk), but this is usually too little to cause intestinal problems, even in most people sensitive to lactose. In those who are truly lactose-intolerant (probably less than 5 percent of the population), this amount of lactose could be a problem.

The curds from milk are used for most cheese making. Cottage cheese is the best example of what curds look like. However, the curd is the protein in milk most people are allergic to when there's a dairy allergy. Newborns and young children are especially vulnerable to curds because their intestine and immune system are too immature to tol-erate this protein.

NOT ALL CASEIN IS THE SAME

"Casein" comes from the Latin word *caseus* or "cheese" and is the main protein found in the milk of mammals including cows, goats, and humans. Four casein pro-teins make up about 80 percent of the protein in cow's milk. One of the major caseins is beta-casein, of which there are several types, but A1 and A2 are the most common. As a protein, A1 behaves like an opiate and has been associated with chronic illness and disease, but A2 has not. If you consume dairy products, it's important to pur-chase those made from milk with little or no A1.

Research shows a strong association between the consumption of A1 casein and various health problems. Numerous studies, including data from the World Health Organization (WHO), have linked A1 with increased risk of heart disease, high cho-lesterol, type 1 diabetes, sudden infant death syndrome, and neurological disorders, such as autism and schizophrenia, and possibly allergies. These health issues are not associated with consumption of A2 casein.

Most people think of black-and-white cows as the source of their milk. These animals, called Holsteins (the U.S. breed) and Friesians (the European version), are the most common sources of milk on the market. These large, high-volume milk producers are most commonly used by big corporate dairy farms. They are typically given bST (bovine somatotropin—a hormone used to increases the cow's milk pro-duction) and provided with special feeds of corn and synthetic vitamins rather than grass. These cows produce milk that contains higher amounts of beta-casein type A1 (red-colored cows, including Ayrshire and Milking Shorthorns, are also in this category and less common.)

The other types of dairy cows are smaller and brownish and white in color. These are called Jersey, Guernsey, and Brown Swiss cows. They produce lesser volumes of milk, are naturally resistant to disease, and convert grass to milk quite efficiently. The level of A1 casein in these animals is very low, and they have higher levels of A2. Their milk is similar to that of other animals including goat, sheep, buffalo, yaks, donkeys, and camels—milk from these animals contain mostly A2 and little A1.

How can you tell which type of animal your milk comes from? Unfortunately, in most cases, the milk from many different herds of cows are mixed by the time it gets to the store as milk or cheese. This makes it impossible to tell what you're getting regarding the kinds of casein it contains.

Short of going to the farm to buy raw milk and seeing the types of cows there, which a surprising number of consumers can do, you will soon have more access to milk higher in A2 and low (or no) A1. New Zealand public company, A2 Corp. LTD, licenses technology that identifies milk with the A2 beta casein protein. The company also sources and supplies A2 milk, with operations primarily in New Zealand, Australia, and now the United States (with plans to soon enter the Asian market).

The Soy Story

While soy is a vegetarian source of a complete protein, it's often a problem for most people. One reason is that most soy in use today is not the natural bean but a highly processed and concentrated food product. Whole green soybeans or edamame are an example of a whole food and a good source of protein (although not as good as eggs, meat, or fish). With a relatively small amount of simple processing, soy can be made into tofu, also a good protein choice. This is how most soy has been consumed for many years, and studies of these populations seem to show that soy has health benefits when consumed as a food.

But most soy is consumed in a highly processed and concentrated form. Soy powders are commonly used in food products and supplements. But they're often so concentrated that a serving or two would be like eating a pound of real soybeans—something most people would never even consider. For this reason, it's best to avoid all processed soy products, especially the most processed forms: soy-protein isolates, caseinates, and hydrolyzed soy.

The more soy is processed, the worse it can be. Monosodium glutamate (MSG), a one-time commonly used powder that makes food seemingly taste better (still used in Chinese and other restaurants), is made by processing soy. The result is that these products containing isolated, caseinated, or hydrolyzed soy also contain MSG (but it is not required to be listed in the ingredients).

Many people, especially children, may be intolerant and even allergic to soy in all forms. In addition, concentrated soy isoflavones, used in dietary supplements, can pose serious dangers, including an increased risk of cancer, particularly for postmenopausal women, the very audience these products are marketed to by the big companies. They may also contribute to hormonal imbalance.

Protein Powders

Soy, milk, whey, egg, and other foods are commonly sold as powders to supplement the diet. These have value when used cautiously. Certainly avoid any of these powders if you're intolerant to those foods. In addition, avoid all powders that have been isolated, caseinated, or hydrolyzed—for the same reasons discussed above. These products are touted as being highest in protein—which is true, but at the expense of being highly processed and containing MSG. Those marked CONCENTRATED are the least processed of the powders and are an acceptable part of a healthy diet.

Egg white powder is the least processed of all the powders. This and whey concentrate are the best and healthiest of all these products. (If you use egg white powder in a blender, it must include a small amount of fat; otherwise, it will create a large volume of foam— great for meringue but not for smoothies and other recipes.)

VEGETARIANISM

Some individuals choose to not eat animal products, including meat and fish, for various reasons. Most people claim ethical, health, religious, political, cultural, or emotional reasons for being vegetarian. Ovo-vegetarians consume eggs but no meat, fish, or dairy. Lacto-vegetarians consume dairy but no eggs, meat, or fish. Lacto-ovo-vegetarians consume both eggs and dairy but no meat or fish. Vegans don't eat any eggs, dairy, meat or fish, and also avoid honey. A strict vegan avoids all forms of exploitation of, and cruelty to, animals for food, clothing, or any other purpose. Vegans say they avoid honey because it exploits the bees that produce it.

About 3 percent of the U.S. population is vegetarian, with only 0.5 percent being vegan.

Those who avoid meat, fish, eggs, and dairy can obtain adequate protein, especially if needs are not high, by carefully planning each meal. At one time it was thought that certain combinations of plant foods had to be eaten at the same meal to ensure sufficient essential amino acids for protein needs. But this type of protein combining is not necessary, as long as a variety of unprocessed plant foods are eaten each day and include legumes, whole grains, nuts and seeds, soy and other beans, and vegetables.

Unfortunately, after evaluating the diets of hundreds of vegetarians throughout my career, this is usually not accomplished even after providing these individuals with proper dietary guidelines.

While the various forms of vegetarianism have shown health benefits, there are many studies that demonstrate ill effects due to malnutrition. I was an ovo-vegetarian for several years in my early twenties, thinking it would improve my health. Initially, I felt better overall. In part, this was due to the required care of shopping for food and creating meals, which resulted in healthier food intake. It was a very difficult—actually impossible—task considering the nutrients not available in a strict vegetarian diet. These included vitamins A, B_{12}, and a number of key amino acids such as cysteine, glutamine, and creatine. These could be obtained from dietary supplements. I attempted to obtain sufficient protein by consuming several whole eggs a day, in addition to nuts and seeds, whole grains, and protein supplements.

Eventually, my energy was not sufficient enough to maintain a busy practice and workout schedule every day, and my muscle mass was declining. I also did not like relying on dietary supplements. In addition, I began craving meat—and when I finally began eating, it felt much better.

I also had many patients throughout my career who followed various forms of vegetarianism. While some were careful about their diets, most were not. The majority consumed too much junk food, including a lot of processed carbohydrates and sweets, and very little vegetables. Most of the vegetarians I saw were extremely unhealthy.

For many years, a variety of published studies showed why. Vitamin B_{12} is usually abnormally low in vegetarians, particularly vegans, because this nutrient can only be obtained in sufficient levels from animal foods such as all meats with some in egg yolks and dairy. The result of low levels of vitamin B_{12} is the rise in a chemical called

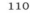

THE POWER OF PROTEIN

homocysteine, which significantly increases the risk cardiovascular disease, including heart attack and stroke.

While mushrooms, tempeh, miso, and sea vegetables are often reported to provide some vitamin B_{12}, they will not prevent deficiency. These foods contain an inactive form of B_{12} and which can interferes with the normal absorption and metabolism of the active form of B_{12}.

Another nutrient that tends to be low in vegetarians is iron. Vegetable sources of iron (called nonheme iron) are not well absorbed by the body while heme forms from meat are well absorbed. In addition, certain foods can impair the absorption of both forms of iron. These include tea and coffee (which contain tannins) and phytates found in whole grains and legumes. (Zinc absorption is also impaired by phytates.)

Studies have shown that bone density is lower in those adhering to a vegetarian diet, especially in vegans, compared to meat-eaters. However, this has not shown that fractures are more common in vegetarians.

To be a healthy and fit vegetarian, an individual will require a high level of care to obtain high-quality food and carefully preparing daily meals. Unprocessed protein supplements, along with other dietary supplements, are usually required.

Along with good carbohydrates and balanced fats, protein foods are key to optimal health and fitness. Most importantly, when choosing protein sources, look for real food. This includes fresh whole eggs, whole pieces of meat and fish, and raw milk cheeses as tolerated. Avoid the processed protein products—cold cuts, frozen foods, processed cheese, and fake fish. If you need to increase protein intake with a food supplement, use egg white powder or a whey concentrate. Another key food group—which contains thousands of unique nutrients—are vegetables and fruits, the topic of the next chapter.

CHAPTER 7

EAT YOUR VEGETABLES AND FRUITS
Understanding the Importance of Phytonutrients and Truly Going "Organic"

So far we've looked in depth at the three macronutrients—carbohydrate, proteins, and fats—as the basis of good nutrition. Now let's shift gears and take a look at a group of foods that really should have their own distinct classification—vegetables and fruits. These plant foods should make up the bulk of your meals because they not only contain macronutrients but micronutrients as well (vitamins and minerals), but just as important is our source of thousands of compounds called phytochemicals or phytonutrients.

The term "phyto" originally comes from the Greek word meaning "plant." Phytonutrients refer to those organic components of plants that are known to promote health and immune function—and there are literally thousands of them. Unlike the traditional nutrients—carbohydrates, protein, fat, vitamins, and minerals—phytonutrients are composed of chemical compounds such as carotenoids, which are the red, orange, and yellow pigments in fruits and vegetables.

Scientists believe that phytonutrients may have an even more important role than the plant's vitamins in promoting health and preventing disease in humans.

Basically, all vegetables and fruits should be considered plant foods. Generally, fruits are foods that contain a seed or seeds inside, whereas vegetables have separate seeds usually not contained inside but found on a stalk or other part of the plant. Both vegetables and fruits contain some carbohydrates, some high enough for those who are carbohydrate intolerant to avoid. These include most potatoes, corn, watermelon, and pineapple (these are less natural as they've been genetically modified through the years to produce much higher levels of starch and sugar). All types of dried fruits, including raisins, are also very concentrated carbohydrates that may be problematic for those sensitive to carbohydrates.

Some foods that are technically fruits are usually thought of as vegetables: avocados, tomatoes, eggplant, peppers, and squash. What's important to know is that vegetables and fruits should make up the bulk of your diet. Most people don't eat enough vegetables and fruits, and there are very few who eat too much of this good thing. I often recommend as a general guideline that adults try to eat at least ten servings of vegetables and fruits per day. Many of these should be raw and most, if not all, should be fresh.

So what is one serving? Traditionally, many have considered a serving to be a half cup. More recently, however, many dietary guidelines have recommended different approaches for measuring servings. For instance, a serving of lettuce might be a cup and a half, a serving of carrots might be one medium carrot, a serving of broccoli is one medium stalk, and a serving of asparagus is five spears. Using guidelines like these will help you to eat more vegetables than using the traditional half-cup serving. Combining servings into one dish make it easier to eat more vegetables. Consider soup as a meal, which can easily include two or three servings of vegetables—homemade tomato soup takes less than five minutes to prepare by first blending fresh tomatoes, cilantro, and carrots.

Eat Your Vegetables

Consider vegetables as an important part of each meal. Including a spinach-and-tomato omelet at breakfast; a large salad of lettuces, carrots, cucumbers, and onions at lunch; and some lightly cooked mixed vegetables with dinner can easily provide you with adequate intake. Even a favorite food like meat loaf can be made so that up to half of it is vegetable content; add chopped onions, red or yellow bell peppers, zucchini, fresh parsley, and garlic.

"PHYTO" FACTS

Scientists have isolated about twenty-five thousand phytonutrients. They can be divided into three main groups of plant compounds that include phenols, terpenes, and nitrogen-containing alkaloids. Within these groups, some of the names are familiar—they include carotenes (including alpha and beta and lycopene), bioflavanoids (including hesperetin and lutein), and a variety of isothiocyanates, which includes the anticancer sulforaphan. While most people are familiar with alpha tocopherol (vitamin E), there are seven other related phytonutrients in the vitamin E family that include three additional tocopherols and four tocotrienols. But don't be concerned about remembering all these names—just remember to consume a variety of vegetables and fruits to obtain these vital phytonutrients.

TABLE 3.0: THREE CATEGORIES OF PHYTONUTRIENTS

Terpenes	Phenols	Alkaloids
carotenoids	lignans	isothiocyanates
lutein	sesamin	sulforaphan
lycopene	isoflavones	indol-3-carbinol
zeaxanthin	flavonoids	crambene
limonene	herperetin	cyano-glycosides
tocopherols	diadzein	morphine
tocotrienols	naringin	caffeine

Vegetables, such as lightly steamed greens, are quick and easy to prepare and are tasty. Depending on the season and markets you shop, fresh produce such as kale, mustard greens, rapini, Swiss chard, collards, and common spinach are also some of the most nutritious plants. These bitter leafy vegetables are full of valuable phytonutrients as well as a host of vitamins and minerals. Greens can be served as a delicious bed for just about any protein food from beef to fish or steamed and served with a little butter or extra virgin olive oil and sea salt as a side dish. Also add these and others to homemade soups, with leeks, white or yellow onions, mushrooms, or red and yellow peppers.

It is also important to eat a variety of vegetables because they contain varying amounts of specific nutrients. For instance, a serving of leaf lettuce supplies a high amount of beta-carotene but only a small amount of vitamin C while a serving of brussels sprouts contains high levels of vitamin C with a small amount of beta-carotene.

One of the easiest ways to ensure that you eat enough variety in vegetables is by choosing vegetables in a rainbow of colors. Consider that carrots and winter squash, which are orange, are high in beta-carotene. Many green vegetables, such as broccoli, are high in folic acid. Purple eggplant and cabbage, red peppers, white, green and red onions, white cauliflower, yellow summer squash, brown mushrooms—each of these colorful vegetables contains its own unique set of vitamins, minerals, and phytonutrients.

Ten Servings a Day

Let me return to that number again—ten. As you might expect, I often get questions e-mailed to me that ask, "Do you really mean ten servings of vegetables and fruits per day?" The answer, most definitely, is yes. And it's not difficult to accomplish. If you consider that these plant foods should be the bulk of your diet and each meal can include them, eating ten servings a day is relatively simple. Even healthy snacks and desserts can provide vegetables and fruits! Here's how I do it in a typical day, which often includes eating more than the minimum of "ten."

- Morning begins with a hearty smoothie (or shake). This typically includes an apple, pear and other in-season options, and frozen blueberries, a large serving of raw leafy vegetable (such as kale, spinach, and or parsley), and a medium carrot. (Of course, it also includes eggs, flax and or sesame seeds, and other items along with water.) Vegetable and fruit servings: 2+.
- After working out, and perhaps some chores in the garden, the next meal is about three hours later. I have some type of egg dish, which includes at least two servings of vegetables—such as lightly steamed greens, zucchini, and raw tomato. Vegetable and fruit servings: 2.
- At lunch, the largest single meal, I have a very big salad with a variety of vegetables—lettuce, tomatoes, carrots, homemade pickles, avocados, and other raw items depending on what's in the garden. It's made up of three servings of vegetables (along with dressing and a protein). Vegetable and fruit servings: 3.
- In the midafternoon I have another shake that's similar to the morning version but a bit smaller. Vegetable and fruit servings: 2.
- Dinner is a smaller version of lunch, and includes two servings of vegetables each. Vegetable and fruit servings: 2.
- Now dessert. I typically have either a fruit or vegetable-type homemade treat. This may be green pudding (made with avocado), pumpkin pie (usually made with winter squash), or homemade ricotta

cheese with pears. Vegetable and fruit servings: 1+.

In this typical day's scenario, I get more than a dozen servings of vegetables and fruits. If you're active—I work out about ninety minutes each day—and have made healthy food a priority, this is easy to accomplish. Even if you don't eat or work out as much as I do, you can still easily get ten servings a day. The problem is that many people eat unhealthy items, such as refined carbohydrate foods like cereals, muffins, and bread, eliminating the opportunity to include more plant foods.

Many people often ask about juicing as an option. I don't recommend it. By blending your vegetables and fruits whole rather than simply extracting their juices, you'll get much more nutrition from the foods because you're not wasting all the fiber and other nutrient-rich components that occurs with juicing. When it comes to fruits, the juice is usually higher in glycemic index than the blended version.

I also have to mention that common items such as ketchup, corn, french fries, iceberg lettuce should not be counted as real food. While they have calories, they lack the micronutrients and phytonutrients compared to those foods mentioned above. And of course, many contain other harmful added ingredients such as sugar or bad fats. Avoid them.

OXYGEN RADICAL ABSORPTION CAPACITY— MEASURING ANTIOXIDANTS IN FOOD

Scientists measure the antioxidant effects of foods by measuring what is known as the oxygen radical absorption capacity (ORAC). Foods with the highest ORAC values—those most potent in true antioxidant capacity—include such items as blueberries, plums, garlic, spinach, and cruciferous vegetables like brussels sprouts, kale, and broccoli.

While antioxidants may be the most potent of substances that prevent and treat disease, the antioxidant foods with the highest ORAC values include phytonutrients. In fact, about 80 percent of a food's ORAC power comes from its phytonutrients.

An example of this can be seen in the antioxidant power of one serving of blueberries. It would take six servings—two each of corn, eggplant, and cauliflower—to obtain the same antioxidant potency.

The chart below lists different foods and their ORAC values.

ORAC of Selected Fruits and Vegetables

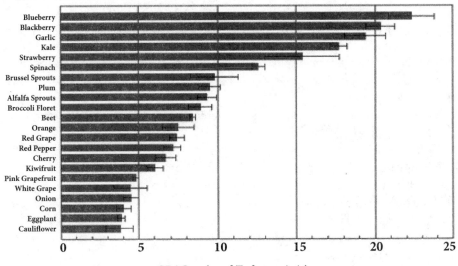

ORAC$_{200}$. (umol Trolox equiv./g)

Vegetables: The Main Course

Many people think of vegetables as little side dish that often not eaten. Instead, consider them as an important part of a main dish. You can even build a meal around your vegetable. Think first what your main course vegetable will be and then create other foods around it—try some steamed kale and carrots with wild salmon or a mixed salad of leaf lettuce, tomatoes, cucumbers, parsley, and onions, with hard-boiled eggs or cheese. More importantly, combine more than one vegetable in a meal. In this way you can make vegetables the bulk of your diet. For instance, a vegetable omelet with onions, red and yellow peppers, and zucchini makes a meal

out of eggs at breakfast. Or how about some organic chicken soup with garlic, leeks, carrots, celery, and chunks of yellow squash—a bowl full of nutrition for lunch or dinner. Even Mom's meat loaf can be adjusted to include up to half vegetables—start with chopped onions, red or yellow bell peppers, zucchini, fresh parsley, and garlic and then add freshly chopped meat and season with sea salt and spices of your choice.

Cooked greens are easy to find in stores and just as simple to prepare. Once you get used to the idea of cooking greens, some meals just won't seem complete without them—truly, cooked greens can be served as a delicious bed for just about any protein

117

RIPE VERSUS UNRIPE?

I always suggest eating red and yellow peppers, but not green. That's because green peppers are not yet ripe. For years, retailers have forced farmers to pick certain crops unripe, such as green tomatoes, so they will have much longer shelf lives. One problem with this is many phytonutrients are not as high in unripe foods as compared with ripe ones. Another is taste—most people know how much more delicious a fresh vine-ripened tomato can be over an old store-bought tomato picked green weeks earlier. One reason why taste is so different is that the starch in the plant turns to natural sugar around the time of ripening.

With less starch in a ripe plant food, digestion is easier since starch is more difficult to break down in the intestines and natural sugars don't require digestion. Many people say, "I like peppers, but they don't like me." Wrong! It's unripe green peppers that are difficult to digest. And they're not nearly as tasty as the red or yellow ones.

Another commonly consumed unripe plant food includes bananas. They're obviously green before turning all yellow upon ripening. When black spots develop, you know they're most ripe and sweetest.

Even winter squash must ripen to taste and digest best. The skin of an acorn squash should be dark green, often with a yellow or orange spot, and that of butternut squash a golden beige color.

Apples, pears, cherries, apricots, and many other fruits are usually picked unripe. This gives them a more starchy, less sweet taste. Even limes turn yellow when tree-ripened, giving them a much more sweet taste over those with green skins. (The corporate bosses wanted limes to stay green—they're picked early, like green peppers, so they can be easily distinguished from lemons.)

Many of these vegetables and fruits will ripen as they are stored in a cooler, dryer area of your pantry or other areas, but not in the refrigerator, which almost stops the ripening process. But some won't, including green peppers—they may rot before they ripen because they've not matured on the plant long enough.

food, from beef to fish. Greens can simply be steamed and served with a little butter or extravirgin olive oil and sea salt. Or add other vegetables to the mix, such as leeks, chopped white onions, mushrooms, or yellow or orange squash. Cook your greens until they are slightly tender, but be careful not to overcook, lest you lose the vital nutrients and taste. Just when they turn bright green is about right.

A Salad a Day

Salads, large and small, can easily provide more than one or two servings of fresh, phytonutrient-rich raw food. Your salad can be a snack, a side dish, or with some added protein, a meal in itself. Salad is quick and easy to make with minimal cleanup. The base for a great salad, of course, is something green—fresh leaf lettuce, spinach, or even young kale. You can also buy whole heads of green- or red-leaf, romaine, Bibb, and endive lettuces. Clean a whole head of lettuce, dry the leaves well (spinning works great), and refrigerate them in an airtight container with a piece of paper towel. A really quick salad will be ready to go when you need it.

A variety of other raw vegetables—such as carrots, chopped red and yellow peppers, thin-sliced purple cabbage, tomatoes, and avocados—are also good on a salad but, separately, can be used as an edible garnish for meals that don't contain a salad. And that parsley or cilantro garnish? Yes, you eat that too.

To make your salad into a true meal, add some protein. Lightly grilled tuna, wild shrimp, sliced beefsteak, hard-boiled eggs, and shredded goat cheese are some options. Of course, a great salad requires a delicious dressing. I always make my own healthy salad dressing. It can be as simple as extravirgin olive oil and balsamic vinegar. Or make a basic dressing from scratch. Here's how:

EATING MORE FRUITS

The best way to add fruits to your diet, including berries, is to use them as they are—as a snack, a healthy dessert, or made into recipes such as smoothies. Fruits can also be a delicious part of a salad; try arugula with sliced pears and goat cheese or an apple walnut salad with tender mixed spring greens.

Fruit as a dessert or snack is quick and easy, with many of these foods can be taken along the way to work or on the road. An organic apple in your pocket or travel bag makes an easier, cheaper, tastier, and healthy snack.

Frozen organic blueberries, strawberries, raspberries, blackberries, and cherries are easy to incorporate into smoothies, sprinkle on healthy desserts, or use to make a sauce. After a delicious healthy meal, a quick dessert can be fresh berries, with cream or plain yogurt or mixed with chopped pears, peaches, or other available fruits.

Steer clear of the overhyped so-called miracle fruits. These plant foods include berries and herbs that intensely stimulate your sweet taste buds and make the foods you eat afterward continue to taste sweet for a while. These foods are not particularly nutritious, ridiculously expensive, and more like a magician's trick of the senses rather than a healthy food choice.

- Mix well in a blender the following:
  - 8 ounces extravirgin oil
  - 2 ounces apple cider vinegar
  - 2 cloves garlic
  - 1 tablespoon fresh (or dried) parsley
  - 2 teaspoons sea salt
  - ½ teaspoon mustard
  - Options:
  - 1 to 2 tablespoons plain yogurt, or sour cream
  - An avocado
  - Fresh tomatoes

- Use other healthy oils for variations, such as half sesame or walnut (and half olive).
- Substitute other types of vinegar such as balsamic (grape), red wine, or rice.
- Store in glass jar with tight-fitting lid. Shake well before serving.

Always use your own homemade dressing and avoid the unhealthy ingredients that usually come out of a bottle. These include vegetable oils, low-grade olive oil, sugar, additives and flavoring, and chemical compounds you probably can't pronounce.

Raw Foods—More Than Just Salads

Consuming a significant amount of fresh, raw food is important for optimal health. You need not be obsessed with raw food, but assure you're getting some at each meal and that the majority of foods on your menu are fresh and raw.

Mention raw foods and most people think of a big salad. But there are so many other ways to add not only raw vegetables and fruits to your diet but other foods as well. Here are some raw vegetable and fruit ideas:

- A garnish for any dish—parsley, large leaves of lettuce or cabbage under a cooked piece of meat or fish
- A small serving of fruit between appetizer and entrée to "clear the palate"
- Fruits for dessert or snack

In addition to raw vegetables and fruits, here are some other raw food ideas:

- Use chopped raw nuts or seeds on top of salads and entrées and even healthy desserts
- Raw milk cheese and yogurt
- Olive and coconut oils
- Honey
- Foods that are slightly cooked on the outside but raw on the inside: rare or medium rare beef, lamb or fish, and eggs (lightly fried, poached or soft boiled)

The nutritional quality of many foods are affected by cooking, canning, and freezing. Consider the following:

- Many vitamins are reduced by cooking, including vitamins A, C, thiamin (B_1), riboflavin (B_2), pyridoxine (B_6), and E, as well as biotin, the carotenoids, folic acid, and pantothenic acid (B_5).
- The amino acids glutamine, lysine, and threonine are unstable to heat. The more they are heated, the more is lost.

- When cooking foods in water, significant amounts of nutrient may be lost in the liquids if these are not consumed.
- Compared to fresh foods, both freezing and canning can reduce nutrients. For example, niacin loss in frozen vegetables may be 25 percent and that in canning 50 percent.
- Foods stored for longer periods may lose nutrients, even when they are still "fresh." After forty-eight hours, lettuce may lose 30 to 40 percent of its vitamin C content.
- Ripened foods generally have higher levels of nutrients. Tomatoes have more vitamin C and beta-carotene when ripe compared to unripe; bananas have more vitamin C when ripe (with black spots) compared to medium ripe (while still green).
- Vitamin E is destroyed by cooking, food processing, and freezing.

The raw food movement is popular with some people who passionately believe in eating almost all their food uncooked. They avoid foods heated above 115°F because of the loss of significant nutritional value but claim these foods are also harmful to the body. Heating food above this temperature degrades or destroys certain valuable enzymes, although your own digestive enzymes do this too. A typical raw food diet is comprised of fruits, vegetables, nuts, seeds, sprouted grains, and legumes. But many of these foods are dried, which can also reduce nutrition, and result in a lower amount of water intake of water (drying a food takes out much of its water). In addition, those eating only raw foods tend to leave out many healthy items, such as meat, fish, and eggs, which can lead to a nutritional shortfall in protein, fatty acids, and vitamins.

The Bitter Truth

How many times have you heard that if something tastes good, then it must not be good for you or vice versa? While this is a gross generalization, it's a fact that many people avoid eating bitter-tasting vegetables and fruits, which are particularly high in natural phytonutrients that cause their bitterness. In general, the more bitter the taste, the more phytonutrients.

It's now clear that naturally occurring phytonutrients in vegetables and fruits can help prevent and treat cancer, Alzheimer's, cardiovascular diseases, and a host of functional problems, from fatigue to muscle aches and even chronic inflammation. The actions of certain phytonutrients halt the production of cancer-causing agents in the body, blocking activation of these chemicals or suppressing the spread of cancer cells that already exist. The vegetables and fruits that researchers think are most capable of preventing diseases are green leafy vegetables, broccoli, brussels sprouts, cabbage, onions, and citrus fruit (not the juice). The more bitter, the better.

While healthy for humans, plants use phytonutrients as natural insect repellents and pesticides. Some are even toxic to small animals like birds, mice, and rats, including some compounds in cabbage and brussels sprouts. Generally, higher amounts of bitter-tasting phytonutrients are found in sprouts and seedlings than in mature plants. This provides young plants with a type of natural protection from being eaten at an early stage of life, before the chance of reproduction. But you would have to consume pounds and pounds of vegetables daily to ingest toxic amounts of phytonutrients.

Despite the therapeutic and nutritive value of phytonutrients, the food industry is solving the so-called problem of bitterness in vegetables and fruits by removing these healthful chemicals through genetic engineering and selective breeding. Unfortunately, our culture has associated bitterness with bad taste instead of health promotion. Now many agricultural scientists, who want foods sweeter, are changing our food supply for us—they are literally removing the healthy components from certain foods in order to sell more food products. And they are succeeding. Canola oil contains significant reductions of phytonutrients due to selective breeding. And transgenic citrus fruit is sweeter but now free of limonene, the bitter substance that can help prevent and treat skin cancer.

Cancer researchers propose that a heightened sense of bitterness might be a healthy trait, allowing people to select foods with the highest phytonutrient content. This view contrasts with the food industry's practice of measuring the content of these bitter phyto-nutrients merely as a way of developing new nonbitter, phytonutrient-deficient strains. So while some nutrition scientists propose enhancing phytonutrients in foods for better health, the standard industry practice has been to remove them for better taste. Indeed, the lower amount of bitter compounds in the modern diet reflects the "achievement" of the food industry. The irony is that as agricultural scientists remove more phytonutrients from plants, farmers have to use even more chemical pesticides to protect their crops; thus consumers are left with the double whammy of vegetables and fruits with less nutrition and more harmful pesticides.

In addition to bitterness, an astringent taste is also associated with healthy phyto-nutrients. These tastes can actually be quite attractive. Consider a fine-aged Bordeaux wine or a high-quality green tea. Unfortunately, these are exceptions, and sweetness is a dominant taste preference in our society.

You can get more phytonutrients into your diet by eating foods that have a natural bitter or astringent taste. Zucchini and other squashes, pumpkins, cucumbers, melon, citrus are some. Other plant foods high in phytonutrients are raw almonds, beans, red wine, green tea, and pure unsweetened cocoa.

Making these healthy vegetable choices is just another journey on the road to optimal health and human performance. In addition to variety, the highest-quality vegetables and fruits may be those that are organically grown.

Organic Foods

Today's consumers may find a large variety of certified organic vegetables and fruits to choose from. It's now common to see produce, meats, nuts, seeds, beans, and other organic foods not only in traditional "health food" stores but in conventional groceries as well. However, two questions emerge: (1) Is it worth the extra price to buy organic food versus conventional? (2) Can you trust the sign or labels that says CERTIFIED ORGANIC?

With great hesitation, my answer to both questions is a qualified yes, with a large asterisk. The USDA organic program is part of an international phenomenon. The regulations are better than the previous unregulated organic movement, where anyone could say a product was organic. Many of the guidelines are potentially good for consumers— organic produce must be grown without commonly used pesticides, herbicides, and other chemicals. Many food product ingredients, including additives and preservatives, are not allowed in organic foods. Organic animals must be raised with organic feed, filtered water, and certified organic pastures; and many commonly used hormones, antibiotics, and other drugs can't be used.

And the program is relatively strict, helping to rid the market of dishonest vendors. So if a product has the USDA CERTIFIED ORGANIC label, it means that the USDA is committed, in theory, to oversee and enforce the program, just like the rest of what the agency does for all foods sold to consumers—

for example, ensuring consumers are not sold bacteria-ridden foods or products made from horse meat. Yet enforcement often comes after the fact when tainted meat, poultry, or eggs have already made their way into the nation's food supply, and hospital emergency rooms see a spike in severe intestinal complaints.

But like the rest of our food supply, you still have to be a careful consumer. Without reading labels and being aware of the usual marketing scams by many companies, you can easily be fooled into buying organic junk food, which makes up most of today's organic products. The USDA allows many highly processed foods to be also certified organic. If wheat is grown without pesticides, herbicides, and other organic standards such as clean water then refined into white flour, the end product can be certified organic. The same with sugar and other processed foods. These are obviously unhealthy ingredients, and the organic certification does not make them any less harmful. The result is organic junk food is made from white flour, processed corn, potatoes, white sugar, and vegetable oils.

You can find organic junk food almost everywhere—as chips, bread, cakes, cookies, candy, soda, pasta, and peanut butter. Companies and retail stores attract buyers by inferring that these organic junk foods are somehow healthy to eat, when in reality they are anything but.

Naturally grown food is your best choice, whether officially certified organic or not. Yes, organic vegetables and fruits usually taste better, they've not been genetically altered and contain much smaller amounts of chemical fertilizers, or none at all. Moreover, various published studies, including several from the *Journal of Agricultural and Food Chemistry* in recent years, indicate that organic produce is more nutritious, containing more vitamins, minerals, and phytonutrients. Some of the nutrients analyzed in organic produce had twice the amount of that found in conventional, nonorganic equivalents. These include carrots, cabbage, lettuce, kale, tomatoes, eggplant, and spinach. The increased nutrients found in certified-organic plant foods are most likely due to better care of the soil through organic farming methods, including composting, crop rotation, and cover crops.

I've even conducted my own research and found that some organically grown vegetables, such as kale and spinach, had significantly higher levels—ten times or more—of certain nutrients, such as folic acid, compared to these same nonorganic vegetables tested and listed in the USDA database.

For years, nutritionists insisted that today's conventionally grown foods were as high in vitamins and minerals as the meals of our grandparents. There is now sufficient evidence indicating this is not necessarily the case. Reductions in food quality have taken place since the mid-1940s, when the use of chemical fertilizers and pesticides rapidly became the norm in modern farming. A recent study published in the *British Food Journal* compared the 1930s nutrient content of twenty fruits and vegetables with foods grown in the 1980s. Significant reductions were found in the levels of calcium, copper, and magnesium in vegetables and magnesium, iron, copper, and potassium in fruit. Similar trends can be found in foods produced in the United States, with reductions in some nutrients of as much as 30 percent.

Most foods are farmed with chemical fertilizers and pesticides, with the exception of certified organic foods, which contain significantly less nitrates and heavy metals, both of which can be very harmful, especially to children. Heavy metals enter the plants through certain chemical fertilizers— some of these fertilizers are even derived from industrial waste. As discussed previously, through genetic engineering, valuable phytonutrients have been removed from some common foods to make them less bitter tasting. Organically grown foods don't contain genetically engineered ingredients or genetically modified organisms, making them a better choice.

The Full Spectrum of Fiber and Prebiotics

Vegetables, fruits, and other plant materials contain certain types of food particles that are not digestible or absorbable, but have powerful health-promoting effects. These include fiber and prebiotics, which are nondigestible food ingredients that stimulate the activity of healthy bacteria in the digestive system. Priobiotics were first identified and named by Marcel Roberfroid in

1995, and as research has shown, they have a positive effect on the immune system and colon and helps promote intestinal regularity. Fiber and prebiotics have a symbiotic relationship that is also important to overall body function.

There are various types of fibers with different names, depending on the type of plant and which part they are derived. They include pectin, cellulose, beta-glucans, mucilages, and an assortment of gums including guar, arabic, and locust bean. By eating a variety of natural foods, you can obtain the full spectrum of these fibers, helping the intestine function better.

Pectin is the substance partly responsible for the ripening of fruit. It is especially high in apples, citrus, and most berries, and it is used as a gelling agent in foods such as jam. Applesauce is a high-pectin food that works well as a remedy for diarrhea by adding bulk to the intestinal contents. Cellulose, such as found in wheat bran, is a component of cell walls of most plants. Beta-glucans from oats have become popular because of their positive association with reducing the risk of cardiovascular disease. Mucilages, found in the herb, psyllium, and in seaweed, are very functional fibers also rich in minerals. Natural gums—guar, arabic, and locust bean—have been used for thousands of years as thickening agents and emulsifiers in cooking and food preparation.

It's not so important to remember all the different names of these natural fibers; rather, the key is to eat a variety of plant foods that will provide you with the full spectrum of fiber important not only for your intestines but also for your entire system. These include ten servings of vegetables and fruits and, as needed, additional foods if necessary, such as psyllium, or, if tolerated, whole grain wheat, rye, or oats.

Try to get all the fiber you need by eating a variety of healthy food, especially vegetables and fruits. At least one, preferably two or even three, semisolid bowel movements per day is a general indication that you're eating enough fiber. Drinking enough water helps fiber function in the intestines.

If you still need more fiber after eating a variety of fiber-rich food and being well hydrated with water, you can supplement your diet with additional concentrated sources. Different people respond differently to specific types of fiber, but generally, the psyllium performs very well in most people. This is especially useful in those people who have reduced their intake of grains and other carbohydrate foods. Begin by consuming a teaspoon of plain, unsweetened psyllium in eight to ten ounces of water each day and increase as necessary. Excess bloating or indigestion may indicate that amount is too much.

Physical Aspects of Fiber

Fiber acts as a vehicle, helping to transport food through the intestines at a healthy rate. Sometimes, too little fiber can result in a too-rapid digestion in the intestine, which can reduce digestion and absorption of nutri-

FOODS WITH THE MOST PESTICIDES

On June 1, 2010, the Washington DC–based nonprofit organization Environmental Working Group (EWG) delivered the sixth edition of its *Shopper's Guide to Pesticides* with updated information on forty-nine fruits and vegetables and their total pesticide load. EWG highlights the worst offenders with its "Dirty Dozen" list and the cleanest conventional produce with its "Clean Fifteen" list. See www.foodnews.org.

Analysts at EWG synthesized data collected from the USDA and the Food and Drug Administration (FDA) from 2000 to 2008. Produce is ranked based on a composite score, equally weighing six factors that examine how many pesticides are on the produce and at what levels. All samples are washed and peeled prior to being tested for pesticides, so the rankings reflect the amounts of the chemicals likely present on the food—as opposed to on the surface of the food—when is it eaten.

Here's a list of the top offenders—those with the most pesticides:

- Celery
- Peaches
- Strawberries
- Apples
- Blueberries
- Nectarines
- Bell peppers
- Spinach
- Cherries
- Kale/collard greens
- Potatoes
- Grapes (imported)

ents and increasing a carbohydrate food's glycemic index. In other cases, the lack of fiber can slow intestinal function, resulting in constipation and poor digestion.

The optimal amount of fiber—our specific needs are very individual—allows food to flow through the gut at a proper pace for optimal digestion and to limit the amount of time cancer-causing chemicals are in contact with the intestine's cells. These chemicals may be toxins from water and air pollution, substances used in food preparation, and even naturally occurring during the cooking. These toxins may also attach to the fiber and be removed from the body.

Fiber is also capable of holding water in the intestine, which further helps dilute toxins and prevents constipation.

In the large intestine, fiber provides the proper environment for the growth of "friendly" bacteria, which have a very important function. These microorganisms ferment some of the fiber substances, producing important fatty acids. These fats regulate the acid-alkaline (pH) balance in the large intestine and in turn control the bacteria themselves. Some fatty acids serve as an important energy source for the cells in the lower intestine. One specific fat, butyric, may also play a protective role against cancer by maintaining a low colon pH and directly inhibiting tumor formation.

The process of fermentation also results in intestinal gas (mostly hydrogen and methane). If there's too much gas, causing discomfort or pain, it's a sign that there's a problem; often too much or too little fiber or the type of fiber is not right for you, such as the case with wheat. Some of this gas is actually absorbed via the large intestine into the body and is released through the lungs. Those individuals with bad breath usually have too much fermentation or gas from unfriendly bacteria. In any of these instances, stress (which reduces intestinal function) or the wrong foods (typically too much carbohydrate) can be the cause.

Antibiotic use can quickly kill the friendly microorganisms in the intestine. This destruction of the normal bacteria results in a "recolonization" of the large intestine with unfriendly, unwanted bacteria. Yogurt and other cultured milk products such as buttermilk and kefir and raw cheese also contain friendly bacteria and can be helpful in these situations. Furthermore, eating foods that contain prebiotics helps promote the growth of healthy bacteria in the colon.

The beneficial effects of fiber on bile (from the liver and gall bladder) may also help prevent intestinal cancers. Excess amounts of bile in the colon may cause normal cells to convert to cancerous ones. By eating enough variety of fiber, the concentration of bile in the colon remains lower.

Fiber and Nutrient Absorption

Another important function of fiber is how it affects the absorption of nutrients from your diet. For example, fiber in your meal can slow sugar (glucose) absorption and lower the glycemic index of that meal. Remember that the glycemic index is a measure of the blood sugar response to certain foods or meals. Fiber-rich foods generally have a lower glycemic index and when consumed result in less insulin production. This makes fiber especially important for anyone with carbohydrate intolerance. Pectins, mucilages, and especially gums seem to do this very well.

Absorption of minerals is also influenced by fiber, but in a negative way. Phytic acid, a natural substance present in the fibers of grains and in much smaller amounts in fruits, can inhibit the absorption of calcium, iron, zinc and copper, and possibly other nutrients. This is another reason to limit the consumption of grains.

In addition to their relationship to mineral absorption, some fibers may have an adverse effect on digestive enzymes. Wheat bran, for example, can inhibit the production of pancreatic enzymes responsible for digesting carbohydrates, proteins, and fats. The fiber in legumes may inhibit the enzyme amylase, which is important for carbohydrate digestion. Other studies show that the fiber in many cereals contains pancreatic inhibitors that can diminish protein digestion. In addition, the fiber in unprocessed soybeans can induce an allergy-type reaction in some people, accounting for the intestinal discomfort some may have with soy.

Energy from Fiber

Since fiber is not absorbed, it does not directly count as an energy source. For this reason, if you eat a slice of whole grain bread that contains fifteen grams of carbohydrate, you really can't count it as fifteen grams of usable energy since some of that carbohydrate is fiber. If that slice of bread contains four grams of fiber, subtract four grams from the fifteen grams of total carbohydrate, giving a total of eleven grams of usable carbohydrate.

While the fiber grams are not directly counted as energy calories, the body does indirectly obtain energy from fiber through fermentation by bacteria in the large intestine. As mentioned previously, fiber provides the environment for this bacterial activity. The bacteria produce short-chain fatty acids, typically butyric, acetic, and propionic, which are absorbed and used by the body as fuel. Some fibers, such as pectin, are more capable of producing energy than others, such as fiber

from grains. Approximately two calories of energy can be produced per gram of fiber. This is compared to four calories for other dietary carbohydrates, four for protein, and nine for dietary fats.

Prebiotics—the Other "Fiber"

The functions of fiber and prebiotics overlap. Prebiotics include a group of natural nondigestible carbohydrates called fructans contained in small amounts in most plant foods. The highest levels are found in asparagus, onions, leeks, garlic, chicory, green beans, and bananas. Dandelion greens are one of the highest sources of fructans, as are Jerusalem artichokes or products made from them. Barley, rye, and wheat are also good sources, although wheat comes with its own set of other drawbacks as discussed earlier.

Fructans act similarly to fiber but do not actually create bulk themselves; instead, they promote bulk by encouraging the growth of healthy bacteria in the colon. In many people, prebiotics can actually help healthy colonic bacteria replace unhealthy bacteria that commonly cause disease.

While improved colon health can help prevent constipation, diarrhea, and other functional problems, it can also help prevent intestinal diseases including cancer and serious inflammatory conditions such as ulcerative colitis and Crohn's disease. Other bodywide benefits may include prevention of heart disease, other cancers, and even osteoporosis. In addition, fructans help the colon's bacteria produce certain nutrients, including biotin, vitamin K, and some of the B vitamins. As opposed to some fibers, such as wheat fiber which can prevent calcium, iron, and other minerals from being absorbed, fructans can actually improve mineral absorption. This is the reason for a positive relationship between fructan intake and prevention of osteoporosis.

Cooking can reduce the availability of prebiotics in a food by 25 to 30 percent, so try to eat enough of the raw vegetables containing prebiotics. Loss of fructans occurs in cooking water, so when cooking these foods, be sure to consume the water too.

Fructan supplements have appeared on the market over the last few years as both inulin and oligosaccharides. The natural version of inulin is extracted from chicory root using only hot water, filtration, and drying. Unfortunately, most versions are highly processed and have been synthesized from sugar. Synthesized fructans are also used in the manufacture of fake food ingredients—both for artificial fats and low-carbohydrate foods. For most people, obtaining sufficient fructans can be accomplished by eating more foods containing them.

How Much Fiber and Prebiotics?

By now you should know the answer to this question—it depends on your individual needs.

On average, between fifteen and twenty-five grams of fiber per day is the absolute minimum most people require. This works out to be about ten grams per one thousand calories of food consumed. Many people need more fiber than this, and some people may need twice this much, or even more, to have optimal health. As you determine your carbohydrate needs, balance your fats and start eating ten or more servings of vegetables and fruits per day; you should notice whether your intestines are working better, or if you need more fiber and/or prebiotics.

While there are no specific recommendations for the amount of prebiotics you should consume, Americans eat on average only about one to three grams of fructans daily while our healthier European friends consume three times that amount. This does not necessarily mean that more is better, but most people will benefit by eating more food fructans.

If you don't get enough fiber naturally from foods in your daily diet, you may need a dietary supplement. The best way to do this is to make your own mix of fibers. This may require some experimentation, but it will be worth the effort. For many people, plain psyllium is all that's needed. Others, for example, may try a mixture of psyllium and oat bran mixed with applesauce (also a good source of pectin). A quick analysis of your diet should give you an idea of how much fiber you're getting and how much more you'll need.

Buy Local?

With the problems in the organic industry, including the easing of a strict standard in growing and producing the cleanest and highest quality foods and the added bureaucratic costs due to the certification process, many truly health-conscious consumers once again are looking for other options. Farmers Markets are now part of the urban landscape, attracting weekend crowds. There are community organic cooperatives, roadside farm stands, and pick-your-own fruit and vegetable farms. Internet shopping for organic food is growing, especially in bulk quantity. These modern markets feature products grown in a "green" way—produced in line with the original organic movement. And they often include a "buy local" slogan.

But the underlying problem is that there is no regulation regarding whether it's "green," organic, or beyond organic. One problem is the notion that products that are better than organic—the "beyond organic" movement—should be more expensive. But just because products are grown with care, without chemicals, doesn't mean they should be more expensive. Without the "middlemen"—typically two, three, or more of them taking a share before products get to the retail stores—most of these products should be less expensive than the same or similar products in retail stores.

If you're a careful consumer and talk to the farmers and those producing these products, and even visit their farms, you can usually find high-quality healthy products that are often better than the organic version in retail stores, often for less cost. Supply and demand will help "weed out" the overpriced products.

Here in Southern Arizona, I buy local raw milk to make delicious raw cheeses and butter. For about $5's worth of milk I get about $40 to $50 in cheese and butter. I have fifteen chickens provide almost as many daily fresh eggs whose yolks are deep orange in color due to the many nutritious antioxidant-rich nutrients. I use some cheese and garden greens to barter for certain local fruits and nuts not grown in my garden.

My meat is purchased at the nearby Double Check Ranch—while they don't participate in the national organic program, it is clean, efficient, inspected by local government, and has a philosophy of not just producing healthy food but also incorporates an approach to farming that's good for the land as well. And their animals are not trucked away for processing—that's also done humanely at the farm. This is the best model of modern farming and results in delicious, healthy grass-fed beef at prices much lower than organic beef in the health stores. (Their website provides many informative articles—www.DoubleCheckRanch.com.)

The Organic Movement

No one is precisely sure just when the organic movement first started since that would depend, in part, on how you define "organic." Certainly in the early stages, the word "organic" was not part of it since the actual term would not be introduced until around 1941 by a British chemist Sir Albert Howard. But by then, the movement was decades old

130

SHOPPING AT WHOLE FOODS: WHY IS THERE SO MUCH JUNK FOOD SOLD HERE?

It had been awhile, maybe over a year, since I had last been inside a Whole Foods store. The store closest to my home—in Tucson, Arizona—is over thirty miles away. But I needed to stock up on some bulk items, and so on the Sunday right after New Year's Day 2011, I made the long trip in my Grand Cherokee jeep.

With 291 stores spread across the United States, as well as six in Canada and five in England, Whole Foods has evolved into a unique shopping experience for many believing that they are buying groceries in a health-conscious environment. Unlike a Walmart or Costco, the public perception of Whole Foods is one of a forward-thinking, eco-aware chain dedicated to selling food that is organic, tastier, more natural and nutritious, and less processed. Prices might be higher, but that's okay for the "enlightened shopper."

Yet as reported in a 2010 *New Yorker* magazine profile of Whole Foods's co-founder and chief executive, John Mackey, the chain has been criticized from all sides as either "an overpriced luxury for yuppie gastronomes and fussy label-readers. Or it is Holy Foods, the commercial embodiment of environmental and nutritional pieties. To hard-core proponents of natural and organic food, Whole Foods is a disappointment—a bundle of big-business compromises and half-steps. It's a welter of paradoxes: a staunchly anti-union enterprise that embraces some progressive labor practices; a self-styled world-improver that must also deliver quarterly results to Wall Street; a big-box chain putting on small-town airs; an evangelist for healthy eating that sells sausages, ice cream, and beer."

Mackey, in a moment of open candor, even told the *Wall Street Journal* in August 2010, "We sell a bunch of junk." Judging from my limited experience inside the Tucson store, Mackey is completely right, though he vowed in the interview to reduce the amount of unhealthy products.

Walking through the open front doors of Whole Foods, you're hit with visual and sensory overload. To my right was a display of sale item leftovers from the holidays, including organic candy canes made with organic sugar. A large display of cat and dog food was nearby. On the other side, there was a generous spread of colorful fresh fruits and vegetables. Normally, I avoid the center aisles because that's where the junk food is found, but I was curious. I wandered down some of them to see what was being sold. The first one was lined with cereals boxes. I looked closely at the "nutrition" labels. Almost all contained highly processed wheat, corn, and other processed grains. Sugar seemed to always be high up on the ingredient list. Yet many of these cereals were being marketed as "organic," and almost all were fortified with synthetic vitamins.

Over in the next aisle were cake, brownie, and other boxed mixes. You just need to add water, mix the batter, and turn on the oven. And these too were being sold as "organic," containing sugar and processed flour as the main ingredients.

There seemed to be bakery items perched on display racks at the end of every aisle. Some featured trays of organic cookies made with white flour and sugar. A large glass display had fancy croissants or at least the American or non-French version. A small line of customers were waiting at the main bakery counter, which was full of large cakes, pies, and oversized cookies covered in rainbow sprinkles. I glanced at the ingredient lists of many of these baked goods—white flour and sugar mostly.

I wandered down another aisle, first passing by the frozen section, which contained mostly prepared microwaveable "health-food" versions of TV dinners. There was nothing I would eat even though many said they were organic. (Then again, I don't own a microwave or see the purpose of having one.) As I passed the dairy section, I stopped and checked out the soy yogurt—most were processed soy made with organic sugar.

Nearby were shelves of chips—almost all made with potato and corn. Surprisingly, I didn't see any organic potato chips. In addition to being high-glycemic nonorganic potatoes are among the more toxic foods—they absorb the herbicides, pesticides, and fungicides they're treated with during growing and afterward are treated with chemicals again so they don't sprout. Just as bad were the oils contained within—typically the more unstable vegetable ones: safflower and sunflower oils. It was too painful to walk down the juice, beverage, and soda aisle, so I avoided it altogether.

The bulk food section reminded me of the old co-ops that I sometimes shopped at in the early '70s. Except that here, the bulk section was usually full of highly processed unhealthy products. I even saw the same ingredients that were staples everywhere I turned in Whole Foods—white sugar and white flour. There were also bins filled with white rice and lots of chewable candies.

I did find beans, lentils, whole grain wheat and rye, and other healthy items. These organic real food items are how people can significantly reduce their food bill. If you steer clear of expensive (per-pound price) and unhealthy items—juice and soda, cereal, bread, frozen dinners, packaged sliced meats and cheese, chips, and sweets, whether you buy organic or not—you can drastically cut your costs by buying whole oats, lentils, whole pieces of meat and chicken, eggs, and fresh fruit and vegetables. And to be fair, these expensive junk food items are not unique to Whole Foods— most other health food stores carry them too. But Whole Foods deliberately banks upon the public image of being a place where you buy "whole foods."

At the checkout counter were small boxes of high-fructose energy bars and more candy. When the young cashier asked me if I had found everything I needed, I said, "There's too much junk food and too few organic items." She cheerfully replied, "But we're adding more organic items all the time." "Like what kinds?" I asked. She smiled and said, "I really don't know," and continued ringing up my groceries.

As I drove away, with several bags of groceries in the backseat—filled with lentils, sesame and flaxseeds, extravirgin olive oil, balsamic vinegar, and Granny Smith apples—I reflected on how the health food industry had been taken over by purveyors of junk food. It wasn't always this way.

In the early 1900s, as big corporate farming grew with its pesticides, herbicides, and chemical fertilizers, the mass manufacturing of packaged and processed foods evolved too. While small groups of citizens protested these changes, America's food supply was now different—there was more corporate profit and less nutrition for consumers. The few who saw this as a health problem continued relying on local farmer's markets for fresh, unadulterated, safer food searched out the difficult to find unprocessed whole foods; and the phrase "health food" was born. The movement also attracted vegetarians, those with special dietary needs, such as those allergic to wheat, or diabetics, and others in search of natural living.

Out of this movement came the rise of health food stores and co-ops, where hard-to-find items could be found in one store, although an 1870s Philadelphia-based retail store, Thomas Martindale Company, may have been the first. Originally, health food stores were small retail shops or home-based co-ops that had bulk items such as whole grains, soybeans, dried fruits, and granola. Blackstrap molasses, brewer's yeast, and coffee substitutes became popular. And there were lots of dietary supplements, and unknown to many store owners and customers, they contained virtually all synthetic vitamins made by pharmaceutical companies. Other items were not healthy either, like dried bananas coated with sugar. The word "organic" was used, but casually here and there, as the USDA's organic program had not been conceived yet. What little fresh produce was to be found was usually old, weepy, and double the price of grocery stores. Yet somehow, the health-food store concept survived long enough to grow up, spurred on by the ecology movement of the 1960s.

But many of the small health-food stores couldn't survive when a Whole Foods, or its rival Wild Oats—both were founded in the 1980s—moved into town. They were either bought or went out of business. In 2007, Whole Foods gobbled up Wild Oats for over a half-billion dollars, despite initial resistance from the Bush administration for antitrust violations in a supermarket sector that the Federal Trade Commission artfully designated as "premium natural and organic."

The publicly traded Whole Foods now has sales of over eight billion dollars a year. Of that revenue figure, one wonders just how much is a result of selling junk food.

and had more than one front. There were those who promoted the scientific reasons for farming with a natural process: those who had more spiritual reasons to care for the land, small farmers who were being driven out of business by the larger players, those with strong social attitudes who wanted to help the "small farmers" get a fair share of the profits, and consumers who demanded better and healthier food. But even before the movement was fully noticed in the press, there were those few who made the observations that growing food in the most natural soils produced better food—and made people healthier.

In the 1830s, German chemist Justus von Liebig was formulating his agricultural biochemistry theories, which he published in the 1840s, discussing how plants utilize nitrogen in the soil along with various minerals. Natural fertilizers, he theorized, including manure, would provide these nutrients. This was the beginning of modern farming,

and the movement soon branched into two: one that became big-business farming, with newly developing chemical fertilizers and pesticides, and the other was the organic movement. Sir Albert Howard may be one of the earliest "organic" farmers—he was from a British farming family but learned about natural soil production and organic gardening in India in 1905.

With the influence of Howard's writings— he called the introduction of chemical fertilizers and pesticides a great threat to the future of human health—there was a clear separation of the organic movement and conventional farming. His writing spread throughout Europe and eventually to America.

By the early 1900s, American food manufacturers, as an integral part of the "modern farming" movement, began mass-producing the first packaged foods. Small groups of concerned citizens immediately and openly protested against the mass packaging of

134

food. Some, including Dr. Royal Lee, began growing high-quality food with natural composting and in 1929 began manufacturing the first dietary supplements in America using these foods.

By the 1930s, with the influence of Howard's writings and others in America, the organic movement was organized, albeit small. One person who jumped on board was an engineer named Jerome Irving Rodale. He not only bought a farm and began organic gardening but also started publishing a magazine on organic methods in the 1940s—and who other than Sir Albert Howard would contribute articles. Rodale also started a printing business that would also publish books—a business that thrives today as a multimillion-dollar corporation.

I was introduced to Rodale's books on organic gardening in the 1960s and soon after planted my first organic garden. As a student working part-time in a health-food store and having studied basic chemistry, I realized almost all the vitamins on the shelves were synthetic, not natural as they claimed. Seeing a growing market in the organic industry, the pharmaceutical companies had quietly jumped on board by producing virtually all the synthetic vitamins for the health-food industry, a problem that continues today.

After studying organic gardening and natural health and many different health care philosophies, I decided to go back to college, became a holistic practitioner, and focused on helping people get healthy.

Into the 1970s and '80s, the organic movement continued to expand as well dividing its social, fair trade, and health-oriented subgroups. Even up to the time when the USDA decided to take charge of the movement by creating a National Organic Program (NOP) in 1990 that would define organic and certify growers, manufacturers, and others involved in the organic movement, there continued to be different philosophies associated with organics.

The NOP would spend the next decade gathering information from the organic movement, create standards, rules, regulations, and a system to certify all those it would allow into the organic movement—often for a hefty fee—under the guise that the USDA needed to regulate the process. The result was the "certified organic" regulations, released in 2002, complete with a seal of authenticity. They established three levels of organic food: 100 percent; 95 percent, which allowed 5 percent nonorganic material; and 70 percent organic.

There was one problem: during this decade, big agribusiness lobbied heavily for regulations that would make it easier and cheaper to jump on the "certified organic" bandwagon. Not only that, the large manufacturers of processed foods, the sugar and wheat industry, and large food chains made sure they were part of the process. The result was a massive growth of organic junk food that coincided with the NOP's "organic" launch in 2002.

Just before the NOP became law, I created, in 1999, the first line of certified organic dietary supplements made from real food. I followed the developments of the USDA's certified organic program and prepared my formulas based on what I thought would be the requirements for organic certification. These standards were easily met, but within a few years, my company was squeezed out of the marketplace by the large synthetic vitamin-based companies.

The Organic Trade Association (OTA) evolved from part of the movement that was the political tail. Its goal was to help companies involved in certified organic activities work with other companies and the NOP. Unfortunately, they were a political organization not oriented to health. At their first national trade show in 2001, I was shocked at the number of organic junk food companies represented—you could sample organic cookies made from organic white flour and organic white sugar, eat processed organic corn and potato chips, drink organic beer, and even smoke organic cigarettes. This was the modern health-food industry! But the worst was yet to come.

There were a number of speakers discussing the value of organic certification. A keynote speaker was JI Rodale's granddaughter, Marie, who was an influential figure in the Rodale publishing empire. She was so excited to see the organic movement get this far and be so successful. After her talk, she took questions. I asked, "Are you concerned that the organic industry is made up of so much junk food that adversely affects people's health?" Her answer was an emphatic no. She said that people can make their own choices.

Marie Rodale's grandfather had promoted the relationship between organic farming and optimal health and helped launch the organic movement. But now, companies making organic junk food have become the biggest advertising revenue for the modern Rodale publishing empire. In joining with big business and the USDA, the small farmers and start-up companies making healthy foods were left out.

Meanwhile, consumers jumped in too. They were the ones eating all the organic junk food and obviously becoming fatter. This was evident just by looking—at the owners, employees, and others working in the "health-food" industry, including those in the stores. See my sidebar on "Shopping at Whole Foods." Go into any large health-food retailers and you'll see the shelves full of organic junk. And a large part of the store is the bakery section—complete with white flour and sugar cakes, cookies, and pies.

My level of disappointment in the organic movement has reached a high while my enthusiasm had bottomed. My first article after returning home from the OTA show, "Organic Junk," brought praise by a few but anger from industry people. Making money, it seemed, was the goal of certified organics, even if it contributed to the explosion of obesity not only in adults but also young children. Along the way, the large companies, including manufacturers and grocery stores, along with the health-food chains, successfully pushed for the NOP, regulations to be diluted—many unhealthy foods, food additives, and other ingredients would now be allowed in organic foods. I began writing and lecturing more on the dangers of organic junk food and "beyond organic"—those small farmers, companies, and consumers left out of the original organic movement who were still there hoping for healthy changes. The organic movement had left them behind. And many legitimate farmers, manufacturers, and food companies that were too small to pay the thousands of dollars to be part of the USDA's organic movement were actually creating healthier food.

What does the situation look like now? Not good. With its government-sponsored organic programs, the USDA claimed the word "organic" for itself; products or companies would not be allowed to use the word "organic" unless it was certified by the USDA. In addition, small farms, legitimate companies producing healthy foods, and others involved in the organic movement are even being harassed by federal and local authorities because they have not embraced the movement by jumping on board by becoming certified. The result is that a small but growing movement continues made up of consumers and health care professionals like me, seeking the best food from good and honest people all working together for a healthier planet.

What's most important is to consume ten servings of vegetables and fruits—most of it fresh and raw. Buy the best you can find, grow some of your own. These foods are the only sources of the thousands of important phytonutrients that will help build optimal health and fitness.

LIVING OFF THE GRID: COOKING AND GARDENING TIPS IF YOU REALLY WANT TO "GO GREEN"

If you really want the highest-quality produce, the best option is to grow your own fruit and vegetables. If you have any yard space at all, a small vegetable plot, properly tended, can yield enough vegetables in season for your entire family. Many cities have community gardens where many individuals share in a larger plot of land. By growing your own vegetables, you can ensure their quality, reduce the price of your produce, and revel in the enjoyment of producing your own food, not to mention the extra exercise you get from working in your garden. You can also sprout many different kinds of seeds for daily consumption—millet, mung beans, and broccoli are some that are delicious. Broccoli sprouts are particularly high in the phytonutrient sulforaphan, a powerful anticancer nutrient. And you are noticeably reducing your energy-consumption footprint. And that also includes cooking, but let me detour for a moment and bring up the topic of solar power and energy.

When it comes to energy, I often talk about it in relation to the human body as the most common symptom people experience is fatigue. Thus the discussion here begins with the simple question, where does our energy come from? The answer is the sun. Light energy from the sun reaches the earth and is converted to chemical energy by plants, which are eaten by animals, including us. Our bodies convert the chemical energy to a mechanical form for everyday use. If we're more tired now than when we were younger, it's because something has interfered with this process of energy production.

This same solar energy that our body relies on can also be harnessed for other needs as well. These include heating our homes, cooking, producing hot water, and lighting. But not only is the solar energy alternative still laughed at by many people in the United States (not so in Europe, Australia, and China), the natural "sun-powered" movement also died out and has been replaced by an industry that created another modern scam: solar energy. Today, investing in a solar system for a small household could take a cash outlay of $20,000 or more and take over twenty years to recover the financial costs compared to using standard energy. Yet you still would probably not be off the grid and continue to rely on the electric company for some of your needs. And that's the price tag if you don't run into problems requiring big repairs or replacements. For most people, this cost is prohibitive, and local governments, zoning boards, and your electric company all make it difficult to accomplish. Sure there are often tax breaks on solar equipment—you can save $300 by spending $20,000.

Since most people care more about saving money and less about the environment, let's look at the reality of the energy issue. There's an alternative to alternative energy—a better way for everyone to benefit with immediate and significant up front costs savings.

Not only do I care about the environment, but I also enjoy a cool home in the summer, warmth in the cool winter, and a hot shower to name a few modern luxuries. And I hate giving money to the utility companies. Part of choosing a healthy lifestyle is finding an optimal location. For most people there are many choices all over the globe. Of these geographical possibilities, I settled in the desert mountains of southern Arizona.

Cooking is a major use of energy, but it can cost to cook and to cool from the heat you create. This is good during cold winter days but not the rest of the year. Reducing energy for cooking is simple, and it can save money and time and provide health benefits. First, consider that if you cooked twice the amount of food at once, you'd use a lot less energy than if you cooked half that amount of food on two different occasions. With twice the food, your preparation for meals over the next few days is reduced, saving considerable time. And with food already made, you're less likely to skip a meal, which is very unhealthy, or eat junk food. Moreover, if you bring lunch to work, it's already made.

In summer, I use a slow cooker to make many meals, placing this pot in an outside room (or outdoors) so the heat never gets into the house. Slow cookers (also known as Crock-Pots) are inexpensive and use little energy unless you keep them on all day, which is unnecessary. You can make just about anything in these pots, from healthy meat loaf to vegetable lasagna, not to mention cheesecake. You also use an outdoor propane cooker all year-round for quickly grilling meats and vegetables, fish in parchment paper, and other foods. Using no energy other than the sun, I use a simple, inexpensive solar oven, which can reach 350°F with southern sun exposure as their only energy source—it's even effective on sunny days in the winter.

In addition, consuming a lot of raw foods with meals and for snacks—especially vegetables and fruits—requires no cooking and is an important part of a healthy diet.

Growing more of your own food or buying healthy food locally produced, such as in a farmer's market, reduces, sometimes dramatically, one's energy dependency on outside sources. An organic orchard owner once told me that Whole Foods might pay 12¢ a pound for apples and sell them for $2.99 (or more) a pound. In addition to corporate profits, some of the costs passed on to you are for fuel (transporting the apples in trucks) and storage (keeping the apples for months in distribution centers, which requires refrigeration).

Virtually anyone can grow food at home and in any climate. In my case, I have two gardens of about four thousand square feet on the east and west sides of the house, growing over sixty different varieties of vegetables and fruits—from lettuces, spinach, and kale to peaches, blue- and blackberries, and various summer and winter squashes—year-round. In addition to superior taste and better nutrition, this provides me with enjoyable physical activity. Once you get the garden properly organized, maintaining it is easy. The garden saves me hundreds of dollars a month.

Whether you use well or city water, a significant source of this natural resource is free—rain. You just need to collect it. I have several rain barrels that gather thousands of gallons of distilled water during our winter and summer "monsoon" seasons, where every inch of rainfall can bring us over one thousand gallons of water. While some areas in Europe and Australia now require rain harvesting, I was amazed to find out some communities in the United States actually forbid it. You can often recoup the cost of a rain barrel in two years. They're very durable, potable, and made of relatively safe hard plastic with a very long life.

I use rainwater primarily for the gardens, but it provides an emergency source of clean water as well. I also reuse most of our house water. The gray water flows out through irrigation pipes to the western garden (of course, many local governments forbid this).

I have a relatively small gas hot-water heater for the house, which most of the year stays plenty hot with just the pilot light (on "vacation" mode) and more than meets our hot-water needs indoors. The outdoor solar shower, which has both hot and cold water, is a homemade coil of black hose that sits on the southern-sloped roof above the large redwood shower stall that provides plenty of free hot water. It also cleans the exercise clothes while showering. On the few heavily clouded covered winter days that don't heat enough water, I shower the traditional way—indoors. The solar shower water is detoured into a flower garden (I avoid any and all unhealthy soaps and toiletries). Even the septic fields provide water for trees and flowering bushes that beautify the surroundings and keep much-needed birds and bees nearby to help with pollination and insect control.

Nothing is wasted—from overgrown green beans and squash to food not consumed. It either goes to the chickens or garden compost to continually rebuild soil nutrients.

There are many other ways to incorporate healthy living with saving energy while not sacrificing luxury. We don't have a microwave or TV (they're unhealthy when turned on and still use energy when turned off), no clothes dryer (this is Arizona), and only use the dishwasher once every few months for dinner parties. I generate very little disposable garbage (most things are reused or composted). I might have two small kitchen garbage bags a month, so I don't have sanitation pickup (instead, I share with a neighbor).

Needless to say, my current living expenses are the least they've been since college days. Can you create this off-the-grid environment overnight? Probably not. But there's no better time to start than now. It's healthy for you—and the planet.

CHAPTER 8

WATER
The Body's Most Important Nutrient

You can go days without eating and still be alive—though it's not something I'd advise in any circumstance. But you can't go very long without water and expect to survive. In hot climates, going without water for even several hours puts you at severe health risk. Water is what makes the human body function. It can comprise between 70 and 75 percent of one's total body weight. Water has such a simple molecular structure—two hydrogen atoms bonding with a single oxygen atom—yet life on Earth as we know it would cease to exist it without its presence. Water also covers 70 percent of our planet, with 97 percent of that water located in the oceans. (One wonders why both the planet and human body have somewhat similar amounts of water.)

Water is your body's most important nutrient and is involved in every bodily function. It helps you regulate body temperature, aids in digestion, transports valuable nutrients, and flushes toxins from your body.

Drinking clean water is so vital to optimal function that a deficiency of less than 1 percent can begin producing signs and symptoms of dysfunction—from low energy and poor circulation to reduced brain function.

Slightly more dehydration can produce serious health problems that include neurological dysfunction and shutting down of organ and gland activity. The key to maintaining proper hydration is to drink plenty of water throughout the day.

Water is the key ingredient in maintaining chemical balance in your body. This includes transporting nutrients to the cells, maintaining the function of blood, and eliminating wastes from the lungs, skin, and colon. Water also plays a major role in hormone regulation and balancing acid-base levels. More importantly, water is like your car's radiator, cooling the reactions that normally create heat in your body. For example, muscle contraction, digestion, and the processing of nutrients produce large amounts of heat, which must be cooled by water. If this regulation did not occur effectively, your temperature would rise to a level that would destroy your enzymes and other protein-based substances, and you would die. The water literally absorbs the excess heat and carries it to the skin where it is dissipated through evaporation and other means.

Water is distributed unevenly throughout the body, with different areas accounting for various percentages. Here are some examples:

- About 80 percent of your blood, heart, lungs, and kidneys is water.
- Your muscles, brain, intestines, and spleen are about 75 percent.

- Your bones are 22 percent water.
- Fat stores are about 10 percent water.
- One of the biggest problems of dehydration is that it decreases blood volume.

Maintaining blood volume is important because so many vital functions are associated with it:

- Transport of oxygen-carrying red blood cells to the muscles.
- Transport of nutrients, including glucose, fats, and amino acids.
- Removal of carbon dioxide and other waste products.
- Transport of hormones that help regulate muscular activity.
- Neutralization of lactic acid to maintain proper pH.
- Maintenance of efficient cardiovascular function.

Dehydration and Its Remedy

Most of the body's water is contained inside the cells of muscles, nerves, organs, and bones, helping to regulate the intracellular environment. Water also functions in between the cells by helping to carry nutrients and hormones into the cells. One of the most significant functions of water is to regulate the balance of potassium (on the inside of the cell) and sodium (outside the cell). This balance is most important in nerve and muscle cells, producing nervous system function and muscle contraction.

Thirst is how most people remember to drink water. But this is not the best indication that you're dehydrating since the brain's thirst center does not send a message until you are almost 2 percent dehydrated. By then, you're already slightly dehydrated. The kidneys, however, provide you with a better signal that you're dehydrating. They can give you two signs: reduce urine production and color change.

If your urine output is diminished, you're beginning to dehydrate. What is meant by "diminished"? If you're not urinating at least six to eight times each day, you may be dehydrated.

The color of your urine may be the best and earliest indicator that you need more water. Urine should be clear, except for the first urine in the morning because you're mildly dehydrated then and drinking water should be one of the first things you do upon awakening. If your urine has a yellow color, it probably means you need more water. The darker the yellow, the more water you need.

A simple formula is important to remember regarding water balance:

Water input = water output

Water input from drinking must balance loss, which occurs from several areas of the body.

- Most water is lost through the kidneys. This water is used to help eliminate normal waste products from the body. During exercise, the body attempts to conserve water, and loss through the kidneys is very limited.
- Evaporation from the skin, important for controlling body temperature, is also a major source of water loss. Even under cool, resting conditions, about 30 percent of water loss occurs here. But sweating, from exercise or normal daily activity, increases this amount dramatically—during exercise, it's about three hundred times the amount lost during rest!
- Water loss in exhaled air is also significant and a bit less than the skin. The air going in and out of your lungs needs to be humidified.
- A small but significant water loss (about 5 percent) occurs through the intestine.
- The amount of water loss is determined in part by air temperature (the higher the temperature, the more water loss), humidity (drier climates result in more water loss), and body size (the larger the person, the more water loss).

If you're dehydrated, just drinking a glass of water won't immediately solve the problem. Complete water replacement throughout the body may take twenty-four to forty-eight hours no matter how much you drink at one time. Unfortunately, the human body does not function like that of many other animals. By drinking a large volume of water, dehydrated animals can consume 10 percent of their total body weight in a few minutes and rehydrate. Humans need to drink water in smaller amounts much more frequently to correct dehydration and maintain proper hydration.

What should you do to prevent dehydration and maintain proper hydration? Here are some general everyday guidelines:

- Don't wait until you're thirsty to drink water. Drink water every day, throughout the day.
- Drink water between meals, not during meals, as it can interfere with digestion of food.
- Drink smaller amounts every couple hours rather than two or three large doses a day.
- Have a source of water near you at all times and get into the habit of drinking water. Especially keep water near your immediate area during work hours or where you spend much of your time (at your desk, by the phone, in your car).
- Avoid carbonated water as your main source; the carbonation may cause intestinal distress.
- Get used to drinking water before and immediately after exercise. If you exercise for more than about an hour, drink small amounts of water during the workout.
- Learn to drink water without swallowing air—drink slowly and without tilting your head up and back.
- The average person may need about three quarts of water each day.

- Avoid chlorinated and fluoridated water and water stored in plastic bottles.

In addition to the above recommendations, get used to drinking water as your main source of liquid. This does not mean drinking heavily marketed, ridiculously overpriced synthetic, vitamin-enhanced bottled water that is sold as a "healthy alternative" to drinking good, clean water. While it's true you obtain some of your water needs through food and other beverages, most should come from plain water, consumed between meals, not during meals since it can interfere with proper digestion.

Certain drinks such as coffee and tea, which contain caffeine, and alcohol can actually increase your need for water because of their diuretic effect (causing the body to lose water). Even decaf coffee and tea can contain small amounts of caffeine.

So don't count these beverages as part of your daily water intake. The same goes for juices, all colas, and other sodas (which you shouldn't be drinking anyway.)

Just How Safe Is Your Water?

Only 1 percent of the world's water is safe to drink. Today, more people are questioning not only the quality of their drinking water but also the container it comes in. Contaminants in drinking water can be a significant risk to your health and fitness. Surprisingly, millions (if not billions) of people are exposed to unhealthy, unnecessary toxins in drinking water every day. Don't just assume your water is safe to drink—you need to take active steps to find out for sure. And if there is a problem, you need to correct it.

CAN YOU REALLY DRINK TOO MUCH WATER?

You may have read media reports about water intoxication—that drinking too much water can cause serious health problems. While this issue is usually related to more active people, especially athletes of all ages performing long training and racing such as marathons and triathlons, it potentially can occur in others. The problem is not just drinking too much water as the media portrays but consuming larger amounts of water in an unhealthy body.

We're about to come full circle with new water recommendations. For years, suggestions regarding water intake during exercise was "more is better." People started carrying water bottles during their thirty-minute walks and kept water within reach during treadmill, stationary bike, and aerobic dance workouts. Of course, drinking water this often during short exercise sessions is not necessary if you maintain proper hydration.

But then athletes competing in long events started dying and getting seriously ill due to overhydration, and the term "water intoxication" was born. A condition called hyponatremia—abnormally low blood sodium—often accompanied overhydration in these individuals, providing the first clue that there was a cause other than just drinking too much water. The proper regulation of water and that of sodium go hand in hand.

While we know that serious water and sodium problems can occur in some people who exercise for long periods, especially in endurance athletes, it's a question of which came first—too much water or body dysfunction that causes poor fluid regulation. Perhaps a better question is this: can excess fluid intake be an aggravating factor rather than the cause of water and sodium imbalance?

The answer to this question is yes. And new recommendations about to hit the exercise world will be that of reducing water intake. Unfortunately, restricting fluids would be treating the symptom.

One of the causes of water intoxication and that of low blood sodium is hormone imbalance. Another cause may be due to chronic inflammation.

The best recommendation is to maintain proper hydration and be healthy and fit.

Most contaminants in water fall into four categories:

- Environmental chemicals, including pesticides, herbicides, trihalomethanes (from chlorination), and man-made chemicals such as bisphenol A (BPA) that can leach out of plastic bottles
- Heavy metals, including lead, copper and nitrates
- Bacteria, including the most common coliform bacteria
- Radiological pollution, including radon, radium, and uranium

If you're concerned about the water in your home, the first step is to analyze it to find out what, if any, contamination exists. Once any questions about the quality of the water are answered, necessary steps to improve it can be taken more logically. The first question to ask is in regard to the source of your water. For most people, this is either a public water system or a well.

Individuals on public systems have the legal right to ask for and obtain the results of past water tests from their water supplier. The supplier must also inform you of any problems, past or present, in meeting federal requirements for safety. The supplier can also tell you if your water contains chlorine or fluoride. This may be easier said than done as many water companies don't want you to know about past tests or current hazards.

If your source of water comes from a well, you'll have to take the initiative and have the water tested yourself. If you've recently purchased your home, a water test should have been done before the sale. At other times, the health department may do certain tests, especially if there are local pollution problems. Deeper wells generally have less contamination than more shallow, often older, wells. Even if your area has a safe environment, many problems can come from water runoffs and chemical leaks far away from your well.

Whether you drink public or well water, another potential source of contamination is your pipes. The biggest problem is potentially found in older houses. Because lead is a serious health hazard, lead pipes, and lead-containing materials were outlawed in 1986. However, in older houses (built before 1930), the plumbing may include lead pipes, lead-containing solder, or other lead-based materials. These soft dull-gray metal pipes are very dangerous, especially with soft water. Some cities, like Chicago and New York, may have lead connector pipes, which connect the city water supply to homes. The water department or city engineer should be able to tell you whether this is the case with your home.

Copper pipes can also leach copper into your drinking water. High copper levels occur in areas where there is soft water (sometimes referred to as a low pH or high acidity). Although not as serious as lead, excess copper can cause health problems, including disturbances of mineral balance, especially zinc, iron, and manganese, with excess copper being stored in the liver and brain where it can be toxic.

Some homes, especially in the northwestern United States, have older pipes or tanks made of galvanized steel. This metal can leach cadmium, and as with copper, this may pose health dangers.

Corrosion of pipes can also cause excess contamination. This is typical in areas where basements are damp year-round. The most common source of corrosion is from the grounding of a home's electrical system. This is easy to inspect. Electrical ground wires should never be attached to your water pipes, but to a separate ground.

Although the most accurate method of analyzing your water is through a lab, observing the stains in your sink may be a clue to some contaminants. The exception is lead, which won't render any discoloration. Copper, however, will produce a blue-green stain and iron a brown streak.

Having your water tested by a competent laboratory will remove all the guesswork regarding its safety. Samples should be taken from a frequently used source, such as the kitchen sink. A morning sample would generally have the highest levels of mineral contamination as water sitting in the pipes all night tends to accumulate these substances. For this reason, let your water run a few seconds or more in the morning or whenever water has stayed in the pipe more than six hours to allow that water to be discarded. If water sources in your area have been contaminated, or if several members of your household have symptoms related to contaminated water (such as recurring diarrhea or vomiting) the health department may do testing. The health department may also give you names of reputable labs that can test your water. These labs use Environmental Protection Agency (EPA) standards, and although some feel the EPA's ranges of normal are too conservative, at least you are ensured accurate testing. The lab may want to provide you with special collection containers as some samples need to be properly preserved.

In some instances, such as in the case of high lead content, you may ask your doctor about testing the levels in your blood. The EPA has changed the standard for this toxic metal from 50 parts per billion (ppb) to 10 ppb when testing home water. But even at low levels, a long-term buildup in the body is always a possibility. Children are most susceptible to lead toxicity.

If you still have questions about your water, the EPA has a Drinking Water Hotline in Washington DC: 800-426-4791. It can provide you with a list of contaminants and the allowable levels. If you find contaminants in your water supply, there are several things you can do to remedy the problem. If the source can be corrected, such as your septic or lead pipes, this becomes an obvious priority. If the source cannot be found, a water-filtering system can usually solve your problem.

THE ABCs OF BPA

The public is understandably anxious about reducing its exposure to bisphenol A (BPA) following a 2008 federal government report warning that the chemical may be linked to breast cancer, prostate cancer, and other health-related problems. BPA is a man-made plastic component that is found in baby bottles, water bottles, food containers, and even toys. Health advocates have advised against using any containers made with BPA. The potential for toxic contamination is too great to overlook or ignore

The Environmental Working Group at Environment California put together these health and safety guidelines:

- Avoid bottles and other food containers made of clear, hard, polycarbonate plastic (made from bisphenol A), which may be labeled #7 or PC on the underside. Also avoid polyvinyl chloride (PVC), labeled #3, which can contain phthalates.
- Choose plastic food containers, bottles, and cups made of #1, #2, and #4 (polyethylene) and softer, opaque #5 (polypropylene), plastics, or glass or stainless steel.
- Avoid canned foods, including baby formula, which may contain bisphenol A in their lining.
- Avoid foods wrapped in plastic.
- Do not put plastics in the dishwasher and dispose of any plastic containers or dishware that look scratched or hazy.

Fluoride Safety

The issue of fluoride and its safety is a long and complex one, and I won't attempt to cover the complete debate here. But I do want to address the use of fluoride as an additive to drinking water. I'm basically opposed to having fluoride in the water supply because it is a high-dose supplement used out of its natural environment. And we're all forced to consume it, whether it's needed or not. Instead of treating everyone with fluoridated water, an attempt should be made to target those who really need it. In the case of cavity prevention, it would be better to treat susceptible individuals than have fluoridated water be part of an entire city's water supply.

Despite what most people think, fluoride is no longer considered an essential nutrient. Natural fluoride is found in most foods, especially chicken, fish, seafood, and tea; and it's found naturally in most drinking water. Through a healthy diet, enough fluoride can be consumed to have a positive effect on cavity prevention. The National Institutes of Health (NIH) says tooth decay has declined sharply in recent years, even in areas without fluoridated water. British researchers also found, after studying people from eight different countries, that tooth decay was declining equally in both fluoridated and nonfluoridated areas.

Fluoride can also negatively affect other areas of the body—especially the bones. Some studies show that fluoride can substantially increase bone loss, producing bone fractures in the spine, wrist, and arm. Other studies have shown that in communities that have fluoridated water, hip fractures are more common.

Fluoride also interferes with energy production. This occurs in the anaerobic biochemical pathways that convert sugar to energy.

About half the water systems in the United States have fluoridated water. If you wish to avoid this water, filter what comes through the tap. But most water filters don't remove fluoride, so check the manufacturer's information regarding which chemicals its product filters.

Filter Your Water

The first step in considering a water filter is learning what contaminants are in the water. Once you know what needs to be filtered, you can use the appropriate system. Unfortunately, there is no single water filter that will solve all your potential water problems. Keep in mind that toxins also can enter the body through the skin or lungs when bathing or taking a shower—the inhalation or absorption of trihalomethanes, a cancer-causing chemical found in chlorinated water, is a common problem. This can be remedied by using a system that filters all water entering your house. You can also install a water filter on your showerhead or bathtub tap if that's frequently used. Jacuzzis and hot tubs may also pose problems if they use unfiltered water swimming pools that are chlorinated are significant health hazards because evaporating chlorine gas is highest just above water level where it's easily inhaled. Avoid chlorine pools and find alternatives—many other mechanisms are used to keep pool water clean, including infrared, bromine, and salt. It's also relatively easy to convert your pool from chlorine to salt.

The three best water filters include activated-carbon systems, reverse-osmosis systems, and distillation units. Each one will filter specific contaminants.

Carbon filters dating back to the ancient Greeks and Romans trap contaminants as the water passes through the filter. Solid-carbon-block filters are the most effective for this process (as opposed to granular-carbon devices). Carbon filters remove most organic chemicals, such as pesticides and herbicides, chlorine, bacteria, metals (lead, iron, copper), and radon; but they do not remove minerals (so they won't soften water), arsenic, nitrates, viruses, and radioactive particles. Carbon filtration usually improves the taste of the water. Some carbon filters contain silver

Preventing Tooth Decay Naturally

More effective than fluoride in the prevention of tooth decay is maintaining proper oral pH. Some foods, mainly carbohydrates, are acid-forming. Many commercial toothpastes also make the mouth more acidic. An acidic environment in the mouth promotes tooth decay. Conversely, a more alkaline environment prevents decay. Certain foods, such as cheese, some toothpastes, and baking soda as well as natural fats and oils, will leave the mouth more alkaline. Honey is one carbohydrate food that can also make the mouth more alkaline and also help reduce dextran, a sticky substance that enables bacteria to stick to the teeth. Oral pH is especially important before bedtime. For children, a glass of apple juice or milk just before bed can promote tooth decay, and fluoride won't necessarily remedy that problem.

nitrate to prevent bacterial buildup; these filters may have the potential to leak silver, which is toxic. Ideally, the carbon cartridge must be replaced periodically to maintain effectiveness and normal water flow. Small carbon-filter units for water bottles are also available, making safer water possible when you are away from home.

Reverse osmosis has been used for large-scale projects, such as industrial desalination of seawater. Essentially, it's a more complex filtration system that includes carbon. Reverse osmosis removes toxic metals and radiation contamination, except radon, but does not remove many organic chemicals.

Distillation, like carbon filtration, is also an ancient method of treating water. This is the best all-around method as it "filters" more items than any other single device, although it is not technically a filter process (it's more like rainwater, made from evaporating water that becomes clouds). The process involves boiling the water to be treated and capturing and cooling the steam, which gives you cleaner water. Distillation removes toxic metals and radiation contamination, except radon, and also removes minerals and thus softens the water. It may not remove all organic chemicals.

Manufacturers of these different filtering devices can provide you with more information on which contaminants they remove as well as proper use, installation, and maintenance costs. Also, it's well worth testing your water again after installing a water filter to be certain it is performing properly.

Plastic Container Toxicity

Water (and other foods) stored in plastic containers may not be as safe to take as once thought. For many years, plastic has been suspect regarding the possibility that harmful chemicals contained in many plastic materials can leach into water. As research continues showing this is a real hazard, there are a variety of things you can do. Here are some recommendations:

- Avoid using plastic as long-term storage containers for water or other foods. Instead, save all your glass containers to use for food storage.
- Certain foods react strongly with plastic. Avoid buying vinegar, tomato, alcohol, and similar products contained in plastic.
- Remove the plastic parts to bottles containing these foods. For example, some bottles of vinegar contain plastic pouring spouts, which can be removed.
- Use glass or stainless steel bottles for water when you are way from home.

When it comes to water—whether you are drinking it, swimming in it, or showering in it—this life-giving substance remains one of the most potential sources of environmental contamination. Always play it safe with water. Your health depends on it.

CHAPTER 9

DIETARY SUPPLEMENTS
What You Don't Know Will Hurt You

Throughout this book I have emphasized the need to eat real food and avoid processed, synthetic, and artificial products. Consuming a healthy diet full of natural carbohydrates, fats and proteins, vegetables, fruits, nuts, and seeds will often provide sufficient levels of micronutrients, macronutrients, and phytonutrients. But when you feel there is a need to take vitamin supplements due to the inability to obtain certain nutrients in adequate amounts from a balanced diet, you need to know that most dietary supplements, even those sold in health-food stores, are unnatural and unhealthy. They usually contain synthetic vitamins and pharmaceutical-like compounds.

So does that mean all supplements are bad and should be avoided? No. Just the majority is. That is why you should always try to obtain all your nutrients from a healthy, real-food diet, though there might be times when taking a supplement is necessary. But taking a supplement is not so simple or risk free as it might first appear. You need to be extra careful and take some preliminary steps.

Many of the popular dietary supplements available are more than unhealthy; they can even be toxic or dangerous over time. For example, a recent study published in the *American Journal of Clinical Nutrition* showed that common doses of vitamin C—1,000 mg a day—can actually reduce oxygen uptake and significantly diminish human endurance; in other words, your energy and stamina can drop. Other recent studies, including one published in the *Journal of the American Medical Association*, show that popular doses of alpha tocopherol (vitamin E)—400 international units (IUs)—can increase the risk of one dying from various health problems, including heart problems. It's important to note that the same nutrients in a healthy diet will not cause these problems. The fault is in the dietary supplement—and this includes the source (natural versus synthetic) and types of nutrients as well as the dosage. Just remember this: the majority of studies show that supplements don't provide the benefits obtained from the same nutrients in the diet.

Do You Need to Take a Supplement?

Knowing whether you need to take a dietary supplement is obviously the first question to answer. The notion that it "can't hurt," that a supplement is "like an insurance policy," or "your body can eliminate what it doesn't need" is a popular myth perpetuated by companies making supplements and is simply untrue. In addition, many people take supplements because their friend takes them or because they saw ads for them.

A more individual determination of your nutritional needs is the first step in deciding whether you might need a dietary supplement. This can be accomplished in a variety of ways. One is with the help of a health care professional who may determine this through a variety of methods, including a good history, blood and urine tests, and other evaluations. However, with some exceptions, blood and urine tests are generally not the best ways to determine nutritional needs. While they can uncover the more obvious and serious deficiencies, such as low iron levels, they might not detect more subtle dietary shortcomings.

The other methods to determine your potential needs for supplementation include experimentation, diet analysis, and health surveys. Let's consider each of these.

Experimentation

Some people may effectively determine the need for a dietary supplement through careful experimentation. A health care professional might conclude, after evaluating you, that there is a need for a particular nutrient. But the best indication that you need one is if taking it improves some aspect of body function. This may include the successful treatment of a particular problem, such as fatigue or asthma or the elimination of an abnormal finding in a blood test or other evaluation, such as an abnormal C-reactive protein test (a measure of chronic inflammation).

153

In almost all cases, seeing some improvement from a particular supplement may occur within a relatively short time. Let's say that every day you have asthma symptoms and want to see if the nutrient choline can help. Taking this supplement for a month or two will almost always either reduce symptoms or do nothing. If it helps, you may want to continue taking it while you also consume more foods high in this nutrient (in this case, the best food source is egg yolks).

Diet Analysis

An excellent way to determine the need for a dietary supplement is to analyze your diet. It can tell you what nutrients you're not getting from your diet, but the remedy should begin by improving your diet not by first taking a supplement.

Diet analysis is a common tool used by some health care professionals, researchers, and even individuals to evaluate nutrient intakes. It makes use of a computerized program and provides information about your levels of nutrients compared to the recommended daily allowance (RDA) or other standard reference (such as the USDA's Dietary Reference Intakes, or DRIs). Studies using this approach and other methods continue to show seriously low intakes of many nutrients by large numbers of people. One USDA survey estimated that 80 percent of American women did not achieve RDA levels of folic acid, iron, zinc, vitamin B_6, magnesium, and calcium. This problem, of course, is due to poor dietary habits.

I used various diet analysis programs during my years in practice and tested almost all patients. Just as other surveys have shown, many people had serious nutritional imbalances in their diets. Even when I factored in dietary supplements some people took, they were frequently below-RDA levels of various nutrients. Today there are many computerized diet analysis programs available, and the USDA web site (www.usda.gov) provides a simple one that is free.

If a diet analysis shows that specific nutrients are below a minimum level, there are two important steps to take:

- First, improve your diet to include or increase foods containing these nutrients.
- Second, you may need additional nutrients from a dietary supplement—at least temporarily until your nutrient levels return to normal and you can maintain these levels with your diet.

Health Surveys

Another approach that can help determine the potential need for a dietary supplement, and one used throughout *The Big Book of Health and Fitness*, is the use of a health survey. In this instance, it's a group of questions based not on nutrient levels in the body or in the food you eat but on certain signs and symptoms associated with a low level of a particular nutrient. Here's an example: fatigue, excess blood loss, and the habit of chewing on ice may be associated with the

154

need for iron, a micronutrient. Sleepiness after meals, intestinal bloating, and frequent hunger and craving for sweets may be associated with excess intake of carbohydrates, a macronutrient. Surveys are based on commonly defined changes in the body when particular nutrients levels are low.

Hidden Dangers of Dietary Supplements

Unfortunately, many people believe they need dietary supplements due to bad advice and misinformation. The usual persuasive culprits are advertising, anecdotal evidence

---

HEALTH SURVEY

Here is an example of an actual survey I've used in private practice. Use it and see which items apply to you:

- History or risk of heart disease
- History or risk of Alzheimer's disease or other reduced mental capacity
- Female (childbearing age)
- Outdoors often in sun or use tanning salons
- Live in southern climates (below San Francisco or Washington DC)
- Over fifty years old
- History of anemia or other red blood cell problem
- Feelings of depression
- History of taking doses of vitamin C above 500 mg
- Reduced intake of meat, fish, and eggs
- Increased caffeine intake (coffee, tea, soda—more than three per day)
- Increased alcohol intake (more than two drinks per day)

If you check even one or two items, it could indicate a need for more vitamin B$_{12}$ and/or folic acid, with the likelihood increasing significantly as you get past two checked items. The necessary dose cannot be determined from a survey as other follow-up tests as noted above may be necessary; dosing is very individual. While most vitamin B$_{12}$ and folic acid in dietary supplements are synthetic, natural forms are available—and will be discussed shortly.

The following surveys will list specific items for you to check before mentioning what particular nutrient the survey pertains to. By doing so, this helps keep the questioning more objective.

---

from a friend, product websites, and bloggers. At one time the notion was that a dietary supplement could only help and not hurt. It's now known clinically this is not the case, and many studies are showing the potential dangers of many types of dietary supplements. These extra nutrients will not improve body function if the body's need for these nutrients does not exist. In other words, taking more B vitamins because you think they will give you more energy won't help you if your levels of this group of nutrients are already normal.

Do you take supplements because you feel they offer some safeguard against some nutritional deficiency? This could be a problem for at least two reasons. First, it may mean that you're not focusing on eating the best diet possible; dietary supplements usually won't provide all the nutrients you can obtain from a healthy diet. Second, you risk causing other nutritional imbalances—for example, taking too much omega-6 oil can cause an imbalance of fats or taking a supplement with too much copper can reduce your levels of zinc.

The fact that a dietary supplement contains nutrients does not mean it's natural or even safe. The vitamins in most dietary supplements are synthetic. Most are made from artificial chemicals in some manufacturing facility and not obtained from plants grown on an organic farm or in the wilds. In fact, the FDA has no regulation when it comes to differentiating a synthetic vitamin from a natural one.

HEALTH SURVEY: DO ANY OF THE BELOW STATEMENTS APPLY TO YOU?

- Take high doses of vitamin C (above 200 mg)
- Combine vitamin C supplements with iron supplements
- Consume above-moderate levels of alcohol (more than 2 drinks/day)
- Take high doses of vitamin E (above 100 IU)
- Take more than 10 mg of iron in supplements.
- Take more than 800 mg of calcium as supplements
- Take over-the-counter or prescription medication.
- Take vitamin A in supplements (multivitamins, cod liver oil, etc.)
- Take more than 50 mg vitamin B_6 per day from supplements
- Take regular supplements containing omega-6 oils (primrose, borage, black currant).

Possible Implications. Increased risk of side effects such as fatigue, interactions with other supplements or medications, intestinal irritation, chronic inflammation from synthetic or high doses of popular dietary supplements.

HSAIDS: The Most Dangerous Dietary Supplements

Most dietary supplements on the market do not provide vitamins and other nutrients as they naturally occur in real food. Although these supplements may be labeled NATURAL, their vitamins are usually synthetic and often provide doses much higher than foods in nature. Other supplements contain natural nutrients but are separated from the foods where they originated, leaving behind many important associated phytonutrients. I call these supplements HSAIDS, which stands for "high-dose synthetic and isolated dietary supplements." When consumed, HSAIDS act more like drugs in the body than like real food.

HSAIDS are not always bad, although some can be deadly, but they're not what most people think they are—equivalent to the same nutrient counterpart in food. The most important nutrients are those contained in foods, and if you supplement, products made from food are the best and safest choice.

In some instances, such as with the careful direction of a health care practitioner trained in nutrition, HSAIDS may be useful. In the case of anemia, they may be beneficial for a relatively short period of time to correct a specific condition. Others may have long-term needs or require a high dose of a particular nutrient, such as an active form of folic acid, to address a common genetic problem as 30 percent of the population may be unable to absorb synthetic folic acid.

While these issues are not that uncommon, they are the exceptions. Most people do not need HSAIDS.

The primary difference between HSAIDS and products made from real food, which contain truly natural nutrients in food doses, is how the body responds to them when consumed.

Biological versus Pharmacological Responses to Supplements

When one takes a dietary supplement, just like when one eats food or takes a drug, the body has particular physiological responses. In general, nutrients in their natural state and dose have a biological effect, just like eating a healthy meal of real food. HSAIDS, however, have a pharmacological effect in the body, like a drug.

Examples of dietary supplements that clearly act in more of a biological fashion include products made from foods, such as vegetable and fruit concentrates, fish oil, and protein powders made from whey or egg whites. These supplements provide nutrients in a concentrated form, acting essentially the same as when you consume the real food. They provide natural doses of vitamins, minerals, macronutrients, or phytonutrients helping to generate energy, regulate immunity, control aging, and perform countless other functions that improve health and human performance—just like real food.

Nutrients with pharmacological effects generally include HSAIDS and have actions like those of drugs rather than foods. These include synthetic vitamin C (ascorbic acid being one of many common forms), isolated high-dose vitamin E (alpha-tocopherol), and popular B complex supplements (almost all being synthetic). These are almost always in doses much higher than a person could possibly consume during a meal or even a day's worth of food intake—even when consuming foods naturally high in these nutrients. Many contain doses that would take weeks of eating foods rich in these nutrients to get to the same levels—in other words, five, ten, even a hundred times normal amounts. By looking at the labels of supplements, you will see that most, even those labeled NATURAL, contain doses much higher than you would get from real food and much higher than the RDA. These unnaturally high doses are one reason they can be harmful.

Dietary supplements that promote pharmacological activity, like most drugs, are capable of modifying brain and body function, often in powerful ways. This is one reason they are accompanied by the risk of adverse side effects—you just don't have control over how they will act. These pharmacological effects of dietary supplements can vary with individuals, and many are not clearly known. HSAIDS with pharmacological actions can also interfere with other nutrients, whether from the diet or other supplements, or with over-the-counter and prescription drugs.

The Contrasting Examples of Vitamins C and E

As an example of the difference between HSAIDS and truly natural nutrients, consider vitamins C and E. Food sources of naturally occurring vitamin C have biological effects, acting as antioxidants and protecting our DNA from oxygen damage. The dose of vitamin C contained in a high-quality meal of vegetables and fruits may be 100 mg or less. However, the synthetic counterpart (ascorbic acid and the various similar forms), found in almost all dietary supplements, can function differently. High doses of synthetic vitamin C, typically 500 to 1,000 mg tablets, can perform as an antioxidant but can also transform to a deadly pro-oxidant—which can cause excess free radical activity and inflammation.

Another illustration of the difference between HSAIDS and truly natural nutrients is found in vitamin E. A natural dose of vitamin E is really quite small. For example, the amount of naturally occurring alpha-tocopherol in a loaf of whole wheat bread made fresh from wheat berries—a relatively high source of natural vitamin E—may be only 2 to 4 IU. In contrast, vitamin E supplements typically come in extremely high doses of 400 to 800 IU. You'd have to eat two hundred loaves to reach these supplement doses. This unnatural dose of vitamin E can interfere with other more effective antioxidants in the diet. And worse, these doses of vitamin E have been shown to significantly increase your risk of death from various unnatural causes.

Vitamins C and E are often sold under the NATURAL label—as are most others, including all the synthetic vitamins. In nature, these vitamins occur with other chemical components that include a wide variety of phytonutrients. In addition, synthetic supplements have lower bioavailability, which means you can't absorb them nearly as well as the natural versions. With synthetic vitamin C, for example, the body gets rid of it more quickly, in comparison to vitamin C in real foods. Studies have also shown that vitamin C from food is 35 percent better absorbed and excreted more slowly than synthetic vitamin C.

There are also other potential side effects associated with HSAIDS; some include the following:

- Popular doses of vitamin C supplements can be toxic when they react with the iron in the body or iron in dietary supplements. This is because of the powerful free radicals produced by iron.
- Consuming popular doses of iron can result in excess ferritin (the body's storage form of iron), which has been associated with an increased risk of heart disease and liver stress. High-iron intake can also produce damaging excess free radicals and intestinal distress.
- Common preparations of copper, zinc, or selenium supplements can be toxic and can even cause disease.
- Popular doses of vitamin K and B_6 can be toxic.

- Consuming popular high doses of vitamin A can result in bone loss and increase the risk of hip fractures in the elderly.
- Consuming popular doses of beta-carotene has been shown to increase lung cancer risk.

OTHER IMPORTANT CONSIDERATIONS

- None of the nutrients that can cause harm in the body from dietary supplements are harmful when consumed in real food.
- Taking a dietary supplement can promote a false sense of security that you're getting all the nutrients needed for optimal endurance and health.
- While researchers have found for decades that consumption of vegetables and fruits significantly decrease the risk of many diseases, most studies have concluded that dietary supplements containing the same vitamins and minerals do not.

HSAIDS Are Not Whole Foods

Another problem with most dietary supplements, even those made from natural nutrients, is that they have been isolated from foods, causing many valuable nutrients to be left behind—much like the processing of whole wheat berries into unhealthy while flour. Some of these are more important than the one that is isolated. One example are the many phytonutrients that accompany vitamins and mineral in real food—by isolating a particular vitamin in a supplement and leaving the thousands of phytonutrients behind, you're missing out on a lot of nutritional benefits. Another common example is alpha-tocopherol, also referred to as vitamin E. Alpha-tocopherol does not normally exist alone in nature but occurs with three other tocopherols—beta, delta, and gamma—and four tocotrienols—alpha, beta, delta, and gamma. Together these seven other components of the vitamin E "complex" can be more important than alpha-tocopherol alone. Consider that gamma-tocopherol is commonly found in natural foods and is more effective than alpha-tocopherol as an antioxidant. By taking a supplement of only alpha-tocopherol, you can actually lower the levels of gamma-tocopherol in the body, reducing the overall health benefits of the vitamin E complex.

In addition, the tocotrienols are powerful substances that have potent anti-inflammatory and anticancer actions, reduce cholesterol, and perform other vital tasks. But taking too much alpha-tocopherol can interfere with some of these functions. Even moderate amounts, such as 100 IU of alpha-tocopherol, can block the ability of tocotrienols to control cholesterol.

Unbalanced, isolated high doses of alpha-tocopherol can interfere with body chemistry in other ways too. They can have a negative effect on anti-inflammatory chemical production, cause generalized muscle weakness, lower thyroid hormone levels, and slightly increase fasting triglyceride levels. Like high-dose vitamin C, alpha-tocopherol may also become a pro-oxidant—which would be counterproductive to its antioxidant function.

Supplement Hype

Within the dietary supplement industry, the biggest players—those that manufacture the synthetic vitamins and raw materials used to make HSAIDS—are the pharmaceutical companies themselves. The natural foods companies that make real food dietary supplements are generally small and not as welcomed into the natural foods market yet.

HEALTH SURVEY

Check the items that apply to you:

- Low consumption of nuts and seeds (less than one serving/day)
- Takes high dose of alpha-tocopherol (more than 200 IU/day)
- Chronic inflammation
- History of heart disease or cancer
- Smoke cigarettes (recent past or present)
- Over age fifty
- Low-fat diet (less than 20 percent)
- High cholesterol
- Skin problems
- Cataracts

These are items that may indicate a need for more vitamin E complex nutrients and the need to avoid high-dose alpha-tocopherol (vitamin E).

However, the image that "natural" dietary supplements are prevalent, and the marketing of supplements as "real food" is widespread. But most of these claims are untrue when you read the fine print or know how products are actually made.

Because of the wholesome image of "natural foods," some supplements may contain food concentrates such as blueberry, broccoli, or spinach. However, these plant materials are not only added in minuscule amounts; they also are often made from foods cooked at very high temperatures. The reason for their inclusion, as market researchers tell us, is that it looks "healthy" and "good" on the label; an ad or commercial can even say the product contains real food, or some other claim about being made from fruits and vegetables. But a careful look at the label shows that the vitamins in these products are usually synthetic, they were added separately, and are not from those "real" foods. Discerning and uncovering these hidden tricks is often not easy for the average consumer.

Another gimmick commonly used in the supplement industry is the use of yeast that's been fed synthetic vitamins. The technique is simple: feed a nutrient such as synthetic vitamin C to living yeast (which are living microorganisms in the fungus family) then dry the yeast and add it to a dietary supplement as a source of vitamin C. Now call it "natural." A trick of the trade. In the case of minerals, it may be a useful process and claims of "natural" can be honestly made since all minerals—from calcium and magnesium to manganese and zinc—exist on earth in its original form. But feeding a synthetic vitamin made to yeast and then adding the yeast to a supplement to call it "natural" and "real food" is grossly misleading and deceptive.

Most companies don't produce supplements made from whole foods. It's difficult and costly to find foods dried with a low-heat process that preserves heat-sensitive nutrients, including the phytonutrients. It's even more difficult to find supplements made from certified organic materials. In addition to these issues, many dietary supplements contain unwanted added ingredients. These fillers, binders, and other chemicals are very common; avoid products containing casein, gluten, soy, wheat, artificial colorings, artificial flavorings, and especially sugar (even if it's labeled organic!).

What is the best alternative to low-quality and often-harmful dietary supplements? Create your own from real food.

Nutrients for Optimal Health and Fitness

Let's now look at some of the important nutrients and groups of nutrients commonly used to help the body build and maintain specific areas of health and fitness. In particular, I want to recommend that you make these foods part of your meals and snacks every day.

To begin with you can make tasty and nutrient-potent health shakes. I *have* two each day.

THE WELL-STOCKED KITCHEN AS APOTHECARY

An apothecary was common during the Middle Ages. It was a shop where a trained person prepared and sold medicines. Of course, these medicines were mainly herbs, roots, and lotions. The modern-day equivalent is the pharmacy, but it's not often the best place to seek a remedy for illness or injury, even its doctor-prescribed pills. There's the cost factor, the harmful side effects, and the potential for addiction. Moreover, your primary health concern should be with finding the cause, not treating the symptoms. Many times, the cure can be found right there in your kitchen.

My kitchen is a well-stocked apothecary. It's a convenient place where many dozens of different foods are found in various forms, from fresh, just-picked vegetables and fruits to raw whole nuts and seeds. Foods like cucumbers, onions, and carrots are sometimes pickled. During the winter months there are more dried and powdered materials made from these same foods. Year-round herbs for adding spice to meals are plentiful—from fresh cilantro and parsley, garlic, oregano, and tarragon, to many dried forms including rosemary, basil, caraway, turmeric, and cayenne. Fresh ginger and peppermint are always available for cold tea in the summer and hot versions in winter.

Some foods are stored whole in the freezer during periods of high yield, including tomatoes, lemons, and limes, with many more kept in glass jars. Various red and white wines are available for cooking and drinking, with distilled liquors used as a base for citrus peel infusions.

All the items are easily within reach during meal preparation—a little of this, a bit of that—depending on the meal or snack, the day, our cravings, the season, and how you feel. A kitchen should always be an apothecary. I will go so far as say that the kitchen should be a sacred place to prepare food as the natural medicine it should be. That means no microwave oven or cupboards full of junk food. Your kitchen should home to therapeutic nutrition—delicious, easy-to-make, beautiful meals and snacks obtained from a well-stocked supply of healthy ingredients.

PHIL'S SHAKE—THE ULTIMATE HEALTHY BEVERAGE

I've been drinking this high-powered healthy smoothie called Phil's shake for years. I usually have one in the morning for breakfast and another midafternoon as a snack.

If you very lightly soft-boil a dozen eggs at a time and keep them refrigerated, preparation for this shake is about five or six minutes. Use a variety of healthy foods, depending on your nutritional needs. Here's my large one-serving recipe:

162

Ingredients

2 soft cooked eggs

1 large or 2 small apples, pears, peaches, or the best in-season fruits

About ½ cup blueberries

1 teaspoon plain psyllium

1 tablespoon raw whole sesame and or flaxseeds

½ or one small carrot

Fresh greens: parsley, young kale, spinach, or broccoli sprouts

8 ounces water

Directions

Add all ingredients into a good blender and blend well.

The best blenders will do a decent job on the whole fruits, including the core, seeds, and all vegetables. I blend my shake for about 45 seconds, which is enough to liquefy all the ingredients—there are no chunks of fruit or whole seeds left. Some blenders that are not as powerful may require much more time to thoroughly mix all ingredients. With enough fruit for sweetness, none of the bitter taste from the vegetables is noticeable—you'd never know there were so many healthy ingredients! Modify this ingredient list based on your likes and nutritional needs.

Antioxidants and the Immune System

One of the most important aspects of nutrition during the aging process is associated with the body's antioxidant system. In particular, a variety of nutrients called antioxidants help prevent cancer, heart disease, inflammation, and chronic illness in general.

The wear and tear of life—physical, chemical, and mental stresses—triggers the release of a variety of chemicals that can influence all body function. Produced in high levels, they can disturb muscle function, increase fatigue, promote chronic inflammation, hinder protein and fat metabolism, and slow recovery from even a normal day's activity. They can also reduce immune function, leading to more illness such as infections. They can even be the start of a long process leading to chronic disease, including cancer and heart disease. These chemicals are called oxygen free radicals. Fortunately, the human body is equipped with a system to control these free radicals—the antioxidant system. This system, an important component of aerobic muscle fibers, uses a variety of nutrients called antioxidants to break down oxygen free radicals into safe chemicals. However, in high amounts, these free radicals are not well controlled by our antioxidant system, and they turn harmful.

Our diet must provide the antioxidant system with the raw materials it needs to function well. These are referred to as antioxidants, and include vitamins C and E, beta-carotene, selenium, zinc, and others that are easily obtained by eating a variety of fresh vegetables and fruits, nuts and seeds, and other foods.

Since many people don't eat sufficiently to obtain their antioxidants from foods, supple-

HEALTH SURVEY

Check the items that apply to you:

- Asthma or allergy (all types: food, environment, hay fever, animals)
- Recurrent infections (bacteria, virus, yeast, fungus)
- Colds/flu: more than 1–2 per year, lasts more than a few days.
- History of cancer (any tumor or "growth," benign or malignant) or ulcer.
- High physical, chemical, or mental stress
- Regular hard (anaerobic) exercise or competitive athlete
- "Age" spots (brown pigmented areas on skin)
- Regular work or living in indoor areas without open windows
- Frequent exposure to chemicals at home (cleaners, perfumes, cosmetics, toiletries) or work (cleaners, solvents, gasoline, etc.)
- Low blood cholesterol
- History or increased risk for diabetes, joint problems, heart disease, inflammatory problems, Alzheimer's, or other chronic diseases
- Frequently in sun or tanning salon

These items are associated with oxidative stress due to increased free radicals, reduced antioxidant nutrients, and lowered immunity.

ments are often used. Unfortunately, antioxidant supplements don't provide the same nutrients that are obtained from the diet, even though the names of these nutrients are often the same. And these dietary supplements don't accomplish the task that the dietary nutrients provide. In fact, recent studies show that dietary supplements of antioxidants not only don't prevent illness and disease but can also impair immune function as one of the side effects.

In addition to antioxidants, the immune system relies on other nutrients that are often low in many people. A cold that lasts more than the few days or other recurrent infections, asthma, and allergies are some of the problems associated with poor functioning of the immune system.

Antioxidant nutrients that help support the immune system are many—but the most important and most powerful is a substance called glutathione. You can't take this in supplement form because it's digested in the intestines before you can absorb it; but that doesn't stop companies from making glutathione products (supplements that claim to be glutathione are really the raw materials the body needs to make glutathione). You can do better—use the foods your immune system needs to make this potent antioxidant:

- Natural forms of vitamin C and E, and the nutrient lipoic acid. Vegetables and fruits, along with raw almonds, cashews, and sesame seeds, will provide sufficient levels of these nutrients.

- The amino acid cysteine is even more important and is a component of whey—in powder form it's a common dietary supplement and whey cheese (ricotta) can often be found in stores and is easy to make from organic milk.

- Sulforaphan, a sulfur compound in cruciferous vegetables such as broccoli, kale, brussels sprouts, and cabbage, is very potent in helping the body produce glutathione. Two- to three-day-old broccoli sprouts (before their leaves turn dark green) have the highest levels of sulforaphan. These are easy to sprout at home for use in salads, smoothies, and garnishes.

- Common herbs that contain phytonutrients with powerful antioxidant effects include turmeric and ginger. These can be obtained in their fresh state—ginger, especially, is available as a root in most stores that carry fresh vegetables. These can be used regularly in many different recipes. Ginger tea made with honey is a great refreshing drink that can significantly help immune function—drink it hot or cold.

Omega-3 Fats

An imbalance in fat can trigger chronic inflammation, pain, and risk of chronic illness. The most common problem that causes this imbalance is low levels of (omega-3) fats. The best source is from cold-water fish and fish oil supplements. In my practice, I found through dietary analysis that significant numbers of patients had diets very low in omega-3 fats. It has been estimated that more than fifty million people in the United States alone have this problem. The addition of cold-water fish, especially salmon and sardines, can supply more EPA to help balance fats. (Farm-raised fish contain little if any EPA.)

Unfortunately, freshwater and ocean fish are increasingly being polluted, and eating fish regularly may pose toxin risks. For most people, this is an instance where a dietary supplement of fish oil may be necessary. Choosing the right one is key.

Most fish oil supplements containing EPA are carefully produced without oxidized oils and to remove any heavy metals and other toxins. When buying oil-based dietary supplements, read the labels and make sure the oil has been tested for oxidation and for heavy metals and other potential toxins found in the oceans. A good guide is to use fish oil labeled as containing "0" cholesterol. Many have levels of only 2 or 4 mg of cholesterol, but this may imply that they have not been cleaned of potential toxins.

Some people like taking flaxseed oil as an omega-3 supplement. But since flaxseed oil is extremely susceptible to oxidation when exposed to air or heat, it is best to purchase it in capsules or refrigerate its liquid form. However, flax oil does not contain EPA and its conversion to EPA in the body is not very effective, requiring additional vitamins C, B_6, niacin, and the minerals magnesium and zinc.

165

Also note: Avoid refrigerating capsules of dietary supplements containing oils as the cold environment may cause air to leak into the oil inside causing oxidation and lowering potency.

Omega-6 Fats

The oils from black currant seed, borage, and primrose contain high levels of omega-6 oils. These are popular dietary supplements. They contain high amounts of GLA, which is converted to the group 1 anti-inflammatory eicosanoids. People with allergies, especially in the spring when the body's natural eicosanoid levels are low, often need this supplement. GLA is also essential for carrying calcium to muscle and bone cells. Without it, the calcium in your diet won't be as useful and some may be stored as calcium deposits. It's important when taking any product containing GLA to make sure your fats remain balanced; make sure to also take an EPA (fish oil) or raw sesame seed oil to help prevent GLA from ultimately converting to arachidonic acid, the B fat which promotes inflammation. Both sesame and all the GLA-containing oils are also very sensitive to oxygen and should be purchased in capsule form or, if liquid, kept refrigerated.

Vitamin B Complex

Along with vitamin C, the B vitamins are the most common synthetic nutrients in the marketplace. Almost all B vitamins available in supplement form, whether the whole B complex or single vitamin products, are synthetic. Even those labeled as NATURAL.

In the case of the B vitamins, those that are synthetic are also referred to as inactive—in order for the body to utilize these vitamins they must be converted to an active form. This requires other nutrients and energy, and conversion is not always effective.

As in the case with natural versus synthetic vitamin C, the body may not utilize the synthetic B vitamins as well. For example, up to 30 percent of the population may be

---

HEALTH SURVEY

Check the items that apply to you:

- Spring or fall allergies
- Muscle cramps
- Dry, scaly, or itchy skin
- Psoriasis or eczema
- Frequent muscle tightness
- Intolerance to sun (skin)
- Intestinal ulcers
- Use aspirin or other NSAIDs
- Chronic inflammation
- Increased alcohol intake

These symptoms may indicate the need for GLA from omega-6 fats. When taken internally, use sesame seed oil to prevent the omega-6 fat from converting to saturated fats. For skin problems and for young children and babies, use topically.

unable to utilize synthetic folic acid. The only way for these individuals to obtain folic acid is from the diet (vegetables and fruits, especially green leafy foods) or by taking an active (natural) form of folic acid.

You can usually determine the type of individual B vitamins a bottle contains by reading the labels. Below is a list of some active (natural) forms of B vitamins:

- Thiamin (B_1): thiamine pyrophosphate and thiamine triphosphate
- Riboflavin (B_2): riboflavin-5-phosphate
- Niacin (B_3): nicotinamide adenine dinucleotide (NADH)
- Pantothenic acid (B_5): pantethine
- Pyridoxine (B_6): pyridoxal-5-phosphate
- Folic acid: 5-methyl tetrahydrofolate and folinic acid
- Cobalamin (B_{12}): methylcobalamin and cyanocobalamin

The B vitamins are important for so many functions throughout the body. If levels become low, virtually any body area can break down. Those who don't get enough vitamins B_1 and B_2 typically are low in other B vitamins too.

High doses of the B vitamins are not well absorbed or utilized. So if a supplement is needed, it's best to take lower doses two or three times daily than one larger dose. For B_1 and B_2, doses above 5 mg are considered high.

Foods high in B vitamins vary considerably and are not difficult to obtain in a healthy diet. Good sources include eggs and meats, nuts and seeds, legumes, whole grains if tolerated, and some vegetables such as broccoli, spinach, and mushrooms, which have moderate amounts. Significant losses occur in cooking and freezing, so fresh, raw vegetables are important sources. However, avoid the following foods in their raw state: red chicory, brussels sprouts, red cabbage, clams, oysters, squid, and other mollusks—these all contain the chemical thiaminase which destroys vitamin B_1. Some antibiotics can also destroy thiamine. Light (especially the sun) can destroy B_2 in foods, and sunlight on the skin can reduce some of the body's folic acid.

Calcium

True calcium deficiencies are uncommon in the Western world, regardless of what the dairy industry tells us. The bigger problem is that many people are unable to use the calcium they already have in their bodies. Poor calcium metabolism, rather than a deficiency, is almost at epidemic proportions. The end result is that not enough calcium gets into the muscles, bones, and other tissues, with the remaining excess calcium potentially depositing in the joints, tendons, ligaments, or even the kidneys as stones. (Plaque that clogs the arteries can also contain this calcium.)

In order for your body to properly metabolize calcium and more effectively absorb it from food, you must have sufficient vitamin D. This nutrient is free and plentiful, yet

VITAMINS B₁ AND B₂

Here are two important surveys associated with the need for more B vitamins. The first one specifically relates to B_1 and the second to B_2.

Survey 1: Check the symptoms below that apply to you.

- Carbohydrate intolerance, including diabetes
- Body temperature below normal
- Diuretic use (typically used for patients with high blood pressure and heart problems)
- Regular alcohol use
- Regular caffeine use (coffee, tea, cola)
- Moderate to high levels of training and competition
- Fatigue
- Regular headaches
- Reduced mental productivity
- Heart problems
- Poor appetite
- Tendency toward anxiety, phobia, panic disorder
- Sleep problems

Survey 2: Check the symptoms below that apply to you.

- Skin problems
- Gingivitis (gum problems)
- Discomfort or pain on lips, tongue, or in mouth (nondental)
- Cataracts
- Hair loss
- Anxiety, tension, or personality changes
- Sleep less than six to seven hours per night
- Use of antacids
- Reduce immune function (cold, flu, or other illness more than twice yearly)
- Increased need for antioxidants
- Frequently low hemoglobin or short of breath

The more boxes that apply to you, the more your levels of B_1 or B_2 may be too low, especially if you are over fifty years old.

NATURAL FOLATES

Two of the many naturally occurring forms of folic acid include folinic acid and 5-methyl tetrahydrofolate (5-MTHF), the most common forms found in the foods you eat. Unfortunately, the most common form of folic acid in our food supply is synthetic and not well utilized by the body. Because it is much cheaper, it is used in food fortification and virtually all dietary supplements on store shelves. This synthetic form of folic acid is inactive and must first be converted to an active form to be useful in the body.

A significant number of people are unable to absorb or otherwise utilize synthetic folic acid. The numbers are difficult to determine, but scientists have estimated that perhaps up to 30 percent of the population has this inability (which is genetically determined). These individuals must rely on natural folic acid from food, or the 5-methyl or folinic acid versions in supplements.

Consumption of natural folic acid is not just important for prevention of neural tube defects, one of many types of birth defects. It's a necessary nutrient with body-wide benefits for all adults and children. These include the following:

- Brain function—the natural forms of folic acid are the only ones that can get into the brain. It is especially important for those who don't sleep well or are depressed.
- Intestinal function—it can help food digestion and absorption, heal the intestines, and as studies have shown, prevent colon cancer.
- Liver detoxification of substances like estrogens in both men and women—it removes their harmful metabolites and prevents breast cancer.
- Protein metabolism and for regulation of certain amino acids
- The production of new blood cells
- Cardiovascular health (by reducing homocysteine)

In addition, unlike synthetic inactive folic acid, natural folic acid does not mask anemia if not taken with adequate vitamin B$_{12}$.

many people don't have enough; you just need sunlight! Just remember that without sufficient vitamin D, calcium cannot be properly absorbed and regulated, and that most problems of insufficient calcium are really due to low levels of vitamin D.

Another important issue regarding calcium is to consume enough calcium-rich foods; this is easily done without supplementation through good dietary practices. And it does not necessarily mean eating a lot of dairy foods. (Recall that dairy foods are highest in B fat, and too many can contribute to inflammation.)

Consider the moderate amounts of calcium in the following single servings of non-dairy foods:

- Salmon: 225 mg
- Sardines: 115 mg
- Almonds: 100 mg
- Seaweed: 140 mg
- Rainbow trout: 100 mg
- Spinach: 135 mg
- Green beans: 100 mg
- Collards: 125 mg

Two other important issues regarding calcium are absorption from the intestine (which is significantly influenced by vitamin D) and, after absorption, getting the calcium into the bones and muscles. Absorption is the first step to using calcium in the body.

In general, smaller amounts of calcium are better absorbed than larger amounts, whether from food or supplements. If a small amount of calcium is present in the intestine, 70 percent may be absorbed, for example, while a larger amount of calcium may have only a 30 percent absorption rate. If you're taking calcium supplements, it may be best to take a lower dose several times a day rather than a large dose once daily. Even though vegetables contain smaller amounts of calcium, larger percentages are absorbed compared to milk. So in some situations, a serving of broccoli may result in more calcium getting into the body than a serving of milk.

The stomach's natural hydrochloric acid is also very important in making calcium more absorbable. Neutralizing stomach acid has a negative effect on calcium absorption and a serious impact on digestion and absorption of all nutrients.

Excess phosphorus intake can be very detrimental for calcium use, pulling it out of muscles and bones. Most soft drinks contain large amounts of phosphorus—and the people who drink them risk significant calcium loss from bones and muscles.

The type of calcium supplement may be associated with absorbability. For example, calcium carbonate is more poorly absorbed than calcium lactate or calcium citrate. This is due to the alkaline nature of carbonate and the acidic nature of lactate and citrate.

Taking too much calcium in supplement form can disturb the body's complex chemical makeup. Namely, it can reduce magnesium. More people may be in need of additional magnesium than calcium—it's necessary for most enzymes to work, including the ones important for fat metabolism. And the best sources of magnesium are vegetables.

Taking extra calcium in supplements can also increase the risk of kidney stones.

From the mid-1970s, the intake of calcium from dietary supplements dramatically increased. In part it was due to the marketing of calcium to women to prevent bone loss and osteoporosis. Unfortunately, the studies don't clearly show that taking calcium supplements accomplishes this, but recent studies do demonstrate the risks. Dr. Robert Wallace and colleagues from the Department of Epidemiology, University of Iowa College of Public Health, Iowa, published their recent research in the April 2011 issue of the *American Journal of Clinical Nutrition* ("Urinary tract stone occurrence in the Women's Health Initiative randomized clinical trial of calcium and vitamin D supplements."). During the past thirty-five years, the incidence of kidney stones has increased 37 percent in women. Of course, kidney stones also occur in men.

Kidney stones are not just an annoyance. They often result in hospitalization, are sometimes a cause of secondary infections, and are associated with being overfat and atherosclerosis.

Iron

Most people think of anemia when the mineral iron is discussed. But iron is an important nutrient for all areas of the body, especially the brain and the aerobic muscles; it aids in the production of neurotransmitters in the brain is in the protective covering of nerves and helps carry oxygen in the blood to all parts of the body. Most people can obtain sufficient iron from a healthy diet, especially from beef and other meats. Vegetable sources of iron, such as spinach, are not as well absorbed. If supplements are necessary because of a clear indication of need, such as a blood test that shows a deficiency, a relatively low daily dose such as 10 mg for a month or two may be enough. Higher doses of iron can be irritating to the intestine and very unhealthy for the whole body. If you have a continuous need for iron, something more important may be missing (sometimes riboflavin—vitamin B_2).

Iron is efficiently recycled in the body, with some loss occurring through sweating, or for women, through menstruation. The combination of excess iron loss and decreased intake may produce a serious deficiency.

Choline

Like all essential nutrients, choline is required for most of the body's basic functions, but many people don't get enough from their diet. Choline is critical for proper fat metabolism, is associated with the adrenal glands' regulation of stress, and has anti-inflammatory effects. It also prevents the deposit of fat in the liver, helps transport other nutrients throughout the body, and is important for the brain's production of acetylcholine (a neurotransmitter used throughout the brain, especially for memory). Egg yolks may be the best source of choline in the diet, along with fish.

Asthma is a common condition associated with low levels of choline. Wheezing, coughing from bronchial spasm, and excessive mucous production during exercise and physical activity has been termed "exercise-induced asthma," although the same types of problems occur in those who don't exercise. The body normally dilates the airways to allow for better air passage into and out of the lungs, especially with the onset of increased activity. In those with asthma, the dilation of the airway is followed by excessive narrowing, causing breathing difficulties. Choline can help the nervous system control proper bronchial action. In this situation, a moderate dose of choline may be needed initially: for example, 500 mg several times daily until breathing improves and dietary choline is increased. (In addition, the excess intake of refined carbohydrate can maintain inflammation, which could also contribute to chronic asthma.)

Nutrition for Skin and Hair

The best way to maintain healthy and good-looking skin and hair is proper nutrition. This starts with a great diet, especially balanced fats, adequate protein, good intestinal function, and proper hydration. If your skin or hair is very dry and unhealthy or you have other skin problems, this is usually a sign of reduced health, including the need to improve the diet.

Below are some specific issues pertaining to skin and hair:

For sun protection, a number of nutritional substances from foods can be helpful. These include folic acid, beta-carotene, and lycopene—a variety of vegetables and fruits will provide these. Tocotrienols, from raw nuts and seeds, and a part of the vitamin E complex can help protect the skin directly, and limonene, found in citrus peel, can protect against skin cancer. All the antioxidants (from a variety of vegetables and fruits) can also help with sun exposure since increased free radicals are one harmful effect of too much sun. In addition, fish oil, by mouth, helps protect the skin during sun exposure.

Many skin problems are associated with low or deficient levels of vitamin B_2 (riboflavin).

Pure shea butter is a unique skin-care product made from an African nut extract (similar to a coconut) and has been used for centuries as a beauty product. European studies have shown that shea butter is remarkably active against skin blemishes and irritation. It's also useful as a daily hand, face, or body ointment. As a moisturizer, it is helpful against the damaging effects of the sun and also helps maintain the skin's elasticity.

Pure coconut oil is also great for the skin and is less expensive and more readily available than shea butter. Some people find that extra virgin olive oil also works well on their skin.

The omega-6 fat GLA is perhaps the best remedy for localized skin problems. Breaking open a gel cap of black currant seed oil and rubbing it into the skin is great for dry areas, wrinkles, or even the most stubborn skin problems and is as good if not better than all the expensive skin remedies on the market. It's also good for burns, including sunburn, but only after the skin has been thoroughly cooled. (If you get a sunburn, cool your skin in a cold tub, pool, or shower sufficiently until the pain is significantly reduced, which could take time depending on the severity of the burn.)

Finally, don't put anything on your skin you're not willing to eat! That's because you absorb most ointments, creams, lotions, soaps, and other items commonly used on the skin and scalp. Most especially avoid fragrance, which is listed on the label as such. Use only plain, pure liquid and solid soaps without chemicals—not easy to find when shopping, but these products are available. Some are scented with lemon, peppermint, or other natural oils, which are healthy components.

The most important factor associated with whether you need to take dietary supplements is that you should first focus on obtaining all your nutrients from a healthy diet. Only after you've done the best job with your food intake should a dietary supplement be carefully considered. This may best be accomplished by evaluating your diet so as to provide a more objective view of your nutrient intake and to determine if any nutrients are low. A health care professional may also be of assistance in performing certain tests that may help determine the need for a dietary supplement. Just be wary of all those heavily marketed supplements promising great, unsubstantiated results. There are of dietary supplements that come and go in the industry. To keep up to date on the latest information, see my website: www.philmaffetone.com.

CHAPTER 10

THE SUN AND VITAMIN D
Why You Need Both to Stay Healthy

In his encyclopedic and vastly entertaining book *Chasing the Sun*, British author Richard Cohen served up many interesting facts about our life-giving star. "The sun is 32,000 light years from the center of its galaxy of a hundred billion stars. There are at least a hundred billion galaxies, each harboring a similarly huge number of stars." One prominent ancient Greek astronomer thought the sun was about the size of a shield and that a new one must rise every day. The sun has been busy for 4.6 billion years, ever since an immense hydrogen molecular cloud collapsed. Every second, the amount of mass that is converted into nuclear energy is equivalent to 90,000 million one-megaton hydrogen bombs going off. The sun makes up 99.8 percent of the mass of the solar system. The shining star provides all our food and is Earth's primary source of energy. It has been many civilizations' clock and calendar. The sun is critical to myths, religion, art, literature, music (my favorite is the Beatles's "Here Comes the Sun,") science, and yes, our own health. In another five billion years, the sun will enter a much-larger red giant phase as it continues to lose its mass and will incinerate our planet, boiling away all surface water.

Because five billion years is a long time to wait around and see what happens here on Earth, your concern should be with the present. You should respect the sun because you can't be healthy without its presence. The sun offers us vitamin D for free and is the major source of this important nutrient that has powerful effects throughout the body. Vitamin D allows one to more effectively use calcium, improves the immune system, helps prevents cancer, and is important for brain function. Yet millions of people have insufficient levels of vitamin D, and rickets—a once common condition of brittle bones in children caused by vitamin D deficiency that was very rare—has made a big comeback.

Whenever the topic of the sun comes up, many people think of skin cancer. Not until the past few decades has the incidence of skin cancer become such a common problem. This period also corresponds with the development of sunscreen and other products that attempt to block the sun's rays. William Grant, PhD who has published many papers on this issue, says that sunscreen is overrated and gives a false sense of security. Other research shows the use of sunscreen can actually increase the risk of malignant melanoma (the most common and deadly form) and other skin cancers. Grant and other researchers describe the problem this way: Most sunscreens keep out ultraviolet B waves (UVB) effectively, but do not block longer waves as well—the more dangerous ultraviolet A (UVA). The body

HEALTH SURVEY

Check the items that apply to you:

- Female (childbearing age)
- Child
- Men and women over age fifty
- Work or reside indoors most days
- Moderate to dark skinned (natural or tanned)
- Risk or history of bone problems (osteoporosis, fractures, etc.)
- Reside in northern half of continental United States (above 30–40 degrees north) or in a large city
- Generally avoids sun or uses sunscreen often when outdoors
- Pregnant or nursing
- Poor calcium levels (blood or bone scan)
- Overweight
- Reduced fresh fish (not farm raised) consumption (less than three times/week)

These are indications of an increased need for vitamin D.

obtains vitamin D through UVB, and if one blocks them, sun-stimulated vitamin D production is reduced.

The false sense of security that sunscreen gives many people causes some to stay in the sun longer, exposing the skin to

175

more dangerous UVA and increasing risk of skin cancer. The growing list of research supports the notion that you can prevent a significant number of many types of cancers by spending some time in the sun, without sunscreen. This includes the prevention of skin cancer.

Some studies show a relationship between sunscreen use and cancer prevention while others have not. Unfortunately, sunscreen manufacturers and cosmetic companies spend millions on marketing, convincing people through scare tactics to use their products.

Based on many scientific studies published in the past decade, the currently recommended vitamin D levels are inadequate. The average daily need for vitamin D may be about 4,000 IUs, but the most recent recommendation is still only 600 IU for most people (up to 800 IU for older individuals). Recent studies show that more than half the population has inadequate levels of vitamin D—and some of these studies were done in the sunny states of Florida and Arizona.

In addition to calcium regulation and prevention of cancer, vitamin D can also help reduce pain caused by muscle imbalance and bone problems. Normal vitamin D levels may also prevent getting sunburned.

Sunlight Is Good for Eyes and Brain

Seeing the natural light of the sun helps the brain work better. No, not staring into the sun, but allowing the eyes to be exposed to natural outdoor light—contact lenses, eyeglasses, sunglasses, and windows block the helpful sun rays.

In addition to the healthy affect on your skin, sunlight also provides another positive benefit. The human eye contains photosensitive cells in its retina, with connections directly to the pituitary gland in the brain. Stimulation of these important cells comes from sunlight, in particular, the blue unseen spectrum. A study by Drs. Turner and Mainster of the University of Kansas School of Medicine, published in the *British Journal of Opthamology* in 2008, states that "these photoreceptors play a vital role in human physiology and health." The effects are not only in the brain but also the whole body.

Photosensitive cells in the eye also directly affect the brain's hypothalamus region, which controls our biological clock. This influences our circadian rhythm, not just important for jet lag but also for normal sleep patterns, hormone regulation, increased reaction time, and behavior. Most cells in the body have an important cyclic pattern when working optimally, so potentially, just about any area of the body can falter without adequate sun stimulation. Turner and Mainster state that "ensuing circadian disturbances can have significant physiological and psychological consequences." This also includes "increasing risk of disease" as the authors state and, as numerous other studies show, including cancer, diabetes, and heart disease.

The hypothalamus also regulates the combined actions of the nervous and hormonal systems.

The brain's pineal gland benefits directly from the sun stimulation. The pineal produces melatonin, an important hormone made during dark hours that protects our skin. In addition, melatonin is a powerful antioxidant for bodywide use, is important for proper sleep and intestinal function, and can help prevent depression. (Aspirin, however, reduces melatonin production.)

Among the specific effects of the eye's photosensitive cells are helping you get out of bed each morning. The transition from sleep to waking up requires the effects of the body's adrenal glands, influenced by the brain's hypothalamus and pituitary. Exposure to morning sunlight also helps raise body temperature to normal (after a slight reduction during sleep), and numerous brain activities, including increased alertness and better cognition—helping mood and vitality. These changes are often not experienced in many people until their morning coffee kicks in. Taking a peek outside at the dawn's first sunlight is a habit worth implementing.

Aging reduces the ability to benefit from sun stimulation through the eyes, mostly due to eye-related disease development, especially problems such as retinitis pigmentosa, glaucoma, and cataracts. Chronic inflammation and carbohydrate intolerance are two common problems associated with these and other eye illnesses.

Up to 70 percent of those sixty-five years and older have chronic sleep disturbances, with potentially any of the other health problems mentioned above. Turner and Mainster conclude that "light deficiency, whether due to improper timing, suboptimal spectrum or insufficient intensity, may contribute to medical conditions commonly assumed to be age-related inevitabilities."

Inside lighting may provide some eye stimulation if your lightbulbs are the full-spectrum type. But it won't take the place of a regular habit of getting morning sun into unshielded eyes. This routine is even more important with age.

While vitamin D is called a "vitamin," it's really a unique steroid hormone that, in addition to helping control inflammation and immunity, it triggers the work of several thousand genes in promoting health and fitness.

The key factors associated with not getting sufficient vitamin D include the following:

- Using sunscreen that blocks the vitamin D–producing ultraviolet B (UVB) waves of the sun.
- Wearing protective clothing, especially materials that block UVB waves.
- Avoiding vitamin D–producing sun exposure.
- Darker skin. Even many light-skinned people have accumulated enough sun to darken their skin to the point where it

CHILDREN IN THE SUN

Coralee Thompson, MD, an Arizona-based expert on child development, says that "many children, especially those with brain problems, are deprived of vitamin D and some are outright deficient, which severely affects brain function." Disabled children, for example, also have a very high incidence of osteoporosis due to calcium wasting secondary to low vitamin D levels. (The same scenario can occur in anyone at any age.) A common problem that's not often discussed is the fact that bone loss later in life is significantly related to a lack of sun exposure and vitamin D levels during childhood. And most of the damage that causes skin cancer in adults occurs during childhood.

"Kids need to be in the sun without sunscreen for short periods of time based on individual needs," says Dr. Thompson. "This may be 15 minutes building to 30 minutes a day for the average skin type, but never allow a child to get sunburned." Most clothing allows some sun to get through for vitamin D production. Dr. Thompson cautions that "dietary supplements of vitamin D are not as effective because the oral dose is usually too low, and higher levels of vitamin D are potentially toxic." Interestingly, high amounts of vitamin D obtained from the sun are not toxic.

It's important to balance minimizing overexposure to the sun (avoiding sunburn) with obtaining enough sun exposure to allow for sufficient vitamin D production.

reduces their ability to obtain vitamin D from sun exposure. As a result, they need to be in the sun longer to obtain the same amount of D.

Proper fat metabolism is necessary for vitamin D production, and those with too high and too low body fat may be unable to release stored vitamin D, which is especially important in winter and early spring when sun exposure produces much less vitamin D.

People living at more extreme latitudes, such as northern Europe and Canada and southern Australia and South America, have significantly less sun exposure throughout the year.

Sources of Vitamin D

There are five sources of vitamin D available for everyone. Our primary source comes from the sun, with foods providing small amounts. Fortified foods such as milk and many processed foods are not a good source. Dietary supplements are the most viable option for those requiring more, and artificial light can also be a source of vitamin D for those in colder climates where optimal sun exposure is limited. Let's look more closely at each of these sources.

Testing Your Vitamin D Levels

A simple blood test can be performed to monitor your vitamin D levels. The lowest levels of vitamin D are in early spring, a good time to test yourself. While different labs can vary in their "normal" ranges, blood levels should be between 50–80 ng/mL (or 125–200 nM/L) year-round, with lower levels in this normal range following winter and higher levels within this range in late summer. How much vitamin D you need from all sources to maintain normal levels is individual? This is best monitored through taking additional blood tests every few months, adjusting your sun exposure and dietary supplements as needed until you find the right balance. Tell your health care professional to include vitamin D in your next blood test or get an in-home test kit, which is a very accurate, easy, and relatively inexpensive way to test your vitamin D level. These are available through the Vitamin D Council's website (www.vitamindcouncil.org).

Sunshine

It's especially important to obtain adequate vitamin D from sun exposure during the warmer summer months to build stores of this nutrient for the winter. But without sufficient exposure in the spring that brings vitamin D levels in the body to moderate or high levels, the amount stored for winter may be inadequate and additional sources necessary.

How much sun and for how long depends on each person's individual needs? For many fair-skinned individuals, exposing arms and legs to sunlight for twenty to thirty minutes—more in northern climates and less as you get closer to the equator during high sun (between the hours of 10:00 AM and 3:00 PM) throughout the week without sunscreen may be adequate to start the process of building normal vitamin D levels. In a healthy person, this amount of sun can produce up to 5,000 to 10,000 units of vitamin D each day—which is not excessive. Interestingly, you can't overdose on vitamin D from the sun like you can with all other sources, such as from dietary supplements.

Even an overcast day can provide you with some exposure to sufficient sunlight to obtain smaller amounts of vitamin D. But on a cloudy day in Cleveland or Seattle, you might obtain only about half the amount if you're in the midday sun. The denser the cloud cover, the less vitamin D, and when the air is higher in moisture, such on those humid days, even less.

As your skin tans, longer periods of sun exposure will be needed to build vitamin D stores for the winter months. That's because those with darker skin will require even more sun exposure throughout the year to obtain the same amount of vitamin D. Those in more northern (and extreme southern) climates may need much more. In general, more exposure may be better as long as you avoid the most important sun stress—sunburn. And as your levels of vitamin D rise and normalize, the risk of sunburn diminishes.

FOOD SOURCES

The best vitamin D–containing foods are from animal sources, which are utilized more effectively by the body. These foods include wild salmon, sardines, and tuna, which provide moderate amounts, and egg yolks. Vegetable sources of vitamin D are generally poor and less adequately utilized by the body, with shiitake mushroom being a modest source.

FORTIFIED FOODS

Foods fortified with vitamin D are not a good source for several reasons. First, the levels are very low and quite insignificant when compared to what you get from the sun. Relying on the consumption of vitamin D–fortified foods has clearly failed to prevent abnormal low levels and associated disease in the population. The synthetic fortification of milk is a common example. Most people would need ten or twelve glasses a day—or more—to consume adequate amounts of vitamin D, something most would not and should not consume. And this form is vitamin D_2, which is ergocalciferol, a synthetic form of the type found in plants. In addition, the foods that are vitamin D–fortified are usually unhealthy products, such as refined cereal, margarine, and processed cheese.

DIETARY SUPPLEMENTS

The most effective natural dietary supplement is cod liver oil, which provides a concentrated form of vitamin D. Cod liver oil contains the vitamin D_3 (cholecalciferol) form, which is better utilized by the body than the vitamin D_2 form obtained from plants, a common source in other dietary supplements. Vegetarians who are low in vitamin D and won't take animal sources must rely more on the sun. Many supplements of cod liver oil also contain vitamin A, an important nutrient, but avoid those with daily doses above 5,000 IUs. High levels of vitamin A can also be toxic (causing such problems as liver stress, loss of bone density, and hair loss), and it can interfere with vitamin D metabolism.

In some individuals who have dangerously low blood levels of vitamin D, even modest amounts of supplementation may not correct the problem. This usually requires medical attention, and much higher doses may be necessary to correct this deficiency. In some cases, 50,000 IU a day or more for the first week may be the start of optimal therapy. This should be done under the guidance of a health care professional, with carefully monitored blood tests to avoid toxicity while ensuring vitamin D levels return to normal. These very high doses of vitamin D, both in oral and injectable forms, in amounts of 25,000 to 100,000 units, come with a risk of overdose.

Vitamin D toxicity can cause significant mineral imbalance, especially of calcium and phosphorus, and fatigue, constipation, forgetfulness, nausea, and vomiting.

Tanning or sun beds, "happy lights," and other sources of UVB rays can increase vitamin D levels. These are readily available for home use and in tanning salons. I don't recommend using them as a replacement for sun exposure, but they are helpful for those who may be unable to spend adequate time in the sun. This is especially true in winter months in cold climates and for those who work indoors all day. With adequate sun exposure in warm weather, cod liver oil supplements, and a tanning bed once a week, even athletes in Canada, northern Europe, and other sun-deficient areas, for example, can maintain healthy levels of vitamin D.

Other Nutrients Associated with the Sun and Vitamin D

Magnesium is an important nutrient to help the body regulate vitamin D. This mineral is often low in many individuals. In fact, having done a dietary analysis on almost all patients I've seen over decades of work, magnesium is one of the more common deficiencies. The best food sources are organically grown vegetables and raw nuts and seeds. These foods will also help you obtain other nutrients needed for better utilization of vitamin D; they include zinc and the vitamins A and K. In the case of vitamin A, however, you'll need egg yolks and other animal foods such as fish since plant foods don't contain vitamin A (they contain large amounts of beta-carotene which the human body can convert to vitamin A but not as efficiently as other animals). Most cod liver oil supplements also contain vitamin A.

As scientific and medical research continues, we'll find out more about the nutrients that are necessary for sun protection if one must spend a lot of time outdoors Various naturally occurring antioxidants from foods and omega-3 fats, for example, are used by the body in helping to protect us from the possible harm of overexposure, so these nutrients will be needed in adequate amounts especially in sunny seasons. For a long time it's been known that sun exposure reduces the body's folic acid, another reason to consume ten servings of vegetables and fruits each day, which should provide sufficient folic acid.

One observation I made many years ago is that healthy people don't burn nearly as much or as fast as those who are less healthy. This may be due to a variety of reasons, as a proper diet can protect your skin from overexposure to the sun.

Consider these factors:

- Getting roasted by the sun is associated with an inflammatory reaction; the more inflammation, the more severe the burn. But by maintaining a good balance of fats, especially the inclusion of fish oil, you control inflammation and protect yourself better from a long day in the sun.
- A full spectrum of antioxidants—from beta-carotene and lycopene to the vitamin

E complex (all eight components) and natural vitamin C—found in the diet can also help protect the skin during sun exposure; in particular, these help control free radical reactions in the skin.

- Because a long day in the sun can significantly reduce the body's folic acid levels, consuming sufficient vegetables and fruits will help offset this, potentially restoring healthy skin.

- Those with normal levels of vitamin D may not burn as fast or as badly as those with low levels.

The body has natural protection from overexposure to the sun. The skin's production of melanin is responsible for this tanning process by providing protection against excess ultraviolet light. Even if you're gardening or have an outdoor job, it's normal for the skin to redden during higher amounts of exposure, but by day's end, or the next morning, the skin should be back to normal. This does not constitute sunburn, just a sign of high exposure, which should be tolerated by a healthy body. If in doubt about how much burn you have, use cold water immediately after a long period in the sun, which can dramatically speed the healing of the skin. While a cool shower is helpful, getting into cool water, covering all areas of exposure if possible, is ideal.

Even when you're healthy, certain skin areas will be more vulnerable to overexposure of the sun. These include the ears, nose, lips, and head in many geographical areas. Proper clothing, including a hat that shades these areas, is very important. Even the right-length hair can help, especially for the ears and neck. Products such as zinc oxide can also help in extreme cases where you must be in the sun for prolonged periods. Clothing can also help shade other areas such as shoulders and arms.

Of course, maintaining a moderate tan is still one of the best ways to protect the skin from sun damage.

Sun Protection Factor—SPF

It should be noted that the SPF—sun protection factor—listed on sunscreen products indicates how much longer you can stay in the sun without burning compared to not having sunscreen. If your skin is unprotected and burns after thirty minutes, a product with an SPF of 10 would mean you could stay in the sun ten times as long or five hours. Using that same product a few times during your stay in the sun will not prolong the protection—you would actually need to use a sunscreen with a higher SPF to accomplish this. Sunscreens with an SPF of more than 30 may not offer any additional protection despite the marketing hype.

My advice has always been the same: don't put anything on your skin you're not willing to eat! That's because sunscreen, along with so many things people put on their skin, gets absorbed into the body.

Humans have lived in sunny environments for tens of thousands of years. While it's healthy to spend time outdoors, it's important to not abuse the skin—this can contribute to dry skin, wrinkles, and the greatest concern, skin cancer. Certainly skin damage and the risk of cancer are possible if time spent in the sun is abused, especially at an early age and when one is not healthy. Moderation is key. Spend adequate time in the sun to maintain vitamin D levels, stimulate brain function, and build a healthy body.

CHAPTER 11

MAKE LIFE A MOVEABLE FEAST WITH HEALTHY EATING, SNACKING, AND COOKING

I like to cook. Not super elaborate meals but those that are simple to prepare and are nutritious. Yet I am amazed by the indifference so many people have when it comes to food preparation. They would rather have a microwaved dinner or make a quick trip to a local fast-food joint. This approach does an injustice to the world of pleasure and sensual delight that a good meal can provide. With this chapter, I want to show you how easy it is to take better control of such simple tasks as healthy eating, snacking, shopping, and cooking.

But first, let's start with a brief diet survey. Check the items that apply to you:

- Carbohydrate intolerance
- Eating breakfast increases hunger during the day
- Frequent hunger
- Sleepy after meals
- Skip meals often
- Insomnia
- Irritable, moody, or shaky if meals are delayed

- Crave sweets frequently
- Eat fast food/convenient foods often
- Increased total cholesterol or low HDL
- Increased weight gain
- Increased stress

These are common indications in people who require more frequent, smaller meals throughout the day rather than two or three larger meals.

Snacking Your Way to Health

Specifically, eating more frequently or snacking between major meals can improve your health in many ways. In fact, perhaps no other single dietary habit can make a more positive difference in your health than healthy snacking.

In our society, snacks are generally seen as an unhealthful addition of unwanted calories and fat and something to avoid. This can be quite true if you snack on junk food such as candy bars, snack cakes, chips, and crackers that are full of sugar, refined carbohydrates, and unhealthy fats. But healthy, real-food snacks have many nutritional benefits and can help provide you with a continuous supply of the fuel necessary for daily optimal human performance. Research clearly shows that healthy snacking can help you control blood-sugar levels, improve metabolism, reduce stress and cholesterol, burn more body fat, and increase energy levels.

A healthy snack is just a small meal. So the key to smart snacking is to reduce the amount of food eaten at regular meals and distribute this nutritional wealth throughout the day. Eat five or six smaller meals that add up to the same amount of food that you would normally consume in a typical two- or three-meal-a-day routine. This way, you're not adding more calories. The ideal plan is to start the day with a good balanced breakfast such as a vegetable omelet, a bowl of plain yogurt and fresh fruit, or a healthy smoothie. Skipping breakfast may be one of the worst nutritional bad habits, but even more counterproductive is eating a high-carbohydrate breakfast of cereal or a bagel. This is because a high-glycemic breakfast starts the vicious cycle of high insulin / unstable blood sugar that brings hunger soon afterward and is a hard habit to break.

By not eating breakfast, your body's gas tank is on empty, but you still need fuel to properly get through the morning. After a good night's sleep, the body is stressed from a metabolic standpoint. By not eating, you don't replace the stored energy (glycogen) used up throughout the night. So your body steals it by breaking down muscle for the needed energy. You can even store more body fat once you do start eating food later in the day.

From breakfast on, plan to eat every two to four hours, based on your energy and alertness and the health problems you've had. Those under more stress or with blood sugar problems usually need to eat more frequently—especially initially, when eating every two hours can quickly make significant changes in overall health.

185

An example of a daily meal schedule starts with breakfast, a midmorning snack, lunch, a midafternoon snack, a light dinner, and if necessary a small snack (which can be a healthy dessert) later in the evening.

Nutritious snacks can be almost anything you like, just as long as they are made from real, healthy food. For many people, snacks, like regular meals, should contain protein. Experiment to discover how much food you need and which types work best. Some people may need to eat much larger snacks, but others can get by on minimal amounts like just a small handful of raw almonds. Snacks should be just like any other healthy meal, just smaller, and still supplying adequate nutrition. This might include the following:

- Vegetables and fruits such as an apple or pieces of carrot and celery
- Raw almonds or cashews or combine almond butter with apple slices
- Leftovers from a previous healthy meal
- Plain yogurt and fresh fruit
- Cheese and fruit
- A boiled egg or two
- Healthy smoothie

The benefits of healthy snacking are many. They quickly suppress cravings, especially for sugar and other junk foods, they improve physical and mental energy and can even stimulate fat burning by changing your metabolism. Since snacking stabilizes blood sugar and prompts your body to produce less insulin, you'll store less fat and use more of it to fuel all your daily activities from work to play. Many people find that they have much more energy when following a program of healthy snacking.

Snacking can also help your body counteract the harmful effects of daily stress. In this way you reduce the overproduction of the stress hormone cortisol and insulin. Both prompt your body to store more fat.

Snacking also helps to reduce cholesterol. Studies show that eating more frequently can lower blood cholesterol, specifically LDL, the "bad" cholesterol. In addition, studies show a staggering 30 percent increase in heart disease in those eating three meals or less per day.

Make Your Own Energy Bars

While many people buy so-called energy bars to curb hunger or find an instant pickup, most are little more than overpriced candy bars made with high-fructose corn syrup or plain sugar, synthetic vitamins, and other highly processed ingredients. To save money and eat a real-food snack to promote health, make your own. A favorite snack food is my homemade energy bar. Use it as an in-between meal snack, as a meal when traveling, and even as a healthy dessert. It's a complete meal, low glycemic, with healthy carbohydrates and protein and good fats. Here's the recipe:

Phil's Energy Bar
- 3 cups whole almonds
- ⅔ cup powdered egg white

- 4 tablespoons pure powdered cocoa
- ½ cup unsweetened shredded coconut
- Pinch of sea salt
- ⅓ cup honey
- ⅓ cup hot water
- 1 to 2 tablespoons vanilla

Grind dry ingredients in a Cuisinart or other mixer.

Mix honey, hot water, and vanilla—add to dry mix.

Mix all ingredients well (at this point, you may have to mix it all by hand if your mixer isn't real efficient).

Shape into bars or cookies or press the batter into a dish (about one-inch deep) and cut into squares. Sometimes these are better when allowed to dry.

Adjust the water/honey ratio for less or more sweetness.

Keep refrigerated (they'll still last a week or more out of the refrigerator).

For other flavor options:

Lemon: Use fresh grated lemon peel in place of cocoa.

Coconut: Eliminate cocoa and add 4 additional tablespoons of coconut.

DEADLY DOUGHNUTS—JUST SAY "D'OH!" WHEN YOU FIND OUT WHY

Love the taste of doughnuts like Homer Simpson? If you want to get healthy, you need to take your mind off these unhealthy food hazards. Even though some doughnuts claim to be "cholesterol-free," these crispy, deep-fried treats are filled with bad ingredients that include trans fats, sugar, refined flour, artificial flavors and colors, and many other chemicals with names you can't pronounce.

But there's more danger—the ingredients tell nothing of what really gives doughnuts their unique crispy flavor. Most doughnut makers buy oil that other fast-food operations have already used to fry their products. This secondhand oil often has been used to fry other foods for weeks. The intense heat breaks down the oil and turns some of it to soap. This chemical combination gives doughnuts their special crispy taste and texture, something that fresh oil fails to do. There are many other flour products made with used oil out there as well, so beware.

The main problem is that these oils—including trans fats—adversely affect the delicate balance of fats in your body, producing too many cancer-promoting chemicals. Along the way, inflammation, increased blood pressure, and other problems can be triggered too. Even just one doughnut contains enough of these dangerous fats to remain in the body and trigger unhealthy actions for weeks.

Almond: Eliminate cocoa and add about one tablespoon of pure almond extract.

Tips for Healthy Cooking

How and if you cook your food can be just as important as how you select it since even the healthiest ingredients can be reduced in quality through improper kitchen practices. The biggest problems are overcooking, using too-high heat, and overheating certain types of oils. Following are some guidelines that can help make your work in the kitchen become a work of health.

The worst method for cooking anything is deep-fat or high-heat frying, especially using corn, soy, peanut, grape seed, canola, safflower, and other vegetable oils. While many healthy foods may be lightly sautéed in coconut or olive oil or butter, deep-frying overheats the oil and can be deadly. In addition, the high heat may destroy other nutrients in the food itself. Meats, fish and poultry can be grilled, roasted, or cooked in their own juices with sea salt. Less oil or butter is needed for pan-cooking meats because they often contain sufficient fats. Additionally, most people overcook meats and destroy some of the valuable nutrients. It's also important to not use too-high heat for too long. For instance, when grilling a steak, remember to turn it every minute or so to prevent the excess formation of chemicals called nitrosamines that can be harmful to your health. This goes for vegetables as well—if using high heat, turn them often.

Vegetables can be steamed, stir-fried in olive oil, roasted, baked, or grilled. Cook vegetables minimally to avoid destroying vitamins and phytonutrients—they also taste better when not overcooked. If boiling or steaming, use as little water as possible to avoid leaching of nutrients.

Eggs can be soft- or hard-boiled or cooked sunny-side up, overeasy, poached, or lightly scrambled. Use low heat as too hot a pan produces "tough" or rubbery eggs.

When using oils for cooking, it's important to remember that all oils contain varying ratios of monounsaturated, saturated, and polyunsaturated fats. Monounsaturated and saturated fats are not sensitive to heat, but polyunsaturated oils are very prone to oxidizing when exposed to heat. This oxidation produces free radicals, which are related to many health problems, reduced immune function, inflammation, and increased aging. Butter is one of the safest oils for cooking as it contains a low amount of polyunsaturated fat. Olive oil can also be used for cooking, but its polyunsaturated content is a little higher. Another fat you may consider for cooking is coconut oil. In addition, try lard which, contrary to popular belief, may be a healthier choice for cooking than butter.

Eat Raw Foods

Consuming a significant amount of fresh, raw food is very important for optimal health. You need not be obsessed with raw food, but

188

Rediscovering Lard

You've probably been programmed to believe that the absolute "worst" fat you can consume is lard. Well, that's a commonly held belief, but consider the facts. Many people are surprised to learn that compared to butter, lard contains more heart-healthy monounsaturated fat and less saturated fat and cholesterol. A tablespoon of lowly lard contains almost 6 grams of monounsaturated fat compared to about 3 for butter. Lard weighs in at 5 grams of saturated fat compared to 7 for butter. And lard contains less than half the cholesterol of butter—about 12 mg compared to 3 mg. Lard also contains less heat-sensitive polyunsaturated fat than olive oil—around 1.4 grams compared to 2.

For these reasons, lard may be a better choice for cooking than butter or olive oil. Many chefs prefer it for its flavor and its ability to withstand heat. And it's relatively inexpensive too. However, if you decide to use lard for cooking, it's important to seek out an organic source since toxins often accumulate in the fats of animals that are not organically raised.

One way to keep a good supply of lard is to buy organic bacon, cook it, then drain off the fat—which is lard—in a glass jar for use with cooking. Strain it to remove nonfat particles.

make sure you're getting some at each meal and that the majority of foods on your menu are fresh and raw.

Mention raw foods and most people think of a big salad. But there are so many different ways to add not only raw vegetables and fruits to your diet, but other foods as well. Here are some ideas:

- A garnish for any dish—parsley, large leaves of lettuce, or cabbage under a cooked piece of meat or fish
- A small serving of fruit between appetizer and entrée to "clear the palate"
- Fruits or berries for dessert
- Chopped raw nuts or seeds on top of various foods
- Raw milk cheese and yogurt
- Olive and coconut oils
- Raw honey
- Foods that are slightly cooked on the outside, but raw on the inside: rare or medium rare beef, lamb or fish, and eggs (lightly fried, poached or soft boiled)

The nutritional quality of foods are affected by cooking and by deep-freezing and other common factors associated with food storage. Individual nutrients may be adversely affected by a number of factors that reduce their levels in food. Consider the following:

- Many nutrients are affected by cooking, including vitamins A, C, thiamin (B_1), riboflavin (B_2), pantothenic acid (B_5), pyridoxine (B$_6$), and E as well as biotin, the carotenoids, and folic acid.

- Glutamine, lysine, and threonine are amino acids unstable to heat. The more they are heated, the more is lost.
- During cooking, significant amounts of nutrients may be lost in liquids if these are not consumed.
- Compared to fresh foods, both freezing and canning can reduce nutrients. For example, niacin loss in frozen vegetables may be 25 percent and in canning 50 percent.
- Foods stored for longer periods may lose nutrients, even when they are still "fresh." After forty-eight hours, for example, lettuce may lose 30–40 percent of its vitamin C content.
- Ripened foods generally have higher levels of nutrients. Tomatoes have more vitamin C and beta-carotene when ripe compared to unripe; bananas have more vitamin C when ripe compared to medium ripe.
- Some vitamin E is destroyed by cooking, food processing, and deep-freezing.

Kitchen Tips and Equipment

Preparing food should not only be delicious, but also enjoyable. A problem for many people is they are not familiar with real-food preparation or don't have the right kitchen implements to make the work easy and fun. A well-stocked kitchen contains various hand utensils, electric items, and other gadgets to make interesting dishes:

- A simple spiral vegetable slicer can create long thin spaghettilike pieces of raw zucchini. Top it with a beef-and-tomato sauce for a delicious Italian meal.
- A mandolin slicer makes quick, easy, and very thin slices of ginger, garlic, and any vegetables.
- A simple meat grinder—even those powered by hand—are great for freshly ground beef, pork, lamb, and other meats.
- Others include glass bowls for mixing and storing, wooden cutting boards, high-quality knives, a garlic press, a grater, a citrus peel slicer, and a small hand citrus juicer for use in recipes.

In addition, the two most frequently used appliances in my kitchen are a food processor (I use a Cuisinart, but any good brand will work) and a very good blender (I have a Vita-Mix).

Glass and heavy-duty stainless steel pots and pans provide the cookware. Avoid all aluminum, copper, and nonstick products due to the potential for food contamination. Iron cookware is also good except avoid using high-acid foods in them, including tomato and vinegar as this can leach out too much iron into the food.

Avoid hard, toxic detergents on all your cookware (and everything else) but especially your iron pot and pans. Instead, treat them with coconut or olive oil, or lard, which remains in the pan for days and weeks allowing for better cooking and little sticking of food.

Cleaning cookware should be done with hot water and minimal soap (I use plain organic castile soap) and well rinsed so no soap residue remains. Glass pans are much easier to clean than all other cookware and often require just hot water and a vigorous scrub. Avoid pots, pans, and even utensils with nonstick materials since their chemicals slowly slough off through normal use.

Shopping for Health

An important step you can take for better dietary habits is to properly shop for the food items that will bring about the greatest health. Bad food has less of a chance of getting into your body if it never gets into your grocery cart. With proper planning, you can make sure only healthy items get into your cart and your body.

Begin planning your shopping trip before you leave home. Never shop or make a shopping list when you are hungry because you will tend to buy unhealthy items. Instead, have a healthy snack, make a list, and decide which store or stores offer you the healthiest and best choices. Many cities now have health-food supermarkets, and many of the larger traditional chain groceries now carry higher-quality foods, including organic produce and meats. Just beware of organic junk foods that are all over the stores.

In most grocery stores, you will find that the real-food items and fresh produce are usually stocked along the store's perimeter or the outer aisles while the sodas, cereals, pro-cessed, and packaged goods are found in the interior. While making this outer loop, try to buy as few items in packages as possible. If you do, buy items in packages, always be sure to read the label, and study the list of ingredients and nutritional facts. If the item contains anything that does not promote health, it belongs back on the shelf and not in your cart. In addition, choose organic items when available. Stick to your list. Remembering everything on it will keep you focused and help you avoid such dietary pitfalls as the fresh-baked French bread (full of refined white flour and fake vitamins) that grocers place strategically and aromatically at the ends of store aisles.

Your most important stop along the store perimeter is the produce section. Choose a variety of fresh greens and vegetables, avoiding the starchy potatoes and corn. Once again, look for organic produce, especially if you are buying spinach or celery as these crops are often heavily sprayed and can retain high pesticide residues. Also in the produce section are fresh fruits. Minimize the high-glycemic fruits such as bananas and watermelon and instead choose fiber-rich apples, pears, and grapefruits, and phytonutrient-rich berries.

Next stop is the meat section. Seek out natural or organic grass-fed beef, pork, and lamb; free-range poultry; and wild-caught ocean fish. These more-natural meats can be found in many supermarkets and health-food groceries.

191

The bakery is usually located on the store perimeter—pass it right by. The deli counter may have some items that are wholesome and healthy, but most are not, so keep pushing that cart and move on.

Also on the outer edge of the grocery you will find the dairy section. If you must buy milk, consider goat milk. Cream, butter, plain yogurt, and cheese are items to consider. Look for organic items, since toxins such as pesticides and hormones often bind to the fat in dairy products.

Near the dairy section are the eggs. Most stores now carry organic eggs. They cost a

MILKING YOUR HEALTH

A wise old axiom is "Cow's milk is for calves, human milk is for humans." Unfortunately, most people see the "Got Milk?" ads and ignore professional recommendations. Per capita milk consumption is up, and so are the problems created by it. In many people, milk can cause various types of gastrointestinal stress, skin problems, and lowered immunity to infections and allergies. And worse are the potential for unwanted hormones and chemicals, so especially avoid milk and milk products that are not organic.

Milk allergy is common in adults and children. In most people, milk allergy symptoms are delayed and not obvious until it's eliminated from the diet. These delayed reactions come in many forms: eczema, asthma, constipation, chronic nasal congestion, gastroesophageal reflux, and vague intestinal disturbances. In some people, there is an immediate allergic reaction by the body's immune system, usually to the unhealthy A1 casein protein. Symptoms typically include swelling, itching, hives, abdominal cramping, breathing difficulty, and diarrhea. In a severe reaction, hypotension or shock can result.

Lactose, or milk sugar, poses another potential problem with milk as many people have difficulty digesting this sugar and some cannot digest it at all. Those who have difficulty digesting lactose do not produce enough of an enzyme called lactase, which breaks down the complex lactose into simple sugars. In these people, the lactose ferments in the small intestine, producing gas, bloating, cramps, and diarrhea. Lactose-digestion problems are also associated with more serious problems such as irritable bowel syndrome and symptoms beyond the gut, such as premenstrual syndrome and mental depression.

Many people who have problems with cow milk find that they can tolerate milk from sheep and goats much better. Goat milk is widely available in many grocery stores and is lower in lactose. The fat in both goat and sheep milk is made up of smaller fat globules that are easier to digest. And these milks contain health A2 casein.

little more but are still an inexpensive protein bargain.

If you stick to the perimeter of the store, you'll find that you only rarely need venture up an interior aisle. Usually the only food items you'll need there are extravirgin olive oil, raw unfiltered honey, beans, nuts, nut butters, spices, and sea salt.

Wine, Alcohol, and Your Health

Wine is not only the oldest alcoholic beverage but the oldest medicinal agent in continuous use throughout human history. The use of wine dates back more than six thousand years and is attributed to physicians, scientists, poets, and peasants. Even today, wine and other alcoholic beverages are classified as foods and used daily in most cultures. More healthful benefits have been bestowed upon wine than any other natural substance. For instance, drinking wine with meals can help with relaxation and digestion (unlike water and other liquids, which can interfere with digestion).

There are few known unhealthy effects from moderate amounts of alcohol consumption, with negative consequences seen mostly in those who go beyond moderation. In fact, as we've all heard for a long time, there are many positive health benefits associated with wine consumption—especially red, but white too. Drinking wine and other alcohol in moderation significantly lowers the risk of coronary heart disease. Moderate drinkers have healthier cholesterol ratios as alcohol raises the HDL and lowers LDL. This may be one reason for the lower incidence of heart disease in consumers versus abstainers. Another may be that alcohol increases blood flow to the heart. In addition, alcohol reduces the tendency to form blood clots, a major cause of heart attacks and strokes. Alcohol also lowers the risk of Alzheimer's disease and other types of dementia. Moreover, those who don't drink actually have greater risk for heart disease. Some scientists say that people who have one or two drinks per day may add three to four years of life expectancy as compared to those who don't drink.

Scientists also say that red wine may be a potent cancer inhibitor. Resveratrol, a substance found in red wine grapes (due to the fact that grape skins are used to make red wine, but not white), not only interferes with cancer's development but may also cause precancerous cells to reverse to normal. These actions are probably due to resveratrol's antioxidant and anti-inflammatory properties. (Rely on resveratrol from red wine or red and purple grapes rather than dietary supplements. Other sources include blueberries and strawberries. Use organic sources.)

Most wine contains about 12 percent alcohol. Sweet dessert wines may contain up to 20 percent alcohol. This compares to 40 percent (80 proof) and 50 percent (100 proof) alcohol in distilled products such as vodka and gin. Wine also contains vitamins B_1, B_2, B_6, and niacin, as well as traces of most minerals, including iron. Most red table wine contains iron in the easily usable ferrous form. The pH of wine is low (more acid), like that of the stomach; perhaps one reason wine improves appetite and digestion. Eating natural fats with wine slows the absorption of alcohol and protects the intestine from possible irritation.

Once in the blood, alcohol is broken down in the liver. About 3.5 ounces of pure alcohol can be safely metabolized by the body if spread out over the day. This translates to about a single bottle of wine—much more than the one or two glasses that is considered moderation, and not something I'm recommending. To a European, this may not seem like excess, but to an American it might. In the United States, the average annual per-capita daily consumption of wine is just a few teaspoons while in Italy, it's about a half bottle.

As a group, women are more susceptible to negative effects of alcohol because of their smaller body size and the lesser amount of alcohol dehydrogenase in their stomachs and livers. This enzyme breaks down much of the alcohol—especially in the stomach before it's absorbed.

If you enjoy wine and want the health benefits associated with it, drink only what you enjoy and can tolerate and no more than one or two glasses. The simplest recommendation is a 4-ounce glass or two with meals. For most people a glass of wine will be completely metabolized in about an hour and a half. Some people, however, should never consume alcohol. But a moderate amount for those who can, and want to, is now considered to be 4 to 8 ounces of wine per day.

An obvious side effect of alcohol is that it impairs your senses, so it should be avoided within four hours of driving a vehicle. One drink increases the risk of an accident by 50 percent, two drinks by 100 percent. Also, wine should not be taken with other drugs or by people with certain illnesses—speak with your own physician for details—and is not recommended for pregnant women.

Although wine gives a relaxed feeling, any alcohol can disturb sleep if consumed shortly before bedtime. Studies of biological circadian rhythms in humans show that alcohol is best metabolized between 5:00 PM and 6:00 PM and less effectively later in the evening. If you enjoy wine, be sure to ask your doctor whether it poses any health problems for you.

Caffeine: Coffee, Tea, and Cocoa

Many people use caffeine as a daily drug, as a means of getting more "energy." While its stimulating effect can improve brain function temporarily, it's also addicting. And if you need a drug to give you a pickup, your fat-burning system may not be working very well. Caffeine can also induce adrenal, liver and nervous system stress, and create unstable blood sugar levels. Caffeine is highest in coffee, with smaller amount in many types of tea (and in many colas, but avoid these due to their high sugar content). As with every-

194

thing else, you must determine whether your body can tolerate caffeine. If so, here are some important considerations:

- Buy your coffee beans as freshly roasted as possible; keep enough in your cabinet in a tightly sealed glass container and the rest in the freezer.
- Grind the beans just before you make the coffee.
- The lighter roasts have more caffeine and the darker roasts less. Just as with fruits and vegetables, it's best to choose organic coffee to avoid pesticides and other chemicals.
- Avoid preground coffee as it loses flavor due to the breakdown of its natural oils. (This is one reason people add milk and sugar, and one reason flavored coffee has become popular—to cover the bad overly bitter taste of coffee that's been ground weeks before.)
- Many health benefits have been associated with both green and black tea, including anticancer properties, since they contain a variety of antioxidants and phytonutrients. Once again, organic tea is better than conventional as tea growers may use many pesticides.

Good News for Cocoa Lovers

The evidence is clear that cocoa is a powerful therapeutic food. But not when combined with sugar, bad fats, or other unhealthy ingredients such as milk and chemical additives. This is the case with chocolate candy bars and drinks and most other chocolate products. Only buy pure cocoa—without sugar or dairy—which comes in powder and solid forms, and use it to make your own healthy desserts sweetened with honey.

Including cocoa in the diet may do more than satisfy a craving—it may also help to improve health. Cocoa can help lower blood pressure and improve cardiovascular health. The flavanols found in cocoa (just like in grape skins and tea) can stimulate processing of nitric oxide, a natural chemical that promotes healthy blood flow and blood pressure and cardiovascular health. In addition, flavanol-rich cocoa may work much like aspirin to promote healthy blood flow by preventing blood platelets from sticking together.

Real, unsweetened cocoa typically contains significant protein content of about 7 or 8 grams per ounce. It is also low in carbohydrate—between 8 and 13 grams per ounce, with 50 to 60 percent or more of that carbohydrate coming in the form of fiber. Like other beans, cocoa contains many vitamins and minerals, including folic acid, niacin, zinc, and magnesium. The fats in natural cocoa also have healthy attributes. More than a third of the fat in cocoa is monounsaturated. An equal amount of fat in cocoa is in the form of stearic acid. Though saturated, stearic acid is a good fat, as it can reduce LDL cholesterol. Cocoa also contains the essential fat linoleic acid.

Cocoa has strong antioxidant benefits, which have also been shown specifically to protect against LDL-cholesterol damage. One study showed that when a cocoa snack was substituted for a high-carbohydrate snack, it increased the "good" HDL cholesterol and reduced blood triglycerides. And it did not increase LDL cholesterol despite being a higher-fat snack. Polyphenols in cocoa, similar to those in red wine, provide protection against blood-vessel problems, including heart disease.

Caffeine Content of Some Single-serving Drinks

(Amounts in milligrams of caffeine. Amount varies with how you make it, the particular product, and serving size.)

Regular coffee	85–300
Double espresso	120
Decaf	3–5
Black tea	50–140
Green tea	20–50
Real cocoa	25–50

Most herb teas don't contain caffeine. But some over-the-counter and prescription drugs do in a range of 15 to 300 mgs. The FDA requires products containing caffeine to be listed in the ingredient lists of these medications, as in the case of some stimulants (NoDoz, Vivarin), pain relievers (Excedrin, Midol), and cold remedies (Coryban-D). If unsure, read the ingredients or ask the pharmacist.

Salt of the Sea

If you use this universal ingredient, sea salt can be a flavorful and healthful addition to your food. Sea salt usually tastes better than regular salt and contains other minerals as well. Early humans obtained much of their food from the saltwater ocean, and we still require many of the sea's vital minerals, including sodium.

People have been bombarded with fear regarding salt's sodium content, almost as much as fats. However, like certain fats, sodium is also an essential nutrient. Sodium is necessary for water regulation, the nervous system, muscle activity, adrenal gland function, and many other healthy activities. Most people obtain sodium through a healthy diet, especially from vegetables, with the inclusion of addition salt as spice. There's a very wide range of healthy sodium intake, which varies with each individual.

For those who sweat a lot or perform high levels of exercise, sodium loss can increase dramatically through sweat. Those under excess stress and athletes who are overtrained may have hormone imbalances that can cause too much sodium loss through the urine. These individuals sometimes crave salt and usually need to consume more.

Sodium can increase blood pressure in susceptible individuals. This occurs in about one-third to one-half of those with hypertension (high blood pressure). In these cases, too much sodium can cause edema and/or further elevation of blood pressure. This sensitivity can be discovered through an examination by a health care professional and by avoiding salt and sodium for a week and checking how blood pressure changes. Most patients with high blood pressure can correct the problem when the proper amounts of carbohydrates are determined, especially beginning with the Two-Week Test. This can often reduce or eliminate sodium sensitivity (see chapter 3 for discussion on sodium sensitivity and blood pressure).

Spice Up Your Health

In addition to salt, other spices have been used in food preparation for thousands of years. The right spice, or combinations, can make foods tempting and delicious by boosting the appearance, smell, and taste. Spices also are useful as natural preservatives, and many have powerful therapeutic and health-promoting properties too. In food, spices can prevent the growth of dangerous bacteria and other organisms. And when ingested, they can fight against cancer, heart disease, and other chronic conditions. All these benefits come from the healthy oils, antioxidants, and phytonutrients. Here are some examples:

- Oregano, thyme, and bay leaf can protect against potentially harmful infectious agents such as candida, *E. coli*, salmonella, and staph, and even the potentially deadly Klebsiella pneumoniae.
- Turmeric contains the antioxidant curcumin and, along with rosemary, has powerful anti-inflammatory (and cancer-preventive) properties.
- Ginger also has powerful anti-inflammatory properties and can inhibit the rhinovirus—one of the viruses responsible for the common cold. Hot ginger tea made from fresh ginger and a small amount of honey is one of the best remedies when those around you are getting a cold or you feel it coming on. Ginger's antioxidant properties are at least as effective as those of vitamin C, can be very useful for nausea and motion sickness, and help protect the intestine from ulcers. In addition, ginger may have properties that promote fat burning.
- Capsaicin, found in hot red chili peppers, also has anti-inflammatory properties and can stimulate increased oxygen uptake, which is one reason it may also increase fat-burning capability.
- Wasabi, a hot root used with Japanese foods, also protects against potential food poisoning by bacteria and fungus. It also contains anticancer properties, including powerful antioxidants.
- Parsley and cilantro not only add a visual pleasure to a plate of food but also are full of therapeutic phytonutrients.
- Fenugreek (the seed) contains high levels of flavanoids, which are important antioxidants and has been shown to have cholesterol-lowering capabilities. This spice can also reduce platelet aggregation (important for proper blood flow) and reduce blood sugar in diabetics.

Many other herbs and spices have therapeutic value as well, including cinnamon, allspice, nutmeg, cloves, dill, and basil. These can be found fresh in groceries or can be grown in your garden, window box, or even an inside windowsill. Dried spices can lose not only their flavor but also their therapeutic value over time as many potent substances break down. And since they contain polyunsaturated oils, they can go rancid. Buy spices in small packages and keep them sealed tightly and stored in a cool, dark place.

As you begin finding the right type of foods that best match your dietary needs, eliminating unhealthy ones and adding more fresh vegetables, fruits, and other items, the overall goal of putting it all together is just as important. This means buying the best foods and preparing them in healthy ways—for both meals and snacks. By doing so, not only will your health improve but also the enjoyment and pleasure of healthy eating will be realized.

CHAPTER 12

THE HEALTHIEST DIET
Follow Your Own Nutritional Intuition

When I had my clinic in Upstate New York, I decorated the waiting room walls with posters by Norman Rockwell. The popular artist had painted covers for *The Saturday Evening Post* for many years. They celebrated the warmth and humorous scenes of everyday small-town life in America. One classic cover depicted an enormously overweight baker taking a lunch break in the back room while reading a tiny book entitled *How to Diet*. There were stacks of cakes on the shelf behind where he was sitting. The cook's meal was a small plate of vegetables.

There was a truthful, honest sadness embodied in much of Rockwell's art. Americans could relate to the portly fellow's situation in the diet painting. The desire to lose weight is a shared and universal one. Yet almost all people fail at following the advice found in the pages of diet books. Certainly, some lose weight. But it's short-lived. The weight eventually comes back, often with additional pounds of body fat. The person is then seduced by hearing or reading about yet another new diet book. The vicious cycle can last for decades.

It's no surprise then that diet and weight loss books consistently appear on *The New York Times* bestseller lists. The public is literally starved for the next quick diet fix, that magical way to effortlessly slough off the excess pounds—and have the pounds permanently stay off.

The word "diet" comes from the Greek *díaita*. It refers to a way of living. The first diet book appeared in the mid-1800s, when obese British casket maker William Banting visited an ear, nose, and throat surgeon named Dr. William Harvey who recommended that he needed to change his diet or he'd be the one ending up in one of his coffins. He advocated no starch, sugar, beer, and potatoes. Banting then lost forty-five pounds on a diet of lean meat, fish, vegetables, dry toast, soft-boiled eggs, and a few glasses of wine a day. He eventually wrote a self-published popular booklet called *Letter on Corpulence Addressed to the Public*, which stayed in print until 2007.

Whenever the word "diet" is mentioned, most people immediately think of the latest weight-loss fads. These radically varying regimens have been highly popular for decades. It's a wide spectrum of food choices, ranging from no or low fat, low protein, no meat, low carbs, to high carbs. These diets often come with a celebrity endorsement and are almost always connected with highly processed meal plans dieters are obliged to buy. Everyone is looking for the overnight weight-loss solution. But that's not the best way to bring about positive change with one's own health.

Long before diet books appeared or rather way before man could read or write, 99.9 percent of all humans ate in a similar way. From the Stone Age until the Ice Age ended, up to the time of the agricultural revolution about ten thousand years ago, virtually all humans were lean. This was called the Paleolithic period. Almost none of these people were ever on a diet. Or needed to be. You shouldn't be either.

There are plenty of published studies and commentary about how and what our human ancestors ate throughout their existence. Their physically active lifestyle was made possible by a diet comprised almost exclusively of lots of vegetables and fruits, meat and fish, nuts and seeds. These items provided the right amount of protein and fat and high levels of micronutrients and phytonutrients. There was the occasional honey but no processed sugar or vegetable oils, and virtually no grains.

There's widespread consensus in today's scientific community that we would be better off eating like they did during the Paleolithic period of human history. This would mean a diet that's about 30 percent fat with a balance of omega-6 and omega-3 fatty acids, the need for moderate protein intake, a high intake of vegetables and fruits, and reliance of real food for vitamins, minerals, and phytonutrients. As expected, these ideas have also found their way onto the diet-book bandwagon with catchy names such as the Stone Age diet, the caveman diet, the paleo diet, the hunter-gatherer diet, and evolution diet.

Whatever these diets are called, the foods all humans ate were similar, varying somewhat depending upon the particular period in human history, the geographical location, and seasonal conditions. This is important because it shaped the human genetic makeup—our nutritional needs and daily requirements were formed by this long period of eating almost exclusively vegetables, fruits, meat, fish, nuts, and seeds. The result is that our dietary and nutritional needs are essentially the same today. But what we are eating is different.

"Humans, as a species, have been around for approximately 10,000 generations, and the human genus has been around for more than 100,000 generations. For all but the last 600 generations, our ancestors were hunter-gatherers," Daniel Lieberman, professor of human evolutionary biology at Harvard University, recently wrote in *The New York Times*. "Accordingly, the bodies we inherited are still mostly adapted to a hunter-gatherer way of life, which includes plentiful exercise, and a diet rich in protein and fiber, but low in saturated fat and simple sugars. The bodies we inherited are still mostly adapted to a hunter-gatherer way of life. Today's well-fed children may grow taller than a typical hunter-gatherer, and they have a much lower chance of dying young. But as standards of living rise throughout the world, so do obesity rates and related illnesses that are virtually unknown among hunter-gatherers such as adult-onset diabetes, coronary heart disease and cancer."

Of course, the hunter-gatherers didn't have it easy; life was a constant struggle for survival. Many starved or died from illness or injury. But evolution takes time to manifest

itself. Natural selection needs hundreds of thousands of years to adjust to drastically new dietary habits. Since that has not happened, the effect ultimately has been an explosion of new chronic illness that Lieberman mentioned.

Around thirty thousand or forty thousand years ago, our ancestors left Africa and crossed land bridges into the Middle East. Mesopotamia and the areas around the Mediterranean Sea are where civilization ultimately took shape. Groups of people formed villages. This was also the beginning of agriculture. Instead of gathering wild greens and fruits, humans learned they could cultivate some of them easily. With the Ice Age ending a couple of thousand years earlier, a major climate change affected the region. It was warmer and wetter. The soil was ready for crops to be planted.

One type of food that would be cultivated throughout the region was a wild grass, which produced a seed called barley. In the more northern and eastern areas, the climate was better suited for another type of grass domesticated from wild einkorn and emmet wheat. These forms of barley and wheat were rough, fibrous, and by today's standards, difficult to eat because they were coarse. Yet this harvested food, in particular, would inevitably change the course of human history: one might as well call this the start of the Carbohydrate Age.

The effect of the agricultural revolution meant that there'd be more food for more people, since storing dried grains, lentils, and peas was easier than searching for food during natural periods of scarce supplies. Populations grew. Civilizations rose and fell.

During the much-later Industrial Revolution, starting around the mid 1800s, the mechanized processing of grains began. This eventually brought about the large production of white flour, canned and processed food, and sugary treats. The most significant change in the American diet occurred right after World War II—the automobile, the move to suburbs, the shrinking farm, the increase in supermarkets with huge aisles of packaged food products, and television all played a role in affecting the way people thought about shopping, eating, and exercise. The obesity epidemic of the past several decades is only an accelerated extension of these earlier developments.

To reverse these unhealthy trends, I'm not suggesting that we all become hunters and gatherers living off the land. That's too impractical unless you are living way far off the grid or in remote regions like the sub-Arctic or Amazon rainforest. There is another approach that is equally at home in the modern world.

The Mediterranean Way of Eating

Most people have heard about the "Mediterranean diet." It's usually defined as a menu of the traditional foods that have been consumed for thousands of years in the areas bordering the Mediterranean Sea. This way of eating has been described by modern-day nutrition researchers as "the cultural heritage of all mankind," since this geographical region is where Western civilization began to flourish.

But the Mediterranean diet is often misinterpreted in the media, just as nutrition researchers have created their own food schemes based on it. While a number of weight-loss books and cookbooks now promote the Mediterranean diet, the truth is that it's really not a specific diet. There are no rules, no precise serving sizes, and no special recipes one must religiously follow. Instead, the Mediterranean diet should connote a flexible, lifestyle approach to eating.

"The Mediterranean diet is specific to a certain climate and culture," Walter Willet, chairman of the Department of Nutrition at the Harvard School of Public Health, told *Discover* magazine in 2009. "By paying attention to healthy ingredients rather than specific recipes, anyone can adapt this plan to his own tastes." The end result is better weight management, increased longevity, and improved health with much less chronic illness.

It's also important to dispel the myth that the Mediterranean people avoided eating meat. They ate poultry and lamb, but they didn't shun beef; it just wasn't part of their daily dietary regimen. Cattle didn't even exist there in large numbers and would have been too difficult to domesticate compared to chickens (which also provided eggs), lamb (which also provided wool), and sheep (which also provided milk).

Nor should it be overlooked that the whole grain foods consumed in the Mediterranean region were truly whole grain. Previous to cultivating barley and wheat, grain was all derived from wild grasses. Most people today, especially in the Western world, have never seen or tasted whole grains despite what the label says on most packaged food items. The phrase "whole grain" is primarily a marketing slogan used to persuade consumers into thinking they're eating something healthy when in fact the product is usually highly processed.

As a result of varying climates, lifestyle, and physical environments in the Mediterranean area, different dietary habits evolved in Greece than the foods consumed in, say, Spain. But the people in each of these regions followed a Mediterranean diet. Published descriptions of a distinctive Mediterranean diet first began to appear in the 1950s when health and nutrition researchers began studying eating habits of those living on the Greek island of Crete. These people lived longer and suffered low rates of heart disease and cancer despite having a diet that was high in healthy fat. They ate vegetables and fruits, legumes, cheese, nuts and yogurt, and whole grain barley daily. Each week, eggs, poultry, and fish were consumed, with lesser amounts of other meat. Olive oil was used daily and liberally, and wine was regularly consumed in moderation. In addition, the Cretans led active physical lives.

In 2003, Antonia Trichopoulou and colleagues, from the University of Athens Medical School, published a study that described the essence of the Greek Mediterranean diet. This included vegetables (excluding potatoes), legumes, fruits, nuts, seeds, whole grains, fish, and moderate alcohol consumption. Another study published in the *New England Journal of Medicine* the same year showed that a greater adherence to this traditional Mediterranean diet is associated with a significant reduction in total mortality. The problem is, there never was an actual Mediterranean diet. There are only Mediterranean-type ways of eating—foods consumed by those who live at or near the Mediterranean Sea. Today, there are more than fifteen countries that include those in Europe to the north and west, including Greece, Italy, France, and Spain; Asia and the Middle East to the east, including Turkey, Israel, Lebanon, and Syria; and Africa to the south, including Egypt, Tunisia and Libya.

What is called the Mediterranean diet existed about ten thousand years ago, and from that time it began to gradually change, ultimately in dramatic fashion in recent years, due to the increased cultivation of grains, greater consumption of refined white flour, sugar, and reliance on nonfresh, packaged food products. The traditional daily fare of vegetables, fruits, nuts, and fish began to vanish.

Angelos Vetsis, a computer engineer who lives in Athens, Greece, with his wife and two children, is a subscriber to my website's weekly newsletter. In one e-mail, he wrote me that he and his family eat in the healthy old manner: "But the problem is that under the pressure of the media the majority of Greek people adopted the so-called 'Western lifestyle,' which among other habits means consuming unhealthy and processed foods."

Greece, for example, has one of the highest levels of overweight adolescents aged thirteen to fifteen years in the world, with children in other age-groups following similar trends. The high level of TV viewing, spending time on the Internet, or playing video games has also contributed to the significant reduction in physical activity. Despite hosting the 2004 Olympics, Greece has become a society of sedentary individuals. (Many of the stadiums and arenas built for the games are unused and already falling apart.) This problem has also played a significant role in increasing the numbers of unhealthy overweight and obese people. Nor does it help matters that Greece has one of the highest smoking per capita rates in Europe.

But almost countries all in the Mediterranean region share a similar fate as what's happening in Greece regarding nutritional neglect. Consider this: there are 290 McDonald's in Italy; in Spain, the number is 276. (There are 12,804 McDonald's in the United States.) The modern Mediterranean diet now revolves around fast-food restaurants, packaged sweets, and highly processed sugary snacks.

Making a Change: Create Your Own Diet

Those willing to take the one simple step to break the bad habit of eating poorly will find the traditional healthy Mediterranean diet is easier to adopt than it first appears. As Vetsis wrote to me from Athens, "There are grocery stores in every neighborhood where you can find a great variety of healthy foods—vegetables, legumes, fresh fish and meat, eggs, and of course, olive oil."

In fact, even in the United States, people can adopt healthier eating habits—just like the premodern people of the Mediterranean region. This does not mean going to an Olive Garden Restaurant with its phony old-world Italian decor and then gorging on breadstick appetizers and pasta. Instead, create your own human diet. It's simpler than you think.

The concept of individuality is important, because no one "diet" can work for everyone. And clearly, this book does not recommend a specific diet to follow. Instead, here's how to individualize your own eating plan.

There are simple rules when it comes to eating right. For example, drink adequate amounts of water because even one day of low intake can put stress on many areas of your body. Avoiding processed food is another basic principle, since a small amount of refined white flour or sugar can have a significant adverse effect on your health. Avoiding bad fats is equally critical—a meal with hydrogenated fat can remain in the body and do damage for a couple of months.

Your own health mission should be a life-long process of education and understanding. Unfortunately, the "natural foods" movement has only muddied the waters. Synthetic vitamins, processed and packaged convenience items, and organic junk food is now the norm in so-called health-food supermarkets. For every bad food, it seems like there's a new diet associated with it. While the low-calorie, low-fat, and endless stream of diet plans don't work very well, they're still the most popular. Let's look at some of them and why they're not for you.

Counting Calories

The calorie-counting theory is based on the idea that the calories in the food you eat minus the calories you burn for energy equals the weight you lose or gain. In other words, balancing energy intake and output results in stable weight. If you eat fewer calories than you burn, you lose weight; or if you take in more calories than you use, you gain. The problem with this theory is that it does not work as simply as it seems for most people. This is because everyone has a slightly different metabolism; food is utilized differently, and fat and sugar are burned at different ratios from person to person. For example, some people get 60 percent of energy from fat and 40 percent from sugar, while others are just the opposite. When you hear "burning calories," your question should be, "calories of what—fat or sugar?" In addition to the number of calories consumed, the amount of carbohydrates, fats, and proteins eaten also significantly affects how the body burns

energy. So to use only the total calories as a guide may be misleading.

Calorie counting almost always results in eating less food. When you eat less food, especially less fat, which contains the most calories, one of the significant results can be that your metabolism slows down and you can eventually store more fat, despite your initial (short-term) weight loss. That's why so many people eventually gain more weight and body fat once they leave a calorie-restricted diet. The best way to speed up metabolism is to eat good-quality food every day and be physically active.

Low-fat Diets

One of the most popular and health-damaging diet plans is the low-fat diet. It's built on the fallacy that calorie-dense dietary fat causes the most weight gain. Many people on low-fat diets have a fat phobia. Low-fat diets are popular among calorie counters because they appear on the surface to be an easy way to reduce calories.

There are several problems associated with low-fat diets, many of which are the same as those associated with low-calorie diets. Low-fat diets can slow metabolism and also increase hunger through reduced satiety. People on low-fat diets tend to eat more carbohydrate-rich foods; what they usually do not realize at the time is that 40 percent or more of carbohydrates is directly converted to body fat. With the fat content lowered, many low-fat packaged foods are also higher in sugar to enhance the flavor.

Essential fatty acids are usually deficient in low-fat diets. Women and men who are on or who have been on low-fat diets are especially vulnerable to hormonal imbalances. And finally, contrary to popular belief, low-fat diets do not prevent disease. In fact, some types of fat are associated with prevention of heart disease and cancer.

The Gram Counter

Knowing the weight in grams of each food eaten at a meal can have more practical meaning. Gram counting also includes the popular 40-30-30 diet, which suggests people eat 40 percent of their calories from carbohydrates and 30 percent each from protein and fat. Soon after starting private practice, I used this ratio as a general starting point—not as a specific dietary plan but to help people further determine their individual needs. Fats have 9 calories per gram, and carbohydrates and proteins each have 4 calories per gram. But counting grams, like counting calories, can also turn obsessive. Each time you eat something, you have to think about how much it weighs or you have to look it up in a food table. Most people eventually get tired of doing that and fall off their "diet." There's a better way: follow what makes you feel the best.

A Better Plan

Why strictly adhere to a highly regimented menu plan when you can do what almost every other animal on earth does—eats small amounts often, consumes what its body needs, and stops when it's satisfied?

Unfortunately, none of the popular diet approaches consider how your metabolism responds to your meals. Do these foods make you feel more hunger an hour later? Do you feel sleepy after meals or energized? Pay attention to how your brain and body functions immediately after eating and for the next few hours. These are good indicators of how these foods work for your specific needs. And by taking into consideration many of the other factors discussed in previous chapters, you'll be on your way to knowing what works best for you. What's really happening is that you will be soon developing your own nutritional intuition.

By carefully planning your meals, you'll become much healthier. So let's begin and create a sample day's menu, beginning with the breaking of your all-night fast—the all-important breakfast.

Breakfast

There's no better way to start your day than with a healthy breakfast. This includes real food, including having quality protein. Keeping your carbohydrates to the proper level will help optimize blood sugar, which will give you more physical and mental energy for the day's tasks ahead.

Eggs are the perfect breakfast food. They are easy to prepare—whether poached, scrambled, soft-boiled, fried, hard-boiled, or in an omelet, which can include a serving or two of vegetables. Just sauté some vegetables, drop in some eggs, and cook—sunny-side up, scrambled, overeasy. When you have more time to prepare breakfast, a fancy omelet with a sauce makes for a nice change. Another version of the omelet is quiche, made with vegetables, meat, or fish. Avoid the crust and save time—just butter the dish before adding the quiche mixture. Make one or two ahead of time for another quick breakfast.

I eat eggs every day, and with so many varieties of egg dishes, there's no need to be bored with them. But maybe you still want more variety. Add real ricotta cheese and some fresh fruit on the side.

Lunch

If you eat a good breakfast and a mid-morning snack of, say, fresh fruit and cheese, making it to lunchtime without crawling on your knees from hunger should not be a problem. If you're away from home, packing your own lunch usually makes for a more healthful midday meal. Arrange for that to be done the evening before so it's not another task you need to do in the morning. Plan ahead by cooking extra food at dinner so that you can include some for lunch. Leftovers from a balanced dinner make for an ideal lunch—perhaps a few slices of beef or a chunk of fish with steamed vegetables. Eating more protein and less carbohydrate during lunch will keep you from getting sleepy or losing concentration after lunch.

A large salad is a great foundation of a healthy lunch. Use a variety of different vegetables and dressing made from simple oil and vinegar to more elegant dressings described in appendix A. Make these dressings ahead of time. On different days you can add different proteins: meat, cheese, fish, eggs, or combinations.

If you're going out to a restaurant for lunch, make sure you take enough time so you're not rushed and be careful of what you order. Today, there are more healthy foods, including organic items, to make it easier, but ask about what's used in the kitchen. Don't be afraid to have eggs again as an option; they're a quick meal you can get almost anywhere.

Dinner

If you start the day with a real breakfast, have a good lunch and eat healthy snacks midmorning and afternoon; dinner should be your smallest meal. This is the ideal scenario. Too often, however, people do just the opposite. They skip breakfast, have a skimpy lunch, and then pile on the food in the evening. Your dinner could include items from the refrigerator that you combine for a sampling of tasty leftovers you've accumulated over the past few days. Or once again, eggs can be a great dinner. Or it could be just a small salad and some protein. Either way, dinner should be easy, delicious, and relaxing.

In the appendix, I have listed many healthy recipe ideas. I call them recipe ideas for a reason. I learned to cook by intuition, "throwing ingredients into the pot" rather than by following a recipe right out of the cookbook and precisely measuring each ingredient. I recommend that you do the same—cook by trial and error. It's more fun this way. Over time, you'll make more delicious meals in less time and without the anxiety often associated with sticking to a recipe. I do, however, strongly recommend reading through cookbooks to get more ideas about combining ingredients.

Eating on the Run

The realities of life dictate that you won't always be able to eat the way that's best. When you travel, are late for work, or somehow find you can't get a good meal when you need it, you'll have to find the best alternative. There are some acceptable options. If you're away from home and are having trouble finding good food, consider going to a deli for a chef's salad or just some sliced meats and cheeses. Or go to a diner for some eggs with a side of vegetables. In some restaurants, prepackaged liquid eggs are used for scrambled eggs and omelets, so get them "sunny-side up."

Finding the foods that best match your needs is the goal of improving health. This begins by avoiding processed items,

FOODS FOR CHILDREN

One of the most common dietary questions I have received from people over the years relates to feeding their children. The answer, in principle, is relatively simple. The implementation is not always so easy, mostly due to the marketing of junk foods to children. Let's start at the beginning.

From birth, mother's milk provides everything the baby needs, including water. It's not unusual for a baby to rely exclusively on breast-feeding for all its nutritional needs through six or eight months of age, or longer. I've never seen a situation where the mother was physically unable to breast-feed. If you're a woman expecting a baby and would like more information and support on breast-feeding, contact La Leche League International (http://lalacheleague.org).

The general recommendation is to wait until at least six to eight months of age before introducing outside sources of food for babies (although baby-food companies want parents to think differently). A baby's intestinal tract is not yet developed to process food other than mother's milk, and the immune system could have adverse reactions to foreign foods if they're introduced too early. This could lead to intestinal distress, allergies, and other problems, often for a lifetime. When babies start wanting to experiment with food after six to eight months of age, you can begin trying different foods individually. If you combine more than one food at a time in the beginning and the baby has an adverse reaction, you may not know which food is the culprit. And it's best to give the baby a choice, letting him or her choose from a variety of healthy options.

Babies are born as instinctive geniuses; they know just what they need to be healthy. And when they start eating foods, they can self-select very well, when not influenced by adults or other kids. Studies by Dr. Clara Davis in the 1920s and '30s showed that once children are weaned, they will naturally select the foods their bodies need the most. In Davis's studies, the children developed very different dietary patterns. In the end, the children were psychologically and physically healthier than average.

Practically speaking, most parents are not willing to prepare a smorgasbord for the baby every time he or she wants to eat. But there are some patterns I discuss below that can be followed—mainly that certain foods, like carbohydrates and dairy products, should be postponed until they are more easily tolerated. And always use organic foods.

The best first foods to introduce are vegetables. Letting the baby play with a fresh raw carrot, zucchini, or other raw vegetable (except potatoes since even a small amount of hidden sprout can be toxic) can be a great way to introduce food. Use larger vegetables, or pieces, so the baby can't get it stuck in the mouth. Regardless, you'll want to keep close—infants seem to get any size item into their mouths one way or another. Eventually they'll figure out they can get pieces of the vegetables with their new teeth. Try one vegetable at a time and see which they like, which, if any, they react badly to, and if they really have an interest. Some babies just want to play with food, just as with everything else around them. If they don't seem ready to eat, don't push it. Wait a couple of weeks and introduce some raw vegetables again.

Next, move on to cooked vegetables—peas, squash, carrots, or whatever you're eating. Just mash up the vegetables you cook for yourself and feed them to the baby. Hold off on the butter and salt until several months later. Also keep away from rough or hard-to-digest vegetables like those in the cabbage family, including broccoli, cauliflower, and brussels sprouts. You'll gradually see what your baby likes and dislike, especially when you change diapers.

Once a variety of vegetables are tolerated, start next with fruits. Try a large piece of apple, pear, or peach. Don't forget, the baby's goal is to get it into his or her mouth—whole, of course. Move on to homemade applesauce and try pear and peach sauce too. Avoid using fruit juice; it's too concentrated, and even if you dilute it, you'll increase acidity in the baby's mouth that can have a devastating effect on the teeth, leading to tooth decay later.

Now that the baby is eating fresh vegetables and fruits, you're ready to experiment with cooked eggs. Initially, try the yolk and white separately in case there's a reaction to either. Next up should be organic meats. Buy everything as fresh as possible, avoiding processed meats and canned foods.

Make milk and grains the very last foods you introduce—these produce the most common allergies in children, followed by soy and corn-based products. Why not hold off on these potential problems as long as possible since the baby will get everything he or she needs nutritionally from the other foods? As with adults, milk from goat and sheep is usually better tolerated, with cow milk most stressful. Better yet, by not introducing them at all to milk, your child won't miss out on any nutrition while lowering the risk for allergies, asthma, intestinal dysfunction, and skin problems.

Fermented milk products are usually tolerated very well. These include cheese and yogurt. And cream and butter are mostly fat and have little milk sugar or protein components, making these choices healthy when used minimally. Raw milk fermented products are best.

So much of the food preferences people develop later in life were acquired at an early age from what their parents fed them as babies. Starting off right makes feeding your older, potentially more finicky children much easier. The bottom line is this: if your kids are not eating right, it's usually your fault. In their early years, take the responsibility to buy and prepare all the food they eat. Don't let the processed-food companies and the lure of convenience dictate how your child will eat for the rest of his or her life. The quality of your child's entire life depends on it.

For more information on children and nutrition, read *Healthy Brains, Healthy Children* that I co-authored with Coralee Thompson, MD.

including all refined junk food, and eating like your early ancestors. As important as nutrition is for optimal health and choosing the right foods that provide all the necessary nutrients, physical activity is a vital part of your life as well. This is how you build fitness. In turn, it will further improve your health. How much, how often, and which types of best are the topics of the next section.

Section TWO

Physical Health and Fitness

CHAPTER 13

UNDERSTANDING THE FOUNDATION OF FITNESS
Your Aerobic and Anaerobic Systems

I n this second section of *The Big Book of Health and Fitness*, our attention is now focused on becoming and staying physically active. Eating healthy and regular exercise is a winning combination. A healthy diet will give you more energy for physical activity. Likewise, being fit will encourage you to follow a daily regimen of good nutrition. Too often, I have seen people sacrifice one for another. They are fit but not healthy. Or they might be healthy, but not necessarily fit. Someone who eats healthy but neglects exercise is not being fair to his her body. And someone who works out regularly but fails to eat sensibly is at health risk or won't be able to achieve optimal performance. And then there's the issue of improperly working out, of pushing too hard or overtraining, which can lead to injury and even poor health.

To understand why all these scenarios are quite common, one must take a close look at the body's two energy systems and how they are related. And the best way to look at the important role that fitness plays in being healthy and vice versa is to first understanding these two terms—"aerobic" and "anaerobic." Each has been thrown around like an old pair of running shoes and has been for years. Most people think they know what "aerobic" means, or so they say. When asked, many associate it with breathing, air, or oxygen. Or they confuse it with "cardio" at the gym, where you can also find aerobic dance classes and pool aerobics. (In fact, aerobics is a relatively recent form of exercise. It's not even fifty years old, although humans have been doing it for millions of years. In the late sixties, Dr. Kenneth H. Cooper, an exercise physiologist for the San Antonio Air Force Hospital, Texas, coined the term "aerobics" to describe the system of exercise that he devised to help prevent coronary artery disease. Dr. Cooper originally formulated aerobic exercises specifically for astronauts but soon realized that the same set of exercises such as jogging, running, walking, and biking are useful for the general public as well, especially those suffering from being overweight, who are more likely to develop various heart diseases. He put together all the aspects and methods he founded in his book *Aerobics*, which came out in 1968 and became an immediate national bestseller.)

And what about "anaerobic"? What does this term mean? Being out of breath after short, intense, and hard activity? Sprinting one hundred yards on the track, going full-speed across the length of the pool, doing push-ups until your arms and shoulders ache, or for many, climbing several or sometimes even one flights of stairs?

Once you see the difference between aerobic and anaerobic, this knowledge can help you build better health and fitness. So let's start with a bit of history.

Dutch scientist Anton van Leeuwenhoek was the first to describe the microscopic components of muscle fibers in the middle of the seventeenth century. (He also was the first to observe and describe bacteria.) By the early 1800s, it was clear that two different types of human muscle fibers existed. Through the microscope, one showed a red color and the other white. In humans, muscles are made different than in other animals such as birds. In chickens, for example, whole muscles are either red or white. The red muscles—the "meat"—are found in legs and thighs, while the white make up the breast. In humans, however, most muscles contain both red and white fibers (the exceptions are jaw muscles, which are predominantly anaerobic).

In 1863, French scientist Louis Pasteur coined the words "aerobic" and "anaerobic." He was studying bacteria—and those that live only in the presence of oxygen he called aérobie. "Aerobic" comes from the Greek word *aero*, meaning "air," and *bios*, which refers to life. Some bacteria could not live with oxygen or air, and Pasteur called these anaérobie—anaerobic.

Around the same time in human physiology, the terms "aerobic" and "anaerobic" were used in relation to how the body obtained energy. They referred to two different complex energy transfer processes in cells—one that required oxygen (aerobic) and one that did not (anaerobic). More importantly, the source of energy produced in each muscle fiber was different. The red aerobic fiber used fat as its source of energy. In order to convert fat to energy, this required oxygen—a reason for the large amount of blood vessels in the human body and in these muscle fibers and for the cell components that aided this process, which are called mitochondria. These iron-containing enzymes have a reddish protein called myoglobin.

In the white anaerobic fibers, none of these structures are needed. Energy is quickly generated through a process that uses sugar (glucose) as fuel that does not need oxygen.

As a result of further scientific research, these red and white muscle fibers in humans were also called type I and type II, respectively. The red type I aerobic fibers contract relatively slowly, and these would be called slow twitch. Their slow contraction would enable them to function for long periods—hours and days—without fatigue. This also allows them to support the body's structures, especially the joints, bones, and arches of the feet.

The white type II anaerobic fibers contract two to three times faster, and these were called fast twitch. They provide speed and power. But these attributes come with a price—they fatigue very quickly as their energy lasts only a very short time, a few seconds to about a minute (coincidentally, about as long as you can hold your breath).

In time, it was discovered that there was more than one type II muscle fiber, and these would be considered subdivisions of type II. Some of these fibers are pure fast twitch while others have a combination of both fiber qualities. Today, there are seven different fiber types, and as microscopic techniques improve, more may be discovered. But there are still two main types in humans—aerobic and anaerobic.

The chart below is an overview of the function of each muscle fiber.

Exercise physiologists in particular refer to the aerobic system when discussing the red slow-twitch, fatigue-resistant, fat-burning muscle fibers, and the anaerobic system referring to the white fast-twitch power and speed sugar-burning fibers.

So which system—aerobic or anaerobic—is working in you right now as you're reading these words? The surprising answer is both. It's easy to see that aerobic activity is important all the time—to maintain various functions such as posture and movement, long-term consistent energy, and circulation. But even though we're not sprinting or lifting heavy objects, the anaerobic system is always

> *Aerobic Muscle Fibers*
>
> - Red iron-containing cells and packed with blood vessels
> - Slow-twitch sustains long-term activity
> - Resistant to fatigue
> - Uses (burns) fat for long -term energy
> - Supports the joints, bones, and overall posture and gait
>
> *Anaerobic Muscle Fibers*
>
> - White cells with limited supply of blood vessels
> - Fast-twitch for short-term power and speed
> - Easily fatigued
> - Burns sugar for short-term energy

performing some basic tasks such as burning sugar. In fact, within the complex metabolic pathways of energy production, burning some sugar helps maintain fat burning. In addition, the anaerobic system is always prepared to take action if necessary—humans have a "fight or flight" mechanism waiting to act should the need arise.

The real question is, which system is predominating—which are you relying on? Is your body burning mostly sugar and less fat? If this is so, your anaerobic system is the one turned on more than your aerobic body. While you may not notice this, especially if it's an ongoing problem, but your energy and endurance is not what it should be, you are vulnerable to aches and pains, body fat content is too high, and you're under too much stress as the anaerobic system is connected with our fight-or-flight stress mechanism. In short, your health is compromised.

Instead, you want long-term energy to be free of fatigue, maximum support for your joints and bones, injury-free muscles, good circulation, and increased fat burning to slim down. You want both optimal health and great fitness.

Aerobic versus Anaerobic Exercises

Certain types of exercise will provide benefits that will build the aerobic system long term. I refer to these simply as aerobic workouts, meaning they will provide the stimulus to improve fat burning for more energy, continuous physical support, improved blood flow throughout the brain and body, and reductions in body fat. Easy activities, such as walking, running, biking, swimming, and the many types of aerobics classes can accomplish this if the intensity of these workouts is not too high. Your heart rate is the best indicator—lower heart rate exercise is aerobic while performing the same workout with a higher heart rate would be anaerobic.

This is where the issues get more complicated. In the short term, any activity can help build the aerobic system, even very hard efforts. But continue these kinds of exercise routines for too long and your body will break down from injury, fatigue, and ill health. You'll become a casualty of the fit but unhealthy crowd.

The one important feature that differentiates aerobic exercises from anaerobic type—in addition to lower versus higher heart rate—is time. Just because a workout stimulates the aerobic system to burn more fat doesn't necessarily means you should keep doing it. If maintaining such a workout regularly for, let's say, two or three months, it could suddenly turn on you, reducing aerobic function, lowering fat burning, suppressing the immune system, and causing physical stress with a reduction in aerobic muscle function. Whether it takes two months, two weeks, six months, or a longer time frame, this type of workout program would be an anaerobic one. Anaerobic workouts performed for weeks can temporarily build the aerobic system, but at a cost.

For a workout to be truly aerobic, you should be able to exercise the same way for many weeks and months with continued benefits. And when you're finished each workout, you should feel great—not tired or sore and certainly not ready to collapse on your couch. Nor should you have cravings for sugar or other carbohydrates—your workout should program your body to burn more fat, not sugar. Burning too much sugar during a workout means it's anaerobic, using up stored sugar (glycogen). It can even lower blood sugar. The result is that you crave sweets.

This is a key to differentiating an aerobic exercise program from an anaerobic one. While even a hard weight-lifting session can produce some of these benefits short term, it does not in the long term.

Eventually, even moderately anaerobic workouts soon can reduce fat burning and even lower the number of aerobic fibers your muscles contain. Scientists have demonstrated this fact. They have measured this decline. It's not something based on anecdotal evidence. I have measured it too, in couch potatoes, aerobic dancers, walkers, and professional athletes.

In a laboratory or clinical setting, the process of fat burning can easily be measured with a gas analyzer—a device that assesses the air you breathe. By comparing the amount of oxygen you consume from the air and the carbon dioxide your body expires, one can determine quite accurately the amount of fat and sugar you burn. As exercise improves fat burning long term, it reflects improvements in the aerobic system. Not so with anaerobic exercise.

For most individuals, the best way to determine whether an exercise is truly building your aerobic system is to check your heart rate—this is detailed in the next chapter. For now, know that there are many aerobic workouts you can perform: you could walk, ride a bike, swim, dance, or perform other relatively gentle workouts that don't allow the heart rate to rise too high.

As the heart rate rises too high, it causes your body to switch from being aerobic to anaerobic. So these same workouts can be anaerobic if you do them too fast or too hard. In addition to heart rate, another key aspect of a truly aerobic workout is that when you're done, you should almost feel like you haven't worked out—you should feel great, full of energy and vigor. You should almost feel like you could do it again with ease.

An anaerobic workout, on the other hand, will make you feel fatigued. Sometimes mildly so, other times quite exhausted. This is not

---

Preventing Osteoarthritis: Aerobic Exercise Is Best

Building the aerobic system is best accomplished with easy exercise rather than those that are harder on your body. A recent study presented at the annual meeting of the Radiological Society of North America provides us with another of the many reasons: prevention of osteoarthritis.

Osteoarthritis—OA—is a chronic degenerative joint disorder commonly occurring with aging. It's associated with loss of the cartilage and bone in the knees, hips, ankles, and other joint and is a frequent cause of pain and disability, joint stiffness and loss of range of motion, muscle atrophy, and joint swelling. Muscle imbalance may be one of the primary causes of OA.

Those who are inactive risk reducing their aerobic muscle fibers due to atrophy, which offer the most protection of joints.

The study's lead author Dr. Thomas Link, professor of radiology and chief of musculoskeletal imaging at the University of California, San Francisco, says that risk of OA can be reduced by exercising easy as well as not overdoing it. Link says that middle-aged adults need to be extremely careful—"once cartilage is gone, it's gone forever."

Light or moderate exercise, such as walking and other easy aerobic workouts, can protect against OA while both hard exercise and none at all can accelerate its onset. Those who exercise too hard risk trauma to joints, along with muscles, ligaments, tendons, and bones. The latter problem can separately have adverse effects on joints, contributing to OA.

If you're a runner, it doesn't mean you can't continue—just do it aerobically, avoiding hard workouts. By avoiding strenuous exercise—anaerobic workouts—one can more easily avoid an injury, even a minor one that can initiate a process that ends with painful OA. A knee, hip, or other joint injury significantly predisposes one to OA. In Link's study, "light exercise was associated with more intact collagen structure and lower cartilage water content, which are indicative of healthier cartilage." This also means healthier joints.

---

only unnecessary but also counterproductive if your goal is to build the aerobic system. In fact, too much anaerobic exercise can impair the aerobic system.

In its purest and most original sense, fitness is the ability to perform physical activity. For most of our existence on this planet, humans were extremely active, expending vast amounts of energy just to accomplish the basic tasks that kept them alive, like walking for miles in search of food. Our early ancestors had tremendous endurance based on an aerobic system that was built by their daily tasks of living. Suddenly, in just a short span of a few generations, today's humans have become much less active, and as a consequence, we are much more prone to muscle, joint, and bone dysfunction and disease. Excluding those who are physically active, such as professional athletes, manual laborers and farmworkers, the majority of Americans have poor aerobic systems. And yet of those who do exercise such as marathoners, most get too much of the anaerobic type, which can be stressful, causing injury and recurring illnesses such as upper respiratory infections. And just like with those who don't exercise, many of these "physically fit" individuals also have poorly functioning aerobic systems.

To get your aerobic system working correctly, you must diminish or avoid factors that suppress it and increase the factors that help it. Stress has a negative impact on your aerobic system. The different types of stress and how to control them are discussed in a later chapter. For now it's important just to know that stress of any kind programs your body to burn less fat and more sugar. The more stress, the worse this problem will be. Anaerobic exercise can be another stress that reduces aerobic function.

Dietary or nutritional factors that cause excess stress can especially inhibit aerobic function. The most common of these stresses is eating too much refined carbohydrate foods and products containing sugar. Deficiencies of essential fats or other nutrients can also inhibit aerobic development.

If the aerobic system is impaired, energy needs switch from fat burning toward using more sugar. This is associated with a real deficiency in aerobic function, resulting in a variety of signs and symptoms I call the aerobic deficiency syndrome.

Walking Your Way to Fitness

Nothing is better than walking for overall fitness and health. Of all the types of exercise, walking is the one I recommend the most, and not just for beginners but also for regular exercisers. I've even had professional athletes add walking to their programs.

Walking is the most fail-safe exercise. Scientific studies show that walking burns a higher percentage of fat than any other activity because of its low intensity. Walking activates the small aerobic muscle fibers, which often are not stimulated by higher-intensity aerobic workouts. Walking also helps circulate blood, process lactic acid, and improve lymph drainage (important to the body's waste-removal system).

THE AEROBIC DEFICIENCY SYNDROME—ADS

The ADS is not an epidemic so easily defined that it makes big news each day, like AIDS, cancer, or heart disease, but this problem is destroying the quality of life for many millions of people. It's one of the major reasons for functional illness, leads to common physical problems from aches and pains to debilitating impairments, is a primary cause of the overfat epidemic, and is a significant contributing factor to chronic diseases such as cancer, diabetes, Alzheimer's, and heart disease.

ADS occurs when the aerobic system is not well developed and maintained, and the body only has the anaerobic system to depend upon for energy, movement, and physical support. This becomes a major risk factor for functional illness and disease. It's no different from vitamin C deficiency or being deprived of any other necessity of life. It can cause problems in any area of the body dependent upon the aerobic system, which is most areas. It can affect your body chemistry causing hormonal imbalance; your physical body causing hip, knee, or back problems; or your brain resulting in depression. By now, you know what causes ADS. In general, the two most common causes of ADS are as follows:

- *The underuse of aerobic muscles.* It's the simple rule of "use it or lose it." Only a small percentage of the population is naturally active—their day-to-day work activity is relatively high. And few people perform proper aerobic exercise.
- *The overuse of anaerobic muscles.* Most exercisers overtrain not by volume but by performing too much anaerobic activity, such as weight-lifting, or activities performed at too high an intensity.

Other common causes of ADS include carbohydrate intolerance, low-fat diets, and stress, all of which can significantly impair aerobic function.

The symptoms of ADS are many; the most common ones include the following:

- *Physical fatigue.* The lack of long-term energy can start each morning with difficulty getting out of bed or produce periods of tiredness during the day.
- *Mental fatigue.* This may include poor concentration or lack of creative energy and even feelings of depressions or lack of initiative. Sleepiness while working or driving is also common.

219

- *Brain dysfunction.* From learning problems to cognitive disorders such as Alzheimer's, building a better brain can only happen with sufficient physical activity that develops the aerobic system.
- *Recurrent physical injuries.* Do you know many people who don't have any type of physical complaints? Shoulder and back pain, knee and wrist problems, spinal dysfunction and weak ankles. It's not normal to have any injury at any age, even for people who exercise. When you have an injury, it means something went wrong, typically in the aerobic system whose muscle fibers support joints, other muscles, ligaments, and tendons.
- *Excess storage of fat.* When the aerobic system doesn't work effectively, instead of burning fat, the body stores it. This can occur on the hips, thighs, and belly, and even inside the arteries.
- *Blood sugar stress.* The many symptoms discussed in the chapters on carbohydrate intolerance, including frequent hunger, craving for sweets or caffeine, tiredness after meals, and moodiness, are associated with abnormal alterations in blood sugar. Without adequate fat burning, more reliance on blood sugar causes stress.
- *Hormonal imbalance.* Premenstrual syndrome and menopausal symptoms are common in women with aerobic deficiency. But both men and women can develop hormonal imbalances, including low levels of sex hormones.
- *Poor circulation.* Since so many of the body's blood vessels are found in the aerobic muscle fibers, a lack of aerobic function results in fewer operating blood vessels and diminished blood flow. In those with aerobic deficiency, up to 70 percent of the body's circulation may be inoperative!
- *Reduced immune function.* Much of the body's antioxidant activity occurs in the aerobic muscle fibers—without their activity, the immune system can be impaired leading to frequent infections and illness.
- *Exercise intolerance.* Some people are unable to exercise consistently without getting more fatigued or physically injured. This is usually due to poor function of the body's aerobic muscle fibers.

Many of these signs and symptoms overlap with those of carbohydrate intolerance. That's because they are intricately related to each other—they can each contribute to the other's presence.

In addition to the problems noted above, ADS is associated with an increased production of lactic acid. The body is always making lactic acid, and it's an important chemical product of muscles which is recycled into energy. But the combination of poor aerobic function and an overactive anaerobic system means too much lactic acid. This not only can cause further reductions in aerobic function but also contribute to depression, anxiety, phobias, and even suicidal tendencies. It's been shown that raising lactic acid levels in normal, healthy people can produce these symptoms. This is probably due to the effect of lactic acid on the nervous system. Excess lactic acid can also disturb coordination. It's a cause for concern, especially in those who require a more finely tuned, coordinated body for their work or sport. A high-carbohydrate and low-fat diet can also aggravate high lactic-acid levels as can various nutritional imbalances such as low levels of thiamin (vitamin B).

Other symptoms related to higher lactic acid levels include angina pectoris, seen in patients with certain heart problems. The heart is a muscle, and it's not immune to the damaging effects of lactic acid. High levels of lactic acid create a major stress on the heart and blood vessels and may aggravate existing problems such as high blood pressure and heart disease. This may be one reason for the incidence of heart attacks in people who are running or jogging—a combination of ADS and excess lactic acid. (It should be noted that both aerobic and anaerobic muscles normally produce lactic acid, and when entering the bloodstream lactic acid is converted to lactate.)

Walking is one of the best ways to get started on an exercise program since it's a simple, low-stress workout that is not easily overdone. Walkers generally have little difficulty keeping their heart rates from getting too high, though there are exceptions. If there's a problem with walking, it's that the heart rate won't go high enough once you've developed your fitness. The mechanics of walking results in less gravity stress than you experience in jogging or running, but still enough to give you the important fat-burning benefits and others such as bone-strengthening effects.

We've all heard and read about the many wonderful benefits of exercise. But did you know most studies that demonstrate these great benefits were done using walking? You don't need to make exercise complicated, expensive, or intense. And I'm talking about just an easy walk—not power walking, race walking, or carrying weights. Here are some of the facts about the benefits of easy walking:

- Regular, easy walking increases life expectancy. It also helps older adults maintain their functional independence, an important concern for society. Currently, the average number of nonfunctional years in our elderly population is about twelve. That's a dozen years at the end of a life span of doing nothing: unable to care for yourself, walk, be productive, or just enjoy life.

- Regular, easy physical exercise such as walking can help prevent and manage coronary heart disease, the leading cause of death in the United States, as well as hypertension, diabetes, osteoporosis, and depression. This occurs through improved balance of blood fats, better clotting factors, improved circulation, and the ability to more efficiently regulate blood sugar.
- Regular exercise like walking decreases your risk of developing degenerative disease. The lack of exercise places more people at risk for coronary heart disease than all other risk factors. Aerobic deficiency is an independent risk factor for coronary heart disease, doubling the risk. Inactivity is almost as great a risk for coronary heart disease as cigarette smoking and hypertension.
- Walking is associated with lower rates of illness, injury, and disease, including such problems as colon cancer, stroke, and low-back injury.

Walking Your Way to a Better Brain

In addition to the above benefits, walking may be the best way to improve the brain. Many studies demonstrate this fact. By age fifty, sometimes sooner, many people begin a long decline of normal nervous system function, especially the brain. Aging itself increases your risk of cognitive decline and conditions such as Alzheimer's disease. One of the best ways to prevent the common loss of brain function is with regular walking. Not only can this easy exercise improve the coordination between brain and body to make movements more efficient, including improved balance and gait, but virtually all other parts of the brain benefits too, including those associated with memory, cognition, social function, speech, hearing, behavior, and learning.

Every step you take sends messages from each muscle fiber throughout your body via nerves to your brain. This increases the brain's blood circulation (brining in oxygen and other nutrients), stimulates the growth of new neurons (brain cells), and improves communication between neurons, even making new pathways between the brain and body. The result is that you can build a better brain that takes better care of your body. In fact, walking can significantly increase the size of the brain. Other exercises, such as weight lifting, yoga, and hard workouts, may not accomplish these same incredible benefits.

How long does it take for these changes in the brain to occur? If you're inactive, they begin to happen during your very first walk. In the first few months of regular exercise, researchers have demonstrated the many physical changes that occur in the brain.

All these brain and body benefits can be accomplished with easy aerobic exercise. How easy? The equivalent of a sustained thirty-minute walk, at least four or five times a week. Many Americans are not this active, including children and teens who spend most of their spare time watching TV and playing computer games.

For some people, especially those who have been inactive, overweight, or have chronic illness, even walking may pose overexercise problems. Whether you're twenty-five or sixty-five, if you're beginning an exercise program, or have been inactive for a period of time and now want to start walking, consider using a heart monitor to take the guesswork out of your walk. I've seen too many beginners walking with too high a heart rate. It's often because they're with other people and the instinct to be competitive comes into play. Talking while walking also increases the heart rate, and so does walking up a hill too fast before some level of fitness has been achieved.

The most important thing for a walker to realize is that it's a fat burning and endurance routine. Base your walking on time rather than miles.

Walking is also a useful physical therapy following an injury or a period of low activity. Many people in this situation can begin building their fitness with easy walking.

Sometimes, even walking is difficult due to an injury or some other problem. Try walking in a pool in waist- or chest-high water. Gradually walk in shallower water before trying it on dry land.

As great as walking can be, many people feel uncomfortable about doing it. They somehow feel it's not enough of a workout or it's too easy. It's that no-pain, no-gain feeling

your nervous system has recorded in its memory. It's time to add some new memory.

Walking for the Average Athlete

Surprisingly for many, walking is also valuable to the competitive athlete whose sport may be cycling, running, triathlon, and even tennis or soccer. Walking can be used as part of a warm-up and cooldown. Competitive athletes, when they're in a rush or working out with others, often don't warm up properly. One way to ensure this is done is to walk for twelve to fifteen minutes before each workout. Even if you bike or swim, a walk is a great way to warm up. It turns on your aerobic fat-burning system, increases circulation, and all the other benefits of aerobic function. The same is true for cooling down after your training session—going for an easy walk can help speed recovery. If you make it a habit, you won't feel right missing it.

Walking can also have a cross-training effect on your muscles and nervous system, helping to stimulate muscles you might not normally use in your workout. These are the very small aerobic fibers used during low-intensity activity. Many trained athletes say that initially, their walk routine initially made them a bit sore. That's due to the lack of use of these small muscle fibers, which helps bring more blood and nutrients to the anaerobic fibers.

Former athletes seeking to restore their fitness can benefit from walking; it keeps

TWENTY WALKING TIPS

You can get in admirable shape simply by walking. It can serve as the cornerstone of building an aerobic base for health and fitness. Most people will succeed with walking because it's simple, very inexpensive, and easy. These three exercise aspects resolve the most difficult parts of getting back into shape. Many people will not need or want more than simple walking, but if you do, you can use this base as an essential platform to build more fitness for running, competition, or just higher levels of working out.

Here are some important and simple recommendations:

1. Have a regular routine. People who fit a regular workout into their daily schedule usually stick with it.

2. Work out from or near home rather than driving somewhere. A treadmill at the gym can be intimidating, especially if you're even a bit overweight or out of shape. There are lots of mirrors and sweaty jocks with enlarged muscles. Personal trainers can be okay, but often have their own agenda that may not fit your specific needs.

3. Don't buy special workout attire. Cheap shoes, simple gym shorts, and T-shirts work great.

4. Wear the flattest and most comfortable shoes you can get—these are usually the least expensive. As studies have shown, these won't increase your risk of getting injured.

5. Your workout should be so easy that when you're done, it feels like you haven't done much of anything. The "no pain, no gain" attitude causes injury and is a common reason why people don't remain in a routine. You want to train your body to burn fat. This is accomplished at moderate levels of training intensity, not high levels. A heart monitor serves as a biofeedback device (like a coach), informing you that your level of intensity is too high or low (as indicated by your heart rate). I strongly advise using a heart rate monitor so you don't work out too hard—this topic is addressed in the next chapter.

6. Don't count calories. You want to burn fat, not just calories. Diet (not dieting) and exercise must go together.

7. Keep your walking simple. There's no need to add more stress to your life. There's no special way to walk (some people look like zombies when they walk as a workout). Just walk. Don't exaggerate your gait or carry weights.

8. Work out in a pleasant environment—a park, quiet streets. Don't walk along a busy road.

9. Schedule your workout in the morning if possible, before you start the day. Those who do this generally stay on course. As the day progresses, if you've not done your workout, you keep adding more things to do. Now your workout is in jeopardy because you're too busy. Get it done early in the day, and it's done.

10. Don't eat sweets, refined carbohydrates, or fruit juice before working out. Actually, don't eat sweets at all, but if you eat them before working out, they can reduce fat burning. Sweets can raise the hormone insulin, which could impair metabolism to turn down fat burning, so the calories you burn from your workout (and for some time afterward) are sugar calories not fat calories. This could result in more fat storage.

11. If you drink a small glass of water after waking, there's no need to carry water with you as you can have some immediately upon completion.

12. Make your walking workouts a time of peace and relaxation. That means not chatting on the cell phone or to others around you. It's a time to meditate on your life and dream of getting more fit and healthy (and anything else you want to dream about).

13. Don't work out if you have an elevated temperature, even a half degree. The body raises the temperature when it has to work very hard (to fight an infection, for example). Exercise can interfere with that process. You could stress your immune system even more if you work out when you're getting sick. Your body requires rest at that time.

14. Don't work out in extremes of weather, especially severe cold or heat. Have an alternative when those days arrive: an indoor workout, a mall (better than not working out), or it may be time to buy that treadmill.

15. Don't worry about how far you go. Base your workout on time. Start with twenty minutes, if that feels physically easy. Build from there, as you are consistent, to thirty, then forty-five minutes. No need to exceed an hour unless you love it so much that longer weekend walks are fun.

16. Slowly start your workout with a slower walk to warm-up. After about twelve minutes, maintain a good comfortable pace. End the same way: by slowing down again.

17. Work out at least five or six days a week. Choose your busiest days, such as Monday or Friday, for an off day from exercise. The body needs recovery, and this will help guarantee that.

18. Don't overtrain: Working out with too high a heart rate (which gauges the kind of workout you're having) increases stress hormones and is not unlike other stress reactions. This is an unhealthy condition. Easy, low–heart rate workouts don't trigger stress responses and are examples of healthy fitness.

19. The most difficult part in getting started is making room in one's schedule. Changing habits is always perceived as difficult; it's really just a matter of deciding to do it. Once you do that, the rest is relatively easy.

20. Occasionally, a particular disability might restrict you from doing certain activities (most people complain of things they believe limit them from working out, yet most of these are not valid excuses). Heart conditions, previous surgery, certain medications, and other things may require an adjustment in workout schedule. Ask your doctor if anything could be a problem.

them from being too aggressive early in their training.

Walking While You Play Golf

Walking is also the best way to keep your body limber and prepare yourself for the next golf shot. While many courses actually discourage walking since it slows down play, the use of a golf cart will only generate one mile of actual walking for 18 holes, but walking the same course is equivalent to going five miles on foot. Nor does walking negatively affect performance, as it once was thought; some studies have shown those who ride and those who walk shoot the same scores. The benefits of walking are obvious: you burn calories, it's a mild aerobic exercise, it keeps the blood better circulated as well as keeping the muscles and joints loose.

The Anaerobic Epidemic

Many people rely on the body's anaerobic system trying to keep up with the fast pace of a stressful life, often leaving the aerobic system behind. Anaerobic muscle fibers provide us with the power and speed we sometimes need in the course of the day. When we see great athletes on TV or in ads, it's often their anaerobic qualities that we find so impressive—speed, power, and bulging muscles. The problem is that many people seek out this type of body at the expense of their aerobic systems, and therefore their health. Ideally, a program direct at both health and fitness would begin by developing the aerobic system first and then carefully improving anaerobic function as necessary and if desired.

226

HEALTHY HIKING

Hiking is something I've enjoyed since I was a child. Growing up in the country, I learned the joy of going out my back door and wandering alone through the wooded mountains of New York State. I never strayed too far from home; but as I got older, longer and more rugged treks would follow. Once I had a driver's license, I began to explore trails in state and national parks throughout the northeast—Maine's Cadillac Mountain, the White Mountains of New Hampshire, and of course, the Appalachian trail. Many years later, after hiking up Colorado's Tenmile Range Peak 10 Summit (13,615 feet), I was so in awe at the top that I stayed too long, not realizing that coming down would be longer and more difficult than the ascent. Tom Petty's hit song "Learning to Fly" was just released and remained in my mind, helping me down the rocky trail after dark.

Of all the sports I've participated in, from running, biking, triathlon, and even golf, hiking still remains my favorite. If the weather is cooperating, I try and go for a short hike almost every day. I am lucky that I don't have to go far to reach the trails since I live in southern Arizona and the Santa Catalina mountains are literally right outside my backyard.

Hiking and walking are really one and the same. Though hiking usually means going longer or venturing out in the backcountry—and away from civilization. Because of this, there are a few things to remember to make these hikes—whether for two hours or two days—more enjoyable.

One of the keys to successful hiking is building a great aerobic base. This teaches your body to burn fat as an energy source. With more aerobic muscle function, other optimal training benefits follow, including the ability to walk farther, hike faster when you want with reduced physical wear and tear, and more rapid recovery. It's also the best way to avoid getting tired or bonking. These are just some of the endurance benefits the aerobic system provides.

Optimal aerobic fitness and health also means more capability to carry heavy loads up steep slopes for long periods, better adaptation to higher altitudes, maintain alertness and good judgment after extended periods of exertion, and better acclimate to the extremes of cold or heat. Of course, training in these same environments for shorter periods of time will certainly help your body function better in preparation for longer treks.

Strength and power can also be developed through your training and is best done following the building of a great aerobic system. For most people, I don't believe that strengthening individual muscles, such as by lifting weights, is a necessity. You can adequately train your body during shorter hikes on hilly terrain; you'll more than likely build sufficient muscle function for longer, tougher treks. However, if you don't train your body by regularly hiking steep trails, you won't be able to easily accomplish these tasks during longer trips. In this case, weight lifting may have a place in training, although it won't be as effective as training your muscles by hiking shorter versions of the same terrain. And this anaerobic activity is best done following a proper aerobic development, which could take two, four, or more months depending on your particular needs. In three to four weeks of weight lifting, you'll obtain significant improvement of muscle function.

Nourishment is an important consideration during hikes. This includes foods consumed during a hike and your regular diet. While hikes of two or three hours may not require any food if you burn sufficient body fat, longer treks will require packing food. During a longer trek, healthy dense foods rather than refined carbohydrates will provide for your long-term needs if your aerobic system is working well.

Whether you're climbing the high Colorado peaks or hiking through parts of the Grand Canyon, your body works best by using its internal energy sources rather than rely on external sources. In other words, by burning more body fat as a major energy source, you can hike longer. While humans use a combination of both fat and sugar (carbohydrate) for energy all the time, training your body to use much higher amounts of stored fat offers many more times the energy than sugar. Fat is our endurance energy, and sugar is for short-term power. In fact, a well-conditioned endurance hiker would need much less food during a daylong trek because, even in a lean body, he or she has significant fat available for energy—enough for long-distance hiking over rough terrain.   This is what training is all about—increasing fat burning is accomplished through relatively easy aerobic exercise. This includes such activities as walking, running, and biking—regular hikes will easily accomplish this task. Lower heart rate training will increase your capability to burn more body fat, but higher levels of intensity can reduce fat-burning and increase sugar-burning. In addition to having more endurance energy, this will also help you reduce body fat and lose weight.

Your day-to-day diet when not hiking is also an important part of this equation. Consumption of refined carbohydrates, such as pasta, bread, sugar-containing foods, sports drinks, so-called energy bars, and other low-quality high-glycemic items, can significantly detrain your body by reducing its ability to burn fat—even if your training seems satisfactory.

Both diet and training can provide you with a great aerobic system that can generate high amounts of energy from body fat. The end result is that you can perform more activity with the same or lower levels of intensity, as measured by heart rate. In other words, walking up steep slopes with a pack becomes much easier and faster without fatigue. This is because your slow-twitch aerobic muscles use fat for energy, so their physical ability improves while having almost unlimited energy. Additionally, your food needs during a hike is reduced.

Relying less on food during a hike is important because eating a meal can reduce blood flow to the muscles (much of your circulation is diverted to the intestines for digestion); eating while walking can also impair digestion (and therefore absorption of sugar, fats, and other nutrients). And all the food you must carry means more weight to haul.

With a good aerobic system, whether you perform a short hike, twelve-hour slog, or a multiday trek, you should not require any special food or sports drink other than your regular meals and snacks, plus water. And those you normally consume should be the same nutrient-rich, easily digestible food items you regularly consume—introducing new foods or ones your body is less accustomed to can sometimes cause gut disturbances such as indigestion, gas, diarrhea, or constipation. For most people, effective foods to carry during a long hike might include natural carbohydrates, such as fresh fruits, protein items like hard-boiled eggs and unprocessed meat and cheese (if consumed relatively soon depending on temperature), and other foods high in fats that include raw almonds and cashews.

Whether a longer or shorter trek, you can also make your own trail ration: My Phil's bar recipe—see pages 186-187—has been used by endurance athletes for decades; it provides everything you'll need nutritionally (except water), is very easy to digest, will last a week or more unrefrigerated, and it's delicious. These would be a great addition on any trek lasting more than two or three hours, especially over several days or a week or two.

Companies that manufacture specialty sports drinks and energy bars make wild and false claims about energy and hydration. However, fruit juice, such as apple or grape (avoid citrus), or honey works just as well, if not better, considering that many sports products have to be digested. Fresh fruit, such as apples, pears, and nectarines, along with fruit juice, and honey do not require digestion, so their sugars are more available for energy and don't produce the typical indigestion from bloating (gas) that other carbohydrate products create. In addition, most of these highly processed food items contain unhealthy ingredients.

The concentration or strength of the carbohydrate solution refers to the amount of sugar and water in the drink. This can influence how your intestines handle the drink, which then affects how well you absorb the sugars. Homemade liquid carbohydrate drinks are best because they are simple to make, are made from natural foods, don't contain unwanted or unhealthy ingredients (some are not listed on the label), and you can adjust the amount of water and carbohydrate to your particular needs.

For most hikes, a 6 to 8 percent carbohydrate solution is ideal for most people. A simple drink can be made by adding six to eight grams of carbohydrate (approximately one heaping teaspoon), such as honey, to 180 ml (six ounces) of water. Another option is to use store-bought juice, most of which is 6 to 8 percent carbohydrate, but not the concentrated versions, which are much more condensed and require dilution.

The 6 to 8 percent concentration will not remain in your stomach for too long but will empty into the small intestines at a similar rate as water. Liquids that are concentrated with more than 8 percent carbohydrate can remain in the stomach longer, not allowing the stomach to empty as fast and delaying the absorption of sugar, and cause stomach distress.

Hiking Shoes

Walking long distances, hiking uneven trails, jumping from rock to rock, maneuvering through tall grass or down slippery slopes all requires one important function—being light on your feet. This means maintaining quickness to prevent falls, sensing the ground's ever-changing terrain for stability and being prepared for a last-moment shift in your body's weight to avoid a loose rock or rattler. (I occasionally see them here in Arizona and give them a wide berth on the trail.) In order to accomplish these physical tasks, your feet and brain must be in constant communication. The right shoes will allow this important activity.

Thick soled, oversupported shoes, including most hiking or trail running shoes, can impair your walking performance. In particular, "high-top" type hiking shoes can weaken your ankles. This can occur because the shoe's support around the ankle, like other physical wraps, braces, and supports, can eventually weaken muscles, ultimately causing you to lose stability in the ankle.

While there are many people who hike barefoot—after all, shoes have been around for only the last ten thousand years while man has been around for several million years—and even barefoot hiking clubs, it's not necessary to be completely unshod to maintain good agility and keep your feet stable. Although spending some time being barefoot, even for only fifteen minutes a day, helps strengthen foot and ankle muscles and improve sensation of the ground and communication with the brain, lighter, simpler, and thinner shoes are best for most people.

The minimalist and barefoot running shoe movement has provided a good way to find shoes that work well for most hikers. These are shoes that offer thinner, more flexible soles, and without an oversized heel that can affect one's natural gait.

I hike in perfectly flat, unsupported shoes. I wear a lace-up Puma running shoe that's leather with a sole that's about a quarter-inch thick from heel to toe. A lace-up style helps assure it's snug enough on your foot each time you put it on without excess movement during hiking. Even if I'm climbing some big boulders in tight spots off the trail, these shoes are perfect. The feel of each crevice in my feet helps with maneuverability.

Thick shoes reduce the brain's ability to properly sense the ground and, therefore, the body's ability to most effectively change movements to match varying terrain. This can increase the risk of slipping and falling. And they can slow you down. In addition, on long hikes, the added weight of thick, oversupported shoes require more oxygen—not a significant factor until you're out there for a couple of days. Most importantly, a great hiking shoe should be perfectly comfortable. Not just on the trails but also on walking around while shopping or going for a walk on paved streets. The topic of feet and shoes, and how to find the best fit, is discussed in chapters 16-18.

For those looking for information on how to get into great hiking shape and related nutritional needs, everything in *The Big Book of Endurance Training and Racing* (Skyhorse 2010) can be applied to hiking and mountaineering.

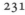

In order for anyone to be both healthy and fit, anaerobic function must be balanced with the aerobic system. Unfortunately, many who exercise focus almost all their attention on their anaerobic systems even at the risk of losing aerobic function. Home gyms, spinning classes, muscle-pumping equipment at the local health club, and the latest fitness rage called CrossFit lure the public into thinking bigger is better. "Go hard, go fast, work those muscles to exhaustion!" This "no pain, no gain" mind-set is injurious to one's health and is a poor way to become fit.

Here's briefly why: The anaerobic system includes the white fast-twitch muscle fibers, along with the related mechanisms used during high-stress activity—speed and power. This includes increased sugar-burning while reducing fat burning; it also adds stress not only to the workout but afterward as well. This throws the body out of whack; it creates a metabolic imbalance.

Interestingly, the same type of imbalance can also occur in someone who is physically inactive. The out-of-shape person must rely on one of the energy systems, but because aerobic function is not turned on, the anaerobic one becomes active with the result of too little aerobic and too much anaerobic function. This imbalance then becomes an additional stress, maintaining a viscous cycle.

Excess anaerobic activity, through some combination of over- or underexercise, work stress or diet, inhibits the aerobic system through several mechanisms:

- Increased anaerobic function can change your muscle fibers, resulting in more anaerobic fibers and fewer aerobic ones.
- Increased anaerobic function produces more lactic acid, which can inhibit the enzymes necessary for the aerobic fibers to function properly.
- Too much anaerobic function can increase stress hormones, reducing fat burning and aerobic function.

It's possible to improve aerobic and anaerobic function, with the result of high levels of both. But the first step must be improving your aerobic system. Since the human body is made up of mostly aerobic muscle fibers, most of your physical activity should be aerobic. There is also a lifestyle factor to consider: for many people, from the time they get up in the morning until they finally drop back into bed at night, they are rushing, hurrying, and continuously under stress. Aerobic exercise, along with good nutrition, can correct common anaerobic system excesses, allowing you to build better health.

An important case history of one of my patients exemplifies the importance of aerobic and anaerobic balance. Gary, a high-level executive in a stressful corporate job, started exercising at his company's gym. At age forty, he felt the need to feel younger, lose the excess fat he was gaining around his waist, and get more energy. At first he felt great. He lifted weights three or four times a week, jogged on the treadmill each day, and played squash once or twice a week. But after three months his shoulder began hurting. Then his knee started aching, and he felt much more tired during the day, unable to concentrate on his work. The company doctor said his examination did not reveal any problems. That's when Gary made an appointment to visit my clinic.

My examination found Gary to be in a state of aerobic deficiency, in part due to every workout being anaerobic. I switched him over to an easy aerobic program of the same training duration, with walking, easy stationary cycling, and swimming; I also told him to avoid all anaerobic exercises. Within three weeks, Gary was much more energetic, and his shoulder and knee problems were gone. After three months of building up his aerobic system, Gary was ready to add weights back to his workout routine and start playing squash again.

Gary had to do two things to improve his fitness and health. First, he had to temporarily stop all anaerobic exercise. By doing this, a significant inhibiting stress was taken off the aerobic system. Second, he had to develop his aerobic system. In Gary's case, it took three months to build his aerobic system to a level that was balanced with his anaerobic system. Only then could he return to anaerobic workouts.

While Gary took three months to build his aerobic system, others may need twice that time frame. Still others are best only performing aerobic exercise for longer periods as they are unable to tolerate even small amounts of anaerobic work.

Anaerobic Exercise and Body-wasting Disease

Some people obtain important benefits from lifting weights or performing other hard anaerobic exercise when performed in balance with aerobic function. However, for most people, ongoing anaerobic exercise creates a physiological state similar to cancer, HIV, or other body-wasting diseases. Studies show that the biochemical changes seen in chronic disease states are similarly found in people who perform anaerobic exercise in as little as three times a week for one hour over a four- to eight-week period. The problems include low amino acids (such as glutamine and cysteine), low T-cell counts (from reduced immune function), and sometimes the loss of lean body tissue (muscle). Even in those who lost weight, it was found that most of what was lost was muscle, not fat. These same problems were not observed in aerobic exercisers.

Another problem common to both anaerobic training and chronic disease is oxidative stress. Normally, there's a significant production of oxygen free radicals produced during anaerobic workouts, which can cause damage to virtually all bodily systems. These dangerous free radicals are controlled by healthy aerobic muscle fibers. This also significantly increases the need for antioxidants, various vitamins, minerals, and phytonutrients discussed in section 1. These are nutrients most people don't get enough of.

Simple "Natural" Strength Training for Bones and Muscles

Outdoor activities such as lifting logs, chopping wood, and building stone walls are a natural way to improve muscle and bone strength, but it must be done in a healthy way. In a similar way, it's one way our ancestors built health and fitness. Unfortunately, the muscle-building trend over the past thirty years has created too many injuries—another example of sacrificing fitness for health. The goal of most of these gym workouts that use free weights, machines, and other devices is to create strength. Instead, the result has been big muscles.

Muscle size is not necessarily related to strength. Bodybuilders who develop huge muscles are not nearly as strong as Olympic weight lifters who don't have nearly as large a muscle mass but are much stronger.

When a muscle is regularly used to lift heavier weight, the nervous system responds by stimulating more fibers, with the result of more strength. Eventually, the muscle itself increases in size, particularly in men. However, both men and women have similar responses to strength training—the *percentage* of increase in muscle mass is similar between the genders. But women don't have nearly the same increase in muscle size. This is due in great part to higher testosterone levels in men which also provided them with more muscle mass to start with, making it easier to further increase it during training.

Overall, there are two general categories of exercise training—strength and endurance:

- Strength training is associated with shorter-duration, more intense workouts usually associated with increased power from both neurological affects that incorporate more muscle fibers, and ultimately larger muscles.
- Endurance workouts are longer with lower intensity resulting in more fat burning capability, and little increases in muscles.
- *Improper* training of any type can contribute to injuries and ill health, and impair endurance.

Like endurance, there are many different philosophies and styles of strength training. But generally, there are two forms—natural and artificial. Natural strength development includes physically working outdoors. In the process of building full body strength, these activities are comprised of two important movements: picking up something heavy and carrying it. Raising an object like a small log above your waist or onto your shoulder relies on muscle contractions throughout the body.

Strength workouts in the gym, whether using free weights or the many available machines, are examples of artificial workouts. Each apparatus, for example, trains a particular muscle or muscle group—such as the pecs, quads, hamstrings, or abdominals. In nature, you would not regularly isolate

NO PAIN, NO GAIN—NO BRAIN!

The media, social myth, and competitive peer pressure associated with "no pain, no gain"—an attitude that more is better regarding more speed, more distance, more weights, more intensity, and so forth—poses both health and fitness problems. Because when you're fully engaged in this approach, you override your brain's common sense—its instincts and intuition—to slow down or take it easier during exercise. Under the faulty pain principle, your body is being forced in the anaerobic zone rather than aerobic zone. This is a problem because it further increases the risk of the aerobic deficiency syndrome adding to injuries and ill health and contributes to the high dropout rate seen in people starting and maintaining a good exercise program.

So when someone tells you to push through the pain, ignore the ill-advised recommendation. The last thing you want to do is not listen to your body and override the brain's better judgment. "No pain, no gain!" is a misguided emotional reaction to being fit and competitive; it's based on sports marketing and media hype. And it's irrational.

One group is most vulnerable to the fallout of the "no pain, no gain" philosophy. It's athletes, and all ages. In fact, this audience is particularly targeted by sports equipment companies, the media, books, and companies that market energy bars and sports drinks. It begins in grade school. Teaching children "no pain, no gain" is an insult on their brain and body. Many of these excessive damaging workouts are encouraged by parents, teachers, and coaches.

Learning bad habits at this age carries poor exercise ethics into adulthood—and sometimes they are turned off to exercise for life. In addition, children and teens have rapidly developing bodies and brains, both of which are more easily damaged by overzealous workouts.

a muscle or muscle group for any length of time. But one could incorporate a natural style program in a gym or home program.

A key factor that differentiates natural from artificial is fatigue. When performing most weight programs, muscles are isolated and worked to the point of fatigue. This is usually not the case with natural outdoor activity, although many people find ways to overstress their bodies.

The Fatigue Factor

Fatigue is often glorified because it's part of the "no pain no gain" image so prevalent in the exercise world. But it defies what most people are attempting to accomplish in a strength training program. This includes better health, stronger muscles and bones, and not impairing endurance and fat burning.

Fatigue diminishes muscle strength by reducing the number of muscle fibers used in an action. It also adversely affects the nervous system, and results in slowing down the action of the muscle—fast actions are less possible, which reduces power. Fatigue also makes one much more vulnerable to injury. Consider these other important factors:

- Fatigue can increase stress hormones and interfere with the fat-burning aerobic system. Natural strength training, where you avoid fatigue, does not create this problem.
- Fatigue can cause muscle weakness. A muscle that's fatigued won't contract as many fibers. You want to train your nervous system to contract larger numbers of muscle fibers to develop higher levels of strength.
- A fatigued muscle will require significantly more recovery time. Traditional weight lifting programs suggest forty-eight hours of recovery before working out again. But natural strength training can be done safely every day (although this is not always necessary).
- Because lifting to fatigue is part of the process whereby muscles get much larger (hypertrophy), the potential for muscle imbalance is high. This is caused by over-

training certain muscles with the result of too much bulk in one particular area (such as the biceps) and not enough in another (such as the triceps). This risk is reduced or eliminated with natural strength training.

- Even when performing what I call truly aerobic exercise—that which is associated with increasingly higher levels of fat burning—fatigue should not be a factor. If done correctly, most workouts should end with a feeling that you have sufficient energy to perform the same workout again. This applies to beginners and professional endurance athletes alike.
- Muscle fatigue can result in poor posture and gait irregularity for many hours following a workout. This is often the first stage of injury—ask a fatigued muscle to continue working and the risk for neuromuscular imbalance, or damage to a related joint, ligament, or tendon increases.
- By not training to fatigue, you'll still achieve the health and fitness results you're looking for—strong bones and muscles.

This is not to say your muscles won't get a bit tired and fatigued when working out naturally—but it's important to avoid significant fatigue. This results in pain and soreness by the next day. Even when moving large stones, chopping wood and other outdoor activities that build full body muscle strength, the same general rule applies.

Many patients used to come to my clinic with problems and complaints about sore, fatigued muscles. Typically, it was a runner with low muscle mass who pushed through every hard run with the result of a stress fracture in the foot or shin, or a triathlete who overtrained with the addition of weight lifting to an already busy schedule. In other cases, it was an inactive person who sustained an overuse injury. John was one of these former patients. With a desk job and no exercise during the past twelve years, John's activity was restricted to walking from home to car, car to office, then back again at the end of the day. One Saturday morning he decided to clean out the garage, which was full of heavy items from power tools, lawn mowers, and inactive exercise equipment, to an old washing machine and cement blocks. After a couple of hours he felt fatigue and muscle aches, and by early afternoon, he was experiencing shoulder and low back pain. By the end of the day, John's forty-five-year-old body was hurting all over. Sunday morning, he could hardly get out of bed and remained on the couch all day. Monday afternoon, his wife and older son helped him into my office.

While John recovered with a couple of treatments using biofeedback to correct muscle imbalance, his story is common in both inactive people and athletes in training. Whether it's too much too soon or the addition of more training into an already full schedule, fatigue is often an indication that you have gone past the point of safety. John's lesson is one even highly trained endurance athletes, and those lifting weights, can follow: avoid working to fatigue. You'll build more strength, get less bulky, recover quicker,

and the risk of injury and overtraining will be greatly reduced. This also translates to increased competitive performance.

Two other factors associated with fatigue are important to note here:

- Rest. Even when your workout is just right, rest is key for recovery, and an essential part of the process. My training equation is an important consideration for everyone: Training = workout + rest.

Nighttime sleeping provides the best rest. All adults need seven to eight hours of uninterrupted sleep, adolescents needs more.

- Pacing. This is associated with resting between lifting stones or barbells. When performing natural outdoor work, pacing is usually natural too. You drag a log or stone to where you drop it on the ground, think about the size of the next one or analyze where the stone will fit. This recovery is important to maintain and enable you to work for one, two, or more hours. In weight lifting, especially if you're in a gym, *faster* pacing is often encouraged by personnel trainers, which can reduce recovery from the previous activity and increase fatigue. After working out on one machine, you usually jump right into another. But resting between each set is essential for the ability of the muscles to recover and fully contract next time. This period of time should be about three minutes or more.

237

This is not to say that all athletic training is easy, although most of the workouts feel that way. And they should be fun. Dedication, discipline, and getting in touch with your body's needs are prime factors for success and are often more difficult than the training schedule itself. The typical image of training to exhaustion, which is, in fact, a common training routine, is a myth.

Another factor that helps avoid fatigue is speed. The muscle's fast-twitch fibers are the ones that provide the most power. Natural strength training involves fast movements. When lifting large stones or dragging logs, you accomplish these tasks more successfully with quick movements. If you've ever tried lifting something heavy with a slow pace, you know it's more difficult. It can also be dangerous as the slow-moving muscle fibers are not as effective and you can hurt yourself due to lack of strength. It's the nervous system that helps regulate the speed of action.

The importance of the nervous system can be seen in a strength program. The most rapid increases in power occur in the early weeks, before the muscles have a chance to get larger. It's the nervous system that's responsible for the increase in strength in part by its fast actions and recruitment of more fast-twitch muscle fibers. For example, in a ten-week program of weight lifting, individuals can significantly increase their strength. But during this period, the increased size of the muscle is not significant. Long-term gains in strength, those that occur after a few months, are due to the addition of increased muscle size that also stimulates more muscle fibers.

How-to: Strong Muscles and Bones

Despite the hype in many magazine articles, websites, and elsewhere, strength training does not guarantee improvements in bone strength. In fact, it can sometimes reduce it. Not to mention the potential for fatigue, overtraining, and injury, all of which are too common. So the first thing to do is keep it simple, safe, and natural.

Instead of images of bodybuilder's bulky muscles, let's take a lesson from Olympic weight lifters. They want the most strength from their bodies without too much muscle weight gain, which can put them into a higher weight category where competition may be more difficult. Apart from the heavyweight and super heavyweight categories, these athletes generally are not bulky but have very strong muscles and bones—more so than bodybuilders.

Lifting heavier weight with fewer repetitions increases muscle strength and bone density better than lifting lighter weights with higher repetitions. *This does not mean more weight is better*. To avoid fatigue, overtraining, or causing an acute injury, the amount of weight that might be appropriate is about 80 percent of your one-repetition maximum weight. This is also the weight you can lift about six times before fatigue develops—you don't want to fatigue your muscles at each workout, so build up slowly to learn your limits.

A heavier weight with less repetition and few activities means a shorter workout. In fact, you may be spending more time resting between reps than lifting! Even more significant is that in the time it takes the average person to travel to a gym and back, he or she could have completed the same workout at home.

For those who are not willing or able to perform regular natural workouts by lifting stones, dragging logs, and chopping wood, consider the alternative of getting some basic equipment for a home workout that will do the same. The plan is to keep it simple and safe. You really only need to perform a couple of routines to build muscle and bone strength, and without interfering with your aerobic system. The two easiest and most effective ones include the dead lift and squat (front, overhead, and/or back). Here are some examples:

- Reps: 1–6 reps in each set.
- Sets: 4 (more if time and energy permit).
- Lifting should be done relatively fast not slow.
- Recovery between sets should be three minutes (timed), more if desired.
- All movements should be smooth and natural.
- As you get stronger, slowly increase the amount of weight rather than repetitions.
- Three times per week, more if time permits.

Here is a sample workout:

- Warm-up: 15 minutes (walk, easy run or other easy aerobic activity)
- Dead lift: 5 reps
- Recovery: 3 minutes
- Squat: 5 reps
- Recovery: 3 minutes
- Repeat above lifts three more times
- Cooldown (same as warm-up)

IMPORTANT!

The most important requirement for performing these workouts is that you are relatively fit and healthy. If you're injured, have frequent colds, flu, asthma and allergies, or other indications of diminished health, wait until you've resolved these issues. In addition, if you don't have a good aerobic system, developing this is the priority—perform easy aerobic training for three months or more before implementing a strength program.

When starting a strength program, even if you're familiar with it, begin with less weight and less reps—be very conservative. Take several weeks to build up. There's no rush. In many cases, use a barbell without added weight so you get used to the movements, then slowly add small amounts of weight every couple of weeks.

If you're new to lifting weights, I recommend getting some one-on-one guidance with a trained professional who can help you with technique. In the meantime, start on some yard work.

239

So say good-bye to isolation exercises—those that attempt six-pack abs and bulging biceps. The bottom line is this: get stronger muscles and bones throughout your entire body. A simple, safe and short routine will accomplish this task. The best way to do it is go natural. Make the outdoors your new gym for a more holistic, natural workout. It's what our ancestors did for eons.

As you can now see, before developing anaerobic function, building the aerobic system is a priority. This is true for everyone—young and old, male and female, competitive athletes and those just wanting optimal health and fitness. Too often, people who have been inactive for a long time rush back into working out without first building an aerobic foundation. As a result, in their hurry to be fit, they get injured, become more prone to illnesses such as chest colds because of a stressed immune system, or are dissatisfied with stagnating results.

In addition, you may unknowingly train the anaerobic system through jogging, running, biking, dance classes, and other seemingly aerobic workouts, including walking. That's because your level of intensity may be too high. Accurately checking your heart rate will demonstrate this problem. There is a simple solution to avoid this potential roadblock in your quest for optimal fitness. It's a device called the heart rate monitor. It's cheap, easy to use, and will help you make amazing fitness gains. It's the subject of the following chapter.

CHAPTER 14

HEART RATE TRAINING
Applying the Basic Principles of Aerobic Fitness

How much time does it take for someone who is relatively healthy to become fit, get in shape for the first time, or come back from injury or illness? I pose these questions simply because over the years, I have been asked them a lot. Based on my own experience, most people try to rush things and end up getting sick or injured. What happens next is fairly common: they give up on the idea of exercise altogether. It's only by gradually building a fitness base that you will be able to achieve success—the healthy long-term kind that will stick around for many years.

Let's then get started. The time necessary to develop the aerobic system is sometimes referred to as establishing an aerobic base, and it's the first step in building your fitness. To do this efficiently and effectively, it will take at least three months or, for many people, up to six months or more. It also takes self-discipline to not work out harder or put in more hours than your aerobic system is ready for. In other words, you must build a base and not go anaerobic. And it's just as important to consider all lifestyle factors related to improving the aerobic system, including diet and stress.

You can walk, jog, run, bike, swim, dance, even play tennis or golf while developing an aerobic base. Unfortunately, these activities can also be anaerobic if the intensity is too high. But you can take the guesswork out of your exercise and be assured you're truly aerobic by understanding your heart rate. And the most useful and least expensive way to do this is with a heart rate monitor.

I began monitoring the heart rates of patients after entering private practice in 1977. I used a crude but effective device that's strapped around the chest and shoulder and sensed the beating heart. It was bulky and oversized. Modern (and much smaller) heart rate monitors would not appear until the early 1980s. Today, many runners, triathletes, and cyclists use these devices.

As one's level of exercise intensity increase, the heart rate also rises. This is necessary to pump more blood that brings additional oxygen and nutrients to the muscles. With a faster-beating heart comes less fat burning and more sugar burning. Overall, higher intensity workouts require quick energy, which comes from sugar. Most importantly, the level of exercise intensity will dictate how your body reacts to that exercise session during the next twenty-four hours. Higher levels of intensity and higher heart rates also train or condition your body to burn more sugar and less fat while easier exercise and lower heart rates do

just the opposite. You can monitor all this by measuring your heart rate.

There are two ways to check your heart rate, either by hand or using a monitor. Trying to obtain your heart rate by stopping to take your pulse, typically on the front of the wrist, is often very inaccurate. If you are just one or two beats off in a six-second count, that's a difference of ten to twenty beats per minute! When you stop to take a pulse, your heart rate also decreases rapidly. In six seconds, the rate may drop by ten, fifteen, or twenty beats per minute. Some try to take a pulse by applying light pressure to the carotid artery in the neck, but this can trigger a more rapid slowing of the heart rate. Besides getting an inaccurate count, you run the risk of fainting—too much pressure on the carotid artery can trigger too rapid a drop in heart rate.

Using a heart monitor is the answer to these problems. These devices strap around the lower chest and sense the heart rate by picking up vibrations of the heartbeat through the rib cage. The heart rate is then transmitted to a special watch worn on the wrist, where you can easily see the number. Monitors usually have an alarm that sounds when you exercise above or below your individually set heart rate.

Other heart monitor devices measure other pulses. These include monitors with sensors that attach to your fingertip or earlobe to pick up pulses. They are less accurate and not as convenient to use for walking or jogging but may be useful for working on a stationary apparatus, such as a bike.

Heart rate monitors are basic biofeedback units, telling you what's going on inside your body. In this case, the goal is to be aerobic to train your body's fat-burning system.

Through years of testing, I measured responses in human subjects to various physiological inputs: sounds, visual effects, and various physical stimulations, including exercise. The observed reactions were evaluated by measuring temperature, blood pressure, sweating, heart rate, and other factors. It became evident that using the heart rate to objectively measure body function was simple, accurate, and useful. Its application in exercise was obvious. This information became important as I developed various biofeedback-based programs including treatment of muscle problems, improving brain function, and individualizing exercise programs.

The 180 Heart Rate Formula

When I began using heart monitors to evaluate the quality of workouts done by patients and correlated these observations with other clinical measurements, even including posture and gait, it led to the development of a formula for determining the best heart rate to use for building the body's aerobic system—the 180 formula.

The 180 formula has been a solid, time-tested method of training the aerobic system in beginners, world-class, and professional athletes and for the rehabilitation of many types of patients since the early 1980s. I arrived at this number through many years of biofeedback research.

You might already be familiar with the 220 heart rate formula, which is a popular number but inaccurate. In any case, here's how it works. You subtract your age from 220 and multiply the difference by a figure ranging from 65 to 85 percent. The resulting number supposedly provides you with an aerobic training heart rate. This formula contains two serious errors. It assumes that 220 minus your age is your maximum heart rate. In reality, most people who obtain their maximum heart rate by pushing themselves to exhaustion (I don't recommend you do this) will find it's probably not 220 minus their age. About a third find their maximum is above, a third will be below, and only a third may be close to 220 minus their age. The second inaccuracy is the multiplier, which can range between 65 to 85 percent. This arbitrary figure doesn't consider a person's overall health or fitness. Do you use 65 or 75 percent? How about 80 or 70 percent? Without a more precise indicator, you are leaving your training heart rate to a very wide range and your fitness to chance.

Or if you don't have access to a heart rate monitor, you might think that the "talk test" is a good alternative. This test assumes you can comfortably talk to an exercise partner during a workout, such as when jogging. If you can carry on a normal conversation, it means you are aerobic. But this test is unreliable and in fact often maintains that someone is in a mild anaerobic state.

So rather than be inaccurate or guess, it's best to use a formula that is not only more sensible but also has a proven success record and is more scientific: the 180 formula. This method also considers physiological rather than just chronological age. (Of course, finding a specialist in an exercise physiology lab who can monitor your fat burning and heart rate changes would be the ideal approach—but it's not practical for most people, and the 180 formula comes very close to what this routine will provide.)

To find your maximum aerobic exercise heart rate, there are two important steps. First, subtract your age from 180. Next, find the best category for your present state of health and fitness, as follows.

Calculating Your Maximum Aerobic Heart Rate

1. Subtract your age from 180 (180–age).
2. Modify this number by selecting one of the following categories:

a. If you have a history of a major illness, are recovering from any surgery or hospital stay, or if you are taking any regular medication, subtract 10.

b. If you have been exercising but have an injury, are regressing in your efforts (not showing much improvement), if you often get more than one or two colds or flu a year, have allergies or asthma, or if you have not exercised before, subtract 5.

c. If you have been exercising for at least two years and four times a week without any injury, and none of the above items apply to you, subtract 0.

d. If you are a competitive athlete, have been training for more than two years without

any injury, and have been making progress in both training and competition, add 5.

For example, if you are thirty years old and fit into category b:

180—30 = 150, then 150—5 = 145 beats per minute

The result of the equation is your maximum aerobic heart rate. In this example, exercising at a heart rate of 145 beats per minute will be highly aerobic, allowing you to develop maximum aerobic function. Exercising at heart rates above this level can quickly add a significant anaerobic component to the workout and stimulate your anaerobic system, exemplified by a shift to more sugar burning and less fat burning.

If you prefer to exercise below your maximum aerobic heart rate, you will still derive good aerobic benefits, but progress at a slightly slower pace.

Note: it always pays to be conservative, so if your resulting number is lower, it's also safer compared to guessing it may be a higher number.

The only exceptions for this formula are for people over the age of sixty-five and those under the age of sixteen, as follows:

1. For seniors in category c or d, you may have to add up to 10 beats after obtaining your maximum aerobic heart rate. That doesn't mean you must add 10 beats. This is such an individualized category, getting assistance from a professional would be very helpful.

2. For children under the age of sixteen, there's no need to use the 180 formula. Instead, use 165 as the maximum aerobic heart rate.

If you're used to exercising, when you first work out at your maximum aerobic heart rate, it may seem too easy. Many people have told me initially they can't imagine it's worth the time. I tell them to not only imagine it will help but to also understand how the body really works. Remember, when you're finished, an aerobic workout you should feel like you could do it all over again.

In a short time, exercise will become more enjoyable, and you'll find more work is needed to maintain your heart rate. In other words, as your aerobic system builds up, you'll need to walk, ride, or dance faster to attain your maximum aerobic heart rate. If you're a runner, your minute-per-mile pace will get faster, cyclists will ride at higher miles per hour at the same heart rate, and even walkers.

Let me give you an example of how a heart rate monitor can help you make great fitness gains. I had a patient named Sally. At age forty and relatively healthy, Sally was dedicated to her exercise routine. She went to aerobic dance class four mornings a week and walked twice weekly with friends. But her time was not well spent, she thought, since her weight and body fat didn't change much in the two years she worked out. She also was tired on the days she did aerobics. I asked Sally to wear a heart monitor during her aerobics class and when she walked. Not surprisingly, her heart rate exceeded 180 beats per minute during aerobics and averaged 155 on her walks. But Sally's maximum aerobic heart rate was 140. Thus she had programmed her body to burn more sugar and less fat.

After seeing that she couldn't physically perform the aerobic routine during an advanced class without her heart rate going over 140, Sally went to an easier class where she was able to control her heart rate at 140. She also began walking on her own, at a much slower pace. Within a couple of months, Sally lost more weight than in the previous two years, and her workouts now gave her energy. In time she was able to go back to the advanced aerobics class and walk with her friends while maintaining a 140 heart rate.

Another former patient of mine, Dave, forty-five, was a former college all-American in football. He was now overweight and feeling the effects of work stress. Since he was in the athletic-apparel business, he wanted to appear more fit. He began walking on the high school track for two miles almost every evening. He got out of breath and tired easily, so he kept his pace relatively slow. After a couple of months with barely noticeable results—he had not lost weight or felt he could increase his distance without more fatigue—Dave came to my office seeking help. I told him to perform his walk as he usually does, but with a heart monitor. To our surprise, he reported back that his heart rate exceeded 170 and stayed there for nearly the entire workout

245

of about fifty minutes. But once Dave began using a heart monitor regularly and kept his rate at the prescribed level of 130, it was only a couple of weeks before he felt some positive results. And within a couple of months, Dave was thinner, losing over ten pounds, had more energy, and was walking faster. Now he was eager to increase the length of his walks.

Using a heart monitor during weight training won't show that you're aerobic or anaerobic; you're always anaerobic when lifting weights or doing push-ups, pull-ups, or sit-ups. When wearing a heart monitor during weight lifting, your heart rate continues to increase as you lift the weight. But before your heart rate reaches its normal peak, your muscle has fatigued and you've stopped the repetition. It's important to understand the weight lifting and similar workouts are anaerobic—avoid them during the period you want to fully develop your aerobic system. Only then can you add anaerobic training to your overall schedule. Otherwise, you won't develop aerobic function as well, and in many cases, not at all. (This issue is discussed in more detail later in the chapter.)

Once you find your maximum aerobic heart rate, you can create a convenient range that starts 10 beats below that number. Most heart monitors can be set for your range, providing you with an audible indication if your heart rate goes over or under your preset levels. Set yours at the maximum aerobic rate you determined. Most monitors also provide for a low setting, which could be 10 below the high. This gives you a comfortable range.

For example, if your maximum aerobic heart rate is 145, then the low would be 135; set the monitor for a range between 135 and 145. It's not absolutely necessary to work out in your range—you just don't want to exceed it. If you're more comfortable exercising under that range, you will still derive good aerobic benefits. But to obtain maximum aerobic benefits, stay within the range during each workout.

The Maximum Aerobic Function (MAF) Test

For many who regularly work out, a common problem (and complaint) is that after a few months, they realize that they aren't making any fitness gains. It's as if they are stuck in one gear. That is why another important benefit of using a heart monitor is the ability to regularly and objectively measure your aerobic progress. A good measure of progress is accomplished using the maximum aerobic function test, or MAF test. (By the way, it's only by sheer coincidence that the acronym is also the same as the first three letters of my last name.)

The MAF test measures the improvements you make in the aerobic system. Without objective measurements, you can fool yourself into thinking all is well with your exercise. More importantly, the MAF test tells you if you're headed in the wrong direction, either from too much anaerobic exercise, too little aerobic exercise, or any imbalance that is having an adverse effect on the aerobic system (such as from stress or poor diet).

PERCEIVED EXERTION

The 180 formula applies to all activities (except weight lifting and other strictly anaerobic training). At the same heart rate, different types of exercise require about the same levels of metabolic activity. So whether you're swimming, biking, running, or walking, many physiological parameters are the same, and the 180 formula applies to all of them. However, there's a difference in how you feel between different activities while exercising at the same heart rate. This is called the perceived exertion; it's a subjective feeling you have about how easy or hard the workout seems. Running at a heart rate of 140, for example, has a perceived exertion that's lower than swimming at that rate. That is, swimming at a 140 heart rate (given the same physical know-how) usually feels more difficult. This difference has to do with gravity stress. The gravity-stress difference between swimming and running is significant; there is very little gravity influence in the water, but gravity maximally affects your body during running, which also requires more muscle activity. A lot of energy may not have to go into countering gravity stress in the pool but just the opposite is true during a run. Another way of looking at this phenomenon is that the heart rate during swimming is lower compared to running at the same effort, since the stress level is diminished in the water.

Riding a bike falls between the two extremes of swimming and running, along with cross-country skiing, skating, and most other endurance activities. In these actions, there is some gravity stress along with mechanical factors, which relates to technique.

Technique can influence the heart rate significantly. For the beginning swimmer, the heart rate is usually much higher. As your technique improves, you waste less energy and the same intensity (pace) results in lower heart rates. Looking at this another way, you need to swim faster to maintain your maximum aerobic heart rate.

The MAF test can be performed using any exercise except weight lifting. During the test, use your maximum aerobic heart rate found with the 180 formula. While working out at that heart rate, determine some parameter such as your walking, jogging, or running pace (in minutes per mile), cycling speed (miles per hour), or repetitions (laps in a pool) over time. The test can also be done on stationary equipment such as a treadmill or other apparatus that measures output.

Let's say you want to test your maximum aerobic function during walking. Go to the local high school or college track and, after

ADJUSTING YOUR TRAINING HEART RATE WHEN ON MEDICATION

For many individuals, reducing the training heart rate is a hard pill to swallow. By lowering the maximum aerobic heart rate by 10 beats, as indicated in the 180 formula, the workout slows even more, further frustrating some people. The common complaint is this: "I can't believe how slow I am going!" But give yourself time. Be patient.

Many people of all abilities, including athletes, coaches, and health care professionals, have frequently asked me for further clarification of the 180 formula. But the math is actually quite straightforward, with the formula containing this caveat: if you are taking any regular medication, subtract 10. Not only is this relevant to prescription and over-the-counter drugs that modify your heart rate during exercise, but it also applies to any medication. The result is a further lowering of the aerobic training heart rate, slowing the intensity of the work out.

There are good reasons for this recommendation. First, some medications slow the heartbeat. This results in false information about how hard the body is working. In other words, you may work out harder but still have a low heart rate—artificially reduced by medication.

A common example is a group of drugs called beta blockers, prescribed for patients with heart problems and high blood pressure. This drug reduces both the resting and exercise heart rate, although not always by the same amount. In some cases, a person can work out much harder without the heart rate elevating even into the aerobic zone. In this case, exercising at 125 beats per minute, for example, may be the same as 155 without the medication—so if your max aerobic heart rate is 140, you can easily be overtraining at 125. In fact, some people are unable to attain their max aerobic heart rate while on a beta blocker.

In this situation, where medication significantly reduces the heart rate, the best suggestion is to work with a cardiologist or other healthcare professional familiar with exercise physiology who can help further individualize a drug's optimal dose and your exercise program.

Antiarrhythmic drugs, calcium channel blockers, and other medications can sometimes reduce exercise heart rate as well. If you're taking any prescription or over-the-counter drug, you should know whether it affects the heart rate.

Some drugs raise the heart rate. These include thyroid medication, Ritalin, and other amphetamines and even caffeine, which is found in certain cold remedies, pain relievers, and of course, coffee, tea, and some colas. These drugs will often cause higher exercise heart rates, forcing you to slow down to maintain your maximum aerobic heart rate. This means that by following your heart rate, you may have to reduce your exercise intensity. But don't increase your max aerobic heart rate because of this—there's another very important factor to consider.

A second reason to subtract 10 beats in the 180 formula for a person on any regular medication has to do with overall health. The fact that a health care professional has prescribed a drug or recommended an over-the-counter one means there's a health problem. In addition, there are the drug's potential side effects.

While people often think many prescription and over-the-counter drugs are perfectly safe or that the health problems associated with their needs are quite innocuous, this is absolutely not the case most of the time. So being more conservative during exercise is important to prevent problems of excessive stress or overtraining from your workouts. There's still a wide range of intensity below the maximum aerobic heart rate that will provide significant benefits. In addition, this will help with optimal development of the aerobic system often to the point where your doctor may reduce a drug's dosage or decide the medication is no longer necessary.

For competitive athletes, progress may be a bit slower, but they'll still get faster at the same heart rate and improve their performances.

Even though many medications don't directly affect the heart rate, the impact on health can adversely affect muscles, metabolism, and other systems of the body that promote health and fitness. An example includes some of the cholesterol-lowering drugs called statins, including Mevacor, Lipitor, and Altocor. These can affect muscle function, sometimes leading to exercise-related injuries. By making the 10-beat adjustment in heart rate, the risk of muscle problems and potential injuries may be reduced.

Another example is aspirin and other NSAIDs, which can interfere with proper recovery after exercise. By working out at a lower heart rate, the stress on the physical body will be reduced along with better recovery.

Even for a woman who is taking birth control pills or hormone replacement therapy, these medications have potential side effects that can adversely affect exercise activity. In this case, the levels of some B vitamins can be lowered, affecting liver function, energy systems, lactate production, and other important body functions necessary for optimal health and fitness.

For those performing higher-intensity workouts, the potential problems of medications and the reasons for prescribing them can be amplified with an increased risk of complications. Consider that increased physical exertion itself is a risk factor that can trigger a heart attack. While lower heart rate workouts generally don't do this and, in fact, protect you from a heart attack or stroke, anaerobic exercise with its associated higher heart rates can increase the short-term risk of death from a heart attack. So does the high intensity associated with athletic competition—it doesn't have to be a 26.2-mile marathon, 5K run, or two-hour bike ride.

A note on caffeine: I don't recommend making further adjustments in the 180 formula for those drinking a large cup (or two) of coffee before working out. Clearly, this can affect the heart rate. But like eating a bowl of junk food cereal or bagel, which can adversely affect endurance performance by reducing fat burning, I choose not to adjust the training heart rate for these habits.

a couple of warm-up laps, walk at your maximum aerobic heart rate. Determine how long it takes to walk one mile at this heart rate. Record your time in a diary or on your calendar. If you normally walk two or three miles, you can record each mile.

Below is an actual example of an MAF test performed by walking on a track, at a heart rate of 145, calculating time in minutes per mile:

- Mile 1 16:32 (16 minutes and 32 seconds)
- Mile 2 16:46
- Mile 3 17:09

During any one MAF test, your times should usually get slower with successive repetitions. In other words, the first mile should always be the fastest, and the last is the slowest. If that's not the case, it usually means you haven't warmed up enough, as discussed below.

The MAF test should indicate faster times as the weeks and months pass. This means the aerobic system is improving and you're burning more fat, enabling you to do more work with the same effort. Even if you walk or run longer distances, your MAF test should show the same progression of results, providing you heed your maximum aerobic heart rate. Below is an example showing the improvement of the same person from above:

Performing the MAF test on a bike is similar. When riding outside, the easiest method is to pick a bike course that initially takes about 30 minutes to complete. Following a warm-up, ride at your maximum aerobic heart rate and record exactly how long it takes to ride the test course. As you progress, your times should get faster. Riding your course today, for example, may take 30 minutes and 50 seconds. In three weeks it may take you 29:23 and in another three weeks 27:35. After three months of base work, the same course may take you 26 minutes. Another option is to ride on a flat course and see what pace you can maintain while holding your heart rate at your max aerobic level. This works best on a stationary apparatus. As you progress, your miles-per-hour should increase. If you start at 12 mph, for example, following a three-month aerobic base you might be riding 17 mph at the same heart rate.

Perform the MAF test regularly, throughout the year, and chart your results. I recommend doing the test every month. Testing yourself too often may result in obsession. Usually, you won't improve significantly within one week.

For those who choose to walk very easy or do other activities that, over time, will not raise the heart rate to the maximum aerobic level, it's possible to do the MAF test without using the maximum aerobic heart rate. Since it's usually too difficult to reach that heart rate, choose a lower rate for your

MAF test. For example, if you have difficulty reaching your max aerobic rate of 150, use 125 during your walk as the rate for your MAF test.

Performing the test irregularly or not often enough defeats one of its purposes—knowing when your aerobic system is getting off course. One of the great benefits of the MAF test is its ability to objectively inform you of an obstacle long before you feel bad or get injured. If something interferes with your progress, such as exercise itself, diet, or stress, you don't want to wait until you're feeling bad or gaining weight to find that out. In these situations where your aerobic system is no longer getting benefits, your MAF test will show it by getting worse or not improving.

Factors That Affect the MAF Test

There are a number of factors that may affect your MAF test results. When walking, for example, the type of track surface may have a slight influence on your pace. The modern high-tech track surfaces result in a slightly faster pace, whereas the old cinder and dirt tracks will slow your pace at the same heart rate. Uneven tracks will give slower times compared to perfectly flat sur-

	September	October	November	December
Mile 1	16:32	15:49	15:35	15:10
Mile 2	16:46	16:06	15:43	15:22
Mile 3	17:09	16:14	15:57	15:31

251

PHASES OF AEROBIC FUNCTION

Many people are aware that the body has periods of progress and plateaus. Losing weight is the example people often are most aware of. Many lose weight for a period of time; then there seems to be a stretch where little or no weight is lost. The aerobic system sometimes does the same thing.

During your exercise program, you could encounter three different phases: progression, plateau, and regression. The first is normal, the second may be normal too but may linger to an abnormal state. The third is not normal. Let's look at these in detail. When you successfully develop your aerobic system, you will have more energy and better aerobic function, with corresponding improvements in your MAF test. This is the progressive phase, and it can and should continue for many years without regression. As you improve, further progression will happen more slowly. For example, the first year your walking may improve from eighteen minutes to thirteen minutes per mile. The second year, your improvement may only go from thirteen minutes per mile, walking, to ten minutes per mile, jogging.

There will also be periods of plateaus. Actually, there are two different kinds of plateaus, one normal and the other unhealthy. With improvement, you will eventually arrive at a normal leveling off—almost as if your body needs a rest from the progress it's making. The many aspects of the body, such as the metabolism with regard to fat burning, or balancing of hormones, requires a period of adjustment, and this may take time. These normal plateaus shouldn't last too long, perhaps a few weeks to a few months in extreme cases. Then progress should resume, as measured by the MAF test. But if you stay in your plateau for longer periods, it may be abnormal.

An abnormal plateau is due to some obstacle that prevents progress. The MAF test can help diagnose an abnormal plateau. Once your test has stayed the same for too long, the next step is to find out why. There could be many factors:

- The most common reason for an abnormal plateau is an excess of physical, chemical, or mental stress. Typically, some lifestyle stress such as an increased nutritional need, an uncomfortable work environment, or even the weather—such as an extreme hot or cold season—may also be a stress that can halt progression.
- Another common reason for an abnormal plateau is the food you're eating. Too much high-glycemic carbohydrate foods are the worst; not enough fats, poor hydration, or any nutritional problems can contribute too.

Even worse than not making progress is regressing. Indeed, that's just what happens if your plateau is prolonged—an abnormal plateau will eventually cause your MAF test to get worse each time you check it. If this happens, something is significantly wrong with your health and or fitness.

If you work out a lot, chances are your body is in a "red alert," and you should be very cautious. This is when you become most vulnerable to injury and ill health. One recommended strategy is to cut your overall exercise time by 50 percent until you find the problem. This will at least ensure you get more rest and recovery. If you don't respect the advice of your body, you may ultimately need to seek first aid advice from a professional. Exhaustion, injury, illness, or some other major breakdown, possibly including mental breakdown, can occur.

faces. On your bike, the roughness of the road surface, varying grades, and traffic can affect your test results. Hills usually result in a slowing of pace, unless there are significantly more downhills. A good option is to use a stationary apparatus on your test days.

To ensure the MAF test is accurate, be consistent; use the same course or method each time you test yourself. If you change your test course, be sure to note it in your diary or chart.

Other factors that could affect your test include weather conditions such as wind, rain, snow, temperature, and humidity; altitude; hydration; and your equipment. Most of these factors can work against you by increasing your physical effort, which raises the heart rate. Since you are working at a specific heart rate, the result is a slower pace.

One other factor worth mentioning is ill health. When you are sick, your body's immune system is working hard to recover,

and it needs all the energy it can get. The last thing your body wants to do at this time is to work out, especially when you have an elevated temperature. Don't exercise if you are ill. If you've ever attempted it and worn a heart monitor, you know what happens: your heart rate elevates, sometimes drastically. The same effect is observed if you are anemic: less oxygen can be delivered to the muscles, and your tests will worsen. For women, menses can also increase heart rate.

By using the 180 formula and regularly performing the MAF test, you will be on the right road for improving health and fitness. But there's one more bonus—warming up and cooling down.

An Aerobic Bonus: Warm-up and Cooldown

Most people think that warming up means stretching. This isn't true. A real warm-up provides many important benefits, most of which stretching can't give. What's more, stretching can often do more harm than good. It can even lead to injury. (See the following chapter.) What you want to do instead is get the slow shifting of blood into the working muscles. The emphasis is on slow. Moving the blood into the muscles too quickly, such as starting off at a brisk pace during walking or biking, can be a significant stress on the rest of the body. Specifically, the blood going into the muscles comes from other important areas of the body including the nervous system, adrenal glands, and intestines. Diverting the blood out of these areas and circulating it into the muscles too rapidly can be much like going into shock. When a warm-up is done slowly, the organs and glands can properly compensate for this normal activity. Warming up provides three important benefits:

- It increases the blood flow, bringing oxygen and nutrients into the muscles, and removes waste products.
- It increases the fats in the blood that are used for muscle energy.
- It increases flexibility in all the joints by gently warming and lengthening the muscles.

The warm-up can be any easy aerobic, low–heart rate activity. Begin your exercise by slowly raising your heart rate from its starting point of, say, 75 beats per minute. Slowly elevate the heart rate, over a twelve- to fifteen-minute period, arriving at your max-imum aerobic level only after fifteen min-utes. At this point, you can maintain your maximum aerobic heart rate until nearing the end of your workout, when you begin to cool down.

The Cooldown

The final twelve to fifteen minutes of your workout are also important; it's vital to slowly reestablish nearly normal circulation without "pooling" blood in the muscles. You want to reestablish the normal circulation in the organs and glands to begin the twenty-four–hour process of recovery and obtaining the benefits from your exercise. This slow lowering of the heart rate from the max-imum aerobic level back to near-resting level is called the cooling down. Carefully bring the heart rate back down by slowing down your activity. Attempt to reach your starting heart rate, which is often not possible—but at least get within 10 beats of your starting heart rate.

Finding Your Optimal Exercise Program

It's clear that regular aerobic exercise is essential for you to attain optimal fitness and health. But I want to reemphasize that I'm not talking about a no-pain, no-gain exercise program that can increase your risk of injury which often falls by the wayside as quickly as you start it. Instead, incorporate into your life-style an ongoing, long-term natural aerobic exercise routine that will greatly improve your energy levels, stamina, and endurance while helping you tone the aerobic muscles and train your body to burn more fat for energy. Physical activity should be something that you look forward to continuing for a lifetime.

Exercise programs are quite individual. Some people just want to stay fit and healthy and keep their weight in check. Others have goals such as training for a local fun run or cycling event. For either of these types, and for everyone in between, many basic principles are the same. All people who exercise want to gradually build up to a specific level, using the 180 formula to improve aerobic fitness. Additionally, anyone on an exercise plan needs to balance this program with everything else in his or her life, including proper rest and recovery.

Balanced Fitness and Health

Working out adds many new dimensions to your life—an important component of optimal human performance. Much like diet and nutrition, each person must find an individualized program to meet his or her particular needs. So start out as simply as possible. You can also consider joining a group to get additional emotional encouragement, as long as you can exercise within your own limits.

There are a number of important factors to consider when starting or modifying your exercise routine:

- *Scheduling.* Create a realistic schedule of exercise that fits in with family, work, and your other commitments. This will allow you to be more consistent and help make it part of a new lifestyle.

THE IDEAL WORKOUT

The graph below shows heart rate changes in relation to time for (a) warming up, (b) maintaining the maximum aerobic level, and (c) cooling down.

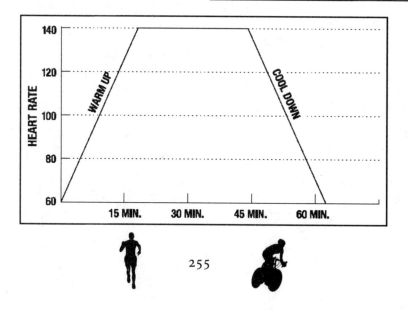

- *Physical factors.* Be sure you can withstand the minor stress of exercise. Do you have some physical imbalances that may be aggravated by exercise? Take into consideration a history of prior injuries or conditions. Grass and dirt surfaces may be safe, but they also can be stressful if they are uneven or too soft.
- *Chemical factors.* The proper nutrients, especially fats, are necessary for aerobic efficiency. High-sugar foods and drinks can be detrimental when consumed before workouts. Proper hydration is a must; drink water all day, not just after working out. Most people don't require water during their workout.
- *Psychological factors.* Studies have shown that people who exercise in the morning find it easier to maintain a regular program. But whether you exercise in the morning, midday, or evening, be consistent. Write out a simple exercise program, if necessary. You are more apt to follow something you can see. Keep a log on a calendar or in a diary to see your success as the days, weeks, and months go by.
- *Set realistic goals.* Some people merely want to progress to exercising thirty to forty-five minutes a day. Be conservative, but don't hesitate to dream.
- *Habit change.* Starting an exercise program is, first of all, a change of habit. And as we all know, a habit change can be the most difficult change to make—even more difficult than the exercise itself. Generally, there are two barriers. One is just getting started, and the other shows up two to four weeks later, when your enthusiasm wears off a bit. (Although being aware of this is usually incentive enough to keep you going.)
- *Time.* Most exercise should be measured in time, and not miles, laps, or repetitions (except when performing your MAF test). At the onset, a minimal time is best, since the purpose initially is to develop an exercise habit. The only exception may be if you progress to anaerobic workouts, such as weight lifting, where a range of measurements should always be used. This gives you more choice, allowing for daily fluctuations in energy level and time restraints. For example, when using weights, the number of repetitions may be ten to fifteen, rather than doing a predetermined exact number based on some program not meant for you.
- *Intensity.* The intensity of your workout is an important consideration, as measured by the heart rate. Make sure you understand how to find your maximum aerobic heart rate using the 180 formula. Base your exercise program on time and intensity (as per heart rate); for example, thirty minutes of walking at a heart rate not to exceed 140 beats per minute, five times per week.

A Word for Beginners

Even if you've never been physically active, aerobic exercise is easy and simple. If you are in reasonably good health and have

256

no serious problems or injuries, it can be done with a simple thirty-minute walk a minimum of four to five times per week. You can do this on your way to work, on your way home, as part of your lunch break, or anytime. It can be performed walking indoors or outdoors. Or you can use a treadmill or stationary bike, either in your home or at the gym. A simple aerobic workout will easily fit into your current work schedule and requires no special equipment, clothing, or gear. Here is a typical starting program for a beginner:

- Thirty minutes easy walking, which includes a warm-up and cooldown
- Heart rate not to exceed the maximum aerobic level
- Monday-through-Friday schedule
- Saturday and Sunday off

Remember, your basic beginning program should be tailored to your specific needs. While most people are capable of at least thirty minutes of walking, perhaps forty-five minutes is a good starting point. The maximum starting point for any beginner is an hour. Still others may benefit starting with twenty minutes per session. If you are recovering from a chronic illness or have been very inactive all your life, you should consider only fifteen minutes of exercise, or even ten minutes, as a start, and also consult your doctor.

Alice consulted me about starting an exercise program. She was about to celebrate her fiftieth birthday and thought it was time to get into shape. Alice was never physically active in sports, although she raised four children. She began a simple program of walking for twenty minutes, Mondays through Fridays, taking Saturdays and Sundays off. After two months, Alice was ready to increase to thirty minutes each day and after another two months progressed to forty-five minutes. After a couple of years, Alice had the desire to take a couple of long hikes a week, gradually working up to about ninety minutes each time.

How rapidly you increase the time period depends on your response. Whatever the starting point, assuming the proper time is chosen, maintain that time for at least three weeks. Listen to your body; it will tell you if and when you can increase. This is also true for any change: maintain the new time for at least three weeks before increasing it if that's desired and there's no difficulty.

Don't increase more than 50 percent at any one time in a program of up to forty-five minutes, and not more than fifteen minutes when the program is forty-five minutes or more. Some people are quite content remaining at forty-five minutes. This is fine, since you can obtain many benefits when exercising at this level five times per week.

Perform the MAF test about every month. If any problems develop, stop. A professional may be helpful in determining what's wrong.

What type of exercise should you do? When starting out, do almost anything, as long as it's aerobic. This may include, besides walking, riding a stationary bike, dancing, rebounding (trampoline), outdoor biking, swimming, hiking, and cross-country skiing. Jogging or running, when done aerobically, can also be a healthy exercise. There is no universally accepted scientific distinction between running and jogging. For the purposes of this book, I refer to jogging when I mean a much slower pace. Running occurs with progression and more speed and involves a slightly different gait. Any combination of these activities is also acceptable, as long as your heart rate doesn't exceed your maximum aerobic level. If you wish, do two or three types of exercise throughout the week, or even in one workout. For example, you can walk for fifteen minutes, ride a stationary bike for twenty minutes, and dance for fifteen minutes. This "cross-training" routine is actually healthier than doing just one exercise each session.

Anaerobic activities, including any type of weight lifting, sit-ups, push-ups, or activities that raise the heart rate above your maximum aerobic heart rate are not acceptable substitutes for aerobic exercise. They shouldn't be started until after you have developed your aerobic system. For the beginner, my recommendation is to wait at least six months, and for those modifying their program, wait at least three to four months before performing any anaerobic work.

Tennis, racquetball, and similar sports often end up being anaerobic for the beginner, because of the type of muscle fibers used and the high heart rates produced. They're fun to do but should be considered "games" and not

exercise unless they're performed regularly; for example, if you walk four times per week, play tennis once a week, or 18 holes of golf once a week. In that case, a proper warm-up and cooldown is important as well as regulating aerobic and anaerobic levels.

Once you have progressed through a certain number of weeks without any problems, you may want to further develop your health and fitness. The following section is for people who wish to take their fitness to another level.

Progressive Fitness Programs

To further increase your level of aerobic fitness, you may wish to spend more time at or just below your maximum aerobic heart rate. Be sure to pay close attention to your heart rate monitor to make sure you are not going over the maximum. If you can't reach your maximum aerobic heart rate by walking, you can jog or run or perform other activities. Other types of aerobic activity, such as biking, swimming, or dancing, can also be used to improve your aerobic fitness. Be conservative and begin this phase slowly.

At thirty-five, a former patient of mine named Kelly didn't like jogging but wanted to do a variety of exercises. She was a work-at-home mother to two young children and primarily wanted to keep in shape and prevent being overfat. After walking regularly for more than a year, she joined an aerobics class. She continued to wear her heart monitor, walking three days a week and going to aerobics three days. After a few months, when the weather turned cold, she bought a stationary bike and rode it instead of walking, only venturing outdoors to walk if the temperature was tolerable. In time, Kelly had no need for her heart monitor; she only was able to get her heart rate to about 130 despite her maximum aerobic level being 145 beats per minute. She still performed her MAF test, but at a lower heart rate. Kelly was happy maintaining her activity at this level. I saw her last when her two children were in college, and she was remaining in great shape and happy with her workout routines.

Basic Fitness Training

For many people, just exercising to be fit and healthy isn't enough. At some point in time this type of casual exercise program crosses over to a training program. Some people train to reach a certain goal, such as walking or running a certain distance or climbing a mountain. Others want to be competitive. While this information goes beyond the scope of this book, here are some basic training guidelines for those who wish to go beyond casual exercise:

- Take at least one or two days off per week for rest and recovery.
- Once per week, if time allows, perform two workouts in one day, preferably one in the morning and one in the evening. Both should be relatively easy, below-the-maximum aerobic level.
- Once per week, do one longer-than-normal workout.

If after several weeks of building more aerobic fitness and your MAF tests are continuing to show improvement, you may wish to add some anaerobic activity. Many people benefit by performing some anaerobic activity, as long as the aerobic system is well developed first, though for some with a high stress level, maintaining an aerobic schedule throughout the year works well. Anaerobic exercise may include lifting light weights, faster running, jogging, dancing, biking, or anything that raises the heart rate higher than the aerobic maximum. The following factors should be considered when scheduling an anaerobic workout:

- For most, one or two anaerobic workouts per week is sufficient.
- Anaerobic workouts should never be on consecutive days.
- Anaerobic workouts should be preceded by a day off or a short, easy aerobic day.
- Anaerobic workouts should be followed by a day off, or a short, easy aerobic day.
- An aerobic warm-up and cooldown should surround anaerobic workouts.
- This anaerobic period should last no more than three to five weeks.

A Word of Caution!

Anaerobic exercise is a common cause of injury, ill health, and overtraining. It is

FROM WALKING TO RUNNING

Many runners started out walking. And after a period of time, many walkers decide they want to go farther and faster. This is not a problem if you follow some basic rules. The transition from walking to jogging means landing on your foot farther forward rather than on your heel like in walking. It's important to feel what this is like before venturing outside for your first jog. Perform this simple experiment in your living room or hallway without shoes. Just jog about ten or fifteen feet. You'll naturally land farther forward on each foot and not on your heels. This is how you should jog. (This issue is discussed in detail chapter 18.)

Go outside, and wearing flat-sole shoes (this means shoes without an overbuilt heel), start out with your normal walking warm-up. After twelve to fifteen minutes, begin jogging slowly. Keep an eye on your heart rate. Most people can jog slowly until reaching their maximum aerobic heart rate. At this point, immediately stop jogging and start walking again at a fast pace. When your heart rate drops below your 10-beat aerobic range, assuming you're physically feeling good, start jogging again following the same heart rate guidelines. Typically, you'll be able to alternate walking and jogging until you're ready to cool down, which you should perform only by walking.

Let's take an example of someone who has been regularly walking five days a week for an hour—and, after several months of this regimen, is ready to jog. The first fifteen minutes is a walking warm-up, the next thirty minutes is a walk-jog pattern as described above, and the last fifteen minutes is a walking cooldown.

As time passes, you'll be able to maintain more jogging and less walking in the middle part of your workout. This occurs because you build better aerobic muscle function that enables you to jog more effectively, and you burn more fat to provide the additional energy needed during jogging.

In time, you'll be able to jog the whole thirty-minute period without having the heart rate exceed your maximum aerobic heart rate. How long this takes depends on your consistency, how strict you are in maintaining the proper heart rates, and your overall levels of health and fitness. In time, more of your warm-up and cooldown can also be accomplished by jogging. Eventually, your pace will quicken and your slow jog will turn to faster runs.

also the most common reason so many who exercise have poorly functioning aerobic systems; they are anaerobic during many, if not most, of their exercise sessions. Be cautious when performing anaerobic workouts. Do your MAF test during anaerobic periods. If you perform too much anaerobic work, you will know it by the results of your MAF test.

Most people don't really need to do anaerobic workouts. Their lives have enough stresses that stimulate the neurological, metabolic, and muscular systems to satisfy the minimal anaerobic requirements of the body. So don't be pressured into anaerobic workouts if you're not absolutely sure you want to.

If, in the course of getting out of shape, you've lost too much muscle, weight lifting can be helpful.

An important rule is worth mentioning here again: Have fun in your workouts. They should be enjoyable and invigorating. If your exercise routine has become stressful, then something is obviously wrong. Maybe it's time to change the time you workout. Or perhaps you feel stressed by trying to keep up with your regular workout partner. Or maybe it's something so simple as not eating well. Whatever the case, if exercise stops being an enjoyable, stress-relieving activity, find out why and correct it.

CHAPTER 15

THE HIDDEN DANGERS OF STRETCHING

In gym class you were probably taught to stretch before exercising. Even people who don't regularly work out think that stretching is a good way to get rid of body aches and pains as well as loosen up tight muscles. Go to any fitness center and you'll see many club members doing all sorts of stretching exercises. Many believe that if they can do deep knee bends or touch their toes, their body is fit and in working order.

Well, all that is wrong.

It's astounding that such huge numbers of people, young and old, athletes and those out of shape, have bought into the notion that stretching is a good idea. This view is widely held despite little, if any, scientific information demonstrating that static stretching is beneficial for most individuals, especially the way it's usually done. As a matter of fact, there's quite a bit of evidence showing that stretching is harmful. One of the most common reasons that people give for stretching is injury prevention. But studies show static stretching can actually increase the risk of injury!

Many exercise buffs believe that flexibility is important and that stretching is the only way to obtain it. While I often recommend that improvements in flexibility be made to prevent injury and create a more stable physical body, those who are much less flexible, or too flexible, have much higher rates of injury. They often have muscle imbalances—

problems that a healthy body can correct, especially with a proper aerobic warm-up and cooldown such as walking.

Before addressing the potential dangers of stretching and increased flexibility, I'd like to outline the two basic types of stretching (there are many versions of these), referred to as static and ballistic, and flexibility.

Static Stretching

This is a very slow, deliberate movement, lightly stretching a muscle and holding it unchanged for up to thirty seconds. When properly done, static stretching promotes relaxation of the muscle fibers being stretched. But static stretching requires that each muscle group throughout the body be sequentially repeated three to four times. It also demands that the activity be done slowly. Note some of the key words: "slow," "deliberate," "lightly stretched." And also note the need to stretch each muscle group three to four times. All this takes time and discipline, which most people just don't think they have or don't make time for.

There are two different types of static stretching, active and passive:

- Active stretching is safer than passive and is accomplished by contracting the antagonist muscle (the one opposite the muscle you're stretching). For example, to actively stretch the hamstring muscles, which are on the back of the thigh, the quadriceps, on the front of the thigh, are contracted.

- Passive stretching uses either gravity or force by another body part or person to move a body segment to the end of its range of motion or beyond—and is one of the primary reasons this type of stretching can easily cause injury. Case in point are football players stretching one leg by having another player lean on it.

Ballistic Stretching

The second basic type of stretching is called ballistic. This is a "bouncing" method and is the most common type done by both beginners and seasoned athletes. It makes use of the body's momentum to repeatedly stretch a joint position to or beyond the extreme ranges of motion. Because this method is more rapid than static stretching, it activates the stretch reflex, which increases tension in the muscle, rather than relaxation. This can result in microtearing of muscle fibers with resultant injury. Ballistic stretching is the type most people say they don't do, but in fact really are doing. That's because most people are in a hurry when stretching.

People who stretch generally are injured more often than those who don't stretch. That's been my observation during more than thirty years of treating patients; it's also the viewpoint of many other health care professionals. In addition, scientific studies support this observation. Halbertsma and Goeken, from the Department of Rehabilitation Medicine, University of Groningen, the Netherlands, conducted a study of men and women twenty to thirty-eight years of age with tight and stiff hamstrings. They found that "stretching exercises do not make short hamstrings any longer or less stiff."

Richard Dominguez, an orthopedic surgeon at Loyola University Medical Center and author of *The Complete Book of Sports Medicine*, also disapproves of stretching: "Flexibility should not be a goal in itself, but the result of . . . training. Strengthening the muscles around a joint naturally increases flexibility. If you can bend a joint beyond your ability to control it with muscle strength, you risk either tearing the muscles, tendons or ligaments that support the joint, or damaging the joint through abnormal pressure on it." Among the specific stretches Dominguez says are most damaging are the yoga plow, hurdler's stretch, toe touching, and the stiff-leg raise. The types of injury created by stretching aren't associated with just the muscle being stretched. The tendons and ligaments associated with that muscle, and even the joint controlled by that muscle, are at risk.

Flexibility

Flexibility refers to the relative range of motion in a joint. This is related to the high or low tension in the muscles around the joint, those that move or restrict the joint. The risk of injury is increased when joint flexibility is increased too much or is greatly diminished, or when imbalance in joint flexibility exists between left and right (or front and back) sides of the body.

When it comes to flexibility, don't assume more is better. There is a consensus among many health care professionals that the least flexible and the most flexible individuals are more likely to get injured compared to those whose joints had moderate flexibility.

Increased flexibility is best accomplished with a proper active aerobic warm-up, such as walking, rather than with stretching. Even patients with debilitating arthritis can improve flexibility with an easy aerobic warm-up of fifteen minutes, such as swimming or walking, and be as flexible as if they had stretched, without the risk.

Given the available scientific evidence that shows stretching may not help prevent injuries or enhance performance, why do people still stretch? In small numbers of serious athletes who require large ranges of flexibility—such as ballet dancers—stretching helps obtain a large range of motion in the joints. But if you're not intent on placing your foot over your head daily, this type of flexibility can greatly hurt you. For the average person who walks, works out out at the gym, runs, bikes, or swims, this kind of flexibility obtained by intense stretching is not recommended; it's unhealthy.

For decades, I've discussed the dangers of stretching, because it's not the best way to warm up and can cause injury. Yet sports medicine professionals and coaches often recommend stretching to athletes and weekend warriors. I first learned about the dangers of stretching in the mid-1970s, and by the early

THE EXCEPTIONS—THOSE WHO NEED MORE FLEXIBILITY

For those who require a wider-than-normal range of motion, proper stretching may be necessary. But these include professional athletes such as football players and ballet dancers—athletes who spend hours a day training. Confusion arises when studies show that these athletes benefit from stretching—but their needs can't be applied to most people who walk, jog, run, and even to endurance athletes such as marathoners and triathletes.

While football players, ballet dancers, martial arts competitors, some track-and-field athletes, and gymnasts may require higher-than-normal levels of flexibility, only by combining careful stretching following an aerobic warm-up will help increase their flexibility. However, with this high level of flexibility comes an increased risk for injury, and these athletes tend to require more physical maintenance from therapists to correct muscle problems as they're created during workouts and competitions. There's a fine line between getting adequate flexibility for walking or jogging and going beyond that point to participate in activities requiring wide ranges of motion such as ballet or football. This is one reason injury rates are high in these sports. I've also had numerous patients in a variety of these sports who did not stretch but were very successful and whose injury rates were much lower.

One of the common scenarios in these athletes is that they are either fully engaged in their activity or standing, resting, and waiting for the next bout of high-intensity activity. Such is the case in professional football players. They may require additional flexibility, which stretching can supply. But like the ballet dancer and gymnast, these athletes are more prone to injury.

In these rare situations, stretching should be a very slow, deliberate movement, where the athlete lightly stretches a muscle or muscle group and holds it statically for up to thirty seconds. While these stretching routines are often done cold—before an aerobic warm-up—they should not; they're best performed after an easy warm-up. Optimal static stretching requires that each muscle group be sequentially repeated three to four times. It also demands that the activity be done slowly and not rushed. Also note that an active static stretch can be safely accomplished by contracting the antagonist muscle, which is the one opposite you're stretching. So if you wanted to actively stretch the hamstring muscles, the quadriceps muscles are contracted, but without moving the hip or low back—just standing in place and tightening the quadriceps muscles will relax the hamstring.

These stretching routines should always be performed following an easy active warm-up of at least twelve to fifteen minutes or sometimes twice this time frame. And a stretching routine that is less risky will require significant care and, most importantly, time—in some cases, it could take an hour or more.

There's another factor to consider. Increases in flexibility obtained from stretching can be short-lived. Some studies show the effects of stretching last for only three minutes. While waiting to get into the game or start performing, the muscles recover from the stretch and return to their normal levels of tension. This is why many of these athletes are frequently stretching during their workouts and competition. This further increases the risk of injury from overstretching muscles.

One reason many professional athletes in sports like basketball or soccer are so vulnerable to injury is that their wide ranges of joint motion are quite unnatural. With intense stretching producing a high degree of flexibility comes a trade-off. A football player, for example, may be more agile from increased flexibility, but his sprint speed will be reduced.

1980s, with more clinical experience, I developed an even better perspective. By that time I had many hundreds of patients for comparison. Many were hikers, joggers, marathon runners, or those who regularly went to aerobics classes. Here's what I found: Those who stretched were often injured often stretched. But in those who did not stretch, injury rates were lower.

Clinicians who evaluated muscle function in athletes observed one outstanding factor: Stretching a muscle could make it longer, the reason it increases flexibility—and this resulted in a reduction in the muscle's function due to a loss of power. In other words,

stretching caused abnormal inhibition—a neurological name referring to a less-efficient longer moving muscle. There was a consensus on this issue by many, although certainly not all, clinicians.

Despite these notions, the tradition of stretching became a difficult one to break for millions of active people—performing it was as ritualistic as reading about the latest exercise equipment or the new diet fad.

Trying to rationalize against the strong tradition of stretching has not been easy. Despite personally having had great success training athletes who no longer stretched, as well as eliminating their injuries by recommending the avoidance of stretching, I was still met with resistance by coaches and those who attended my lectures or read my articles. To counter their arguments, I cited the hamstring muscles as a common example of the increased injury rate in stretchers versus non-stretchers. Studies now show that stretching does not make tight hamstrings less stiff. In fact, overstretching these muscles often contributes to injury. On occasion, a spirited but cordial debate would take place during a sports medicine conference or seminar with other health care professionals. These included various for- and against-stretching doctors citing published and unpublished studies and anecdotal observations.

The '80s saw a dramatic rise in the number of walkers, joggers, runners, and people going to gyms and workout classes. In addition, there were more athletes on university and college campuses, giving researchers what they needed: more test subjects for research. Studies began appearing in scientific journals that showed stretching not only did not reduce injuries or improved performance, but it could also actually cause injuries and reduce performance. But most of these studies were not reported in the general media, and people continued to stretch. The research is ongoing. For the most part, these carefully conducted human studies have continued to demonstrate that stretching decreases a muscle's force production capacity; in other words, it causes weakness and can be measured using electromyo-graphic equipment, dynamometers, or other standard research devices.

While many studies demonstrated that stretching a muscle could damage it, others showed how stretched muscles affected other parts of the body. One particular study, conducted by J. Cramer and colleagues from the Department of Kinesiology at the University of Texas in 2005, compared changes in muscles that were stretched and not stretched in the same person. It concluded that stretching one muscle can also impair another unstretched muscle. This can occur because the nervous system senses the weakness in the first muscle and compensates by impairing another. So by weakening a muscle through stretching, the brain and spinal cord may trigger other muscles that are not stretched to become weak as well. This can even occur in muscles of the left leg when those in the right leg are stretched.

Other studies demonstrated adverse effects on a number of physical abilities, often using younger college-aged individuals, in which stretching has been shown to cause a decline in muscle power, reduced sprinting ability, diminished vertical jump, and a lessening of endurance. Despite these studies, the tradition of stretching continues in related sports:

- Power activities such as weight lifting, wrestling, and boxing
- Track-and-field athletes who sprint and jump
- Basketball players who also jump and sprint

- Endurance sports such as running, biking, and swimming

While the studies show that these abnormal changes induced in a stretched muscle can last for an hour, some clinicians have demonstrated that stretching can cause prolonged muscle problems such as weakness that can last days and even weeks.

Confusion in the public arena of athletes and coaches arises when studies show that ranges of motion or flexibility improve with stretching. While an increased range of motion can occur with stretching, albeit temporarily, what are the negative side effects? One problem caused by stretching is that muscles become too loose, too long—weaker—thus allowing the associated joint to move in a wider range of motion. This increased range of motion and the accompanying flexibility can put more stress on the joint, which is no longer supported properly by the muscle. This is a recipe for injury.

Damaging a muscle through any means, including stretching, will obviously have an adverse affect on the effectiveness of moving posture—gait. A recent study published in 2010 by Jacob Wilson and colleagues from Florida State University showed that stretching resulted in poor running economy, increasing energy consumption, and decreasing performance. The study was performed on seasoned male endurance runners, average age twenty-five.

My recommendation for runners or just those who like walking has always been to include an active aerobic warm-up as part of each workout that lasts at least twelve to fifteen minutes. In other words, start out slow. If you are a runner, walk. Or if you are a cyclist, go slow in an easy gear. In addition to improving oxygen utilization, increased blood flow, greater lung capacity, and fat burning, it increases whole body flexibility in a safe way because you improve muscle function—a muscle that contracts and relaxes properly and is warmed up provides a greater range of motion. Stretching cannot do the same.

Judging from all the e-mails I received on my website after my antistretching article appeared in early 2011, it became apparent that my observations about stretching struck a positive chord with many. Some wrote how relieved they felt because they felt they needed to stretch but didn't feel right about doing it. More recreational and serious athletes, sports medicine professionals, and coaches are quietly changing sides in the stretching-versus-nonstretching debate.

Yoga versus Stretching

Those who seriously practice traditional yoga are sometimes offended by the notion that yoga is a type of stretching. Or that yoga and stretching are even in the same universe. Unfortunately, yoga has been Westernized. Many Americans rush from the stress of work to squeeze in a yoga class, stretch into a few

"BUT I DON'T FEEL WEAK WHEN I STRETCH . . ."

For most people, stretching does not usually feel bad—otherwise, the stretching trend would have died out years ago. Many people still claim that they don't feel weak after stretching. You won't immediately feel weakness or pain unless you over-stretch a muscle so much that you cause significant damage. In fact, if you create a weakness, it's usually asymptomatic—you don't feel it right away.

To better understand this issue, the concept of muscle imbalance is important. Muscle imbalance is the combination of abnormal tightness and weakness—when you have one, you usually have the other. This typically occurs in muscles with opposing function, such as in the hamstrings on the back of the thigh and the quad-riceps on the front of the thigh, or the anterior tibialis muscle on the front of the leg and those in the back of leg that include the gastrocnemius.

If you have muscle imbalance, you tend to feel the tightness but not the weak-ness. If you stretch a tight muscle, it may even result in that muscle feeling looser to you, or less tight. But in the process, you can further damage a weak muscle, or cause a new weakness.

Ultimately, the associated joint controlled by the muscles becomes painful. The joint often becomes inflamed because it's unable to move properly due to muscle imbalance. For example, the hip joint is controlled in part by both the hamstrings and quadriceps muscles, and when they are not balanced, the joint cannot move prop-erly, and inflammation can result.

In addition, stretching could also change pain patterns—in particular, stretching might mask muscle pain. Ian Shrier, MD, a past president of the Canadian Society of Sports Medicine, published a study in the *Clinical Journal of Sports Medicine* in 1999 titled "Stretching Before Exercise Does Not Reduce the Risk of Local Muscle Injury." Among his conclusions were that stretching can produce damage in muscles and can actually mask muscle pain. This may be due to stretching a muscle that's tight, giving the subjective feeling that something is better, when, in fact, the cause of the tight-ness (the weakness) remains.

The feeling many people have of tightness is often a secondary problem whose primary cause is from a muscle weakness—trying to reduce the tightness by stretching is treating the symptom and ignoring the cause. And it can worsen the weakness or create a new one.

In addition, stretching can perpetuate a vicious cycle. By inadvertently stretching a weak muscle (which is already weak and lengthened), an opposing muscle can get even tighter. An example of this occurs in the hamstrings—by continually stretching them, maintaining or even worsening the weakness, the quadriceps can get tighter and tighter. Even if you were to stretch the quadriceps, the cause of the imbalance is weakness of the hamstrings.

positions, dash back to their car, stopping for take-out food, get home to gulp down dinner, and then spend the evening watching TV.

Just the notion of "power yoga" is painful for those familiar with the holistic lifestyle in traditional yoga. This includes being relaxed and avoiding a stress-filled life—far from the notion of "power."

While I'm not a yoga expert, I am very familiar with its holistic teachings. Rather than stretching, the idea is to slowly obtain various whole body postures. This is very different from isolating a muscle group like the hamstrings and quickly stretching it. And yoga's body positions are only a part—actually a small part—of this discipline. Deep breathing, ethical behavior in society, moral obligation to one's self, and spiritual enlightenment are among other equally important aspects of the discipline of yoga.

Bob's Book on Stretching

For many years, people became familiar with Bob Anderson's decades-old classic book, *Stretching*. Some have said that stretching must be beneficial if this book sold so many copies. But the fact is, good marketing reaches people easier than good research. (If you go online to Amazon, you will find that there are over a hundred books on stretching written by many different authors, yet you will be hard-pressed to find a single "antistretching" book.)

I don't know Bob Anderson personally, but I'm sure he's probably a great guy who means well. However, I've seen many patients through the years who visited me with an injury and who brought in Bob's book to show me how they stretch. My first recommendation was usually to stop stretching because what they're doing is harmful, despite following his guidelines. His book is an example of being wedded to a tradition that's hard to break despite the new scientific research going against it. Now in its thirtieth year of being in print, *Stretching* is still going strong despite all the weak evidence to support it. In fact, the picture on the cover (someone lying on their side stretching the lower limb straight up over the head) is a great way to get injured. All I can say is this: Don't try this at home!

Stretching as Treatment

Many people want to know how common injuries, such as shin splints and iliotibial band tightness, to neck and shoulder tension and low-back problems, can be remedied without stretching. Since most mechanical problems are directly or indirectly due to muscle imbalance, addressing this cause of the problem is the short answer. In other words, most ligament, joint, and other physical ailments are usually secondary to muscle imbalance, which consists of a tight muscle and a loose one—you usually feel the tight one as tension or pain while its cause is a weak muscle. Treatment of these common problems must be directed at the cause—the weakness—not the tightness.

Fran, who would eventually become a patient, experienced chronic upper-back and hip pain for over ten years. Its onset was slow, without any trauma or injury, beginning when she was thirty-eight years old. It progressed to a very painful debilitation. In the two years before consulting with me, Fran took significant time off from her job as an office manager and most social activities due to pain. A variety of conservative therapies, including spinal manipulation and acupuncture, were tried with massage helping the most, but the relief was symptomatic in nature as the pain returned within a few days. One of her doctors gave her a stretching routine, which provided symptomatic relief, but if she did not stretch each day, the pain was there. More extreme treatment included a prescription from her medical doctor for a pain-relieving codeine drug, which made her tired and unable to carry on normal daily chores. Fran's doctor ultimately referred her to an orthopedic surgeon, who recommended an operation on her low back. This is when she consulted me.

My evaluation found that Fran had a significant number of muscles that were not balanced—a pattern of weak and tight ones typical of muscle imbalance. While the weak ones appeared to be causing many of her problems, the secondary tight muscles in her upper back and hip are were particularly painful to the touch and to even simple movements. Lying down was also accompanied by severe pain from a few painful tight muscles. (These tight muscles are often referred to as spasms.)

Chronic pain can be the start of a vicious cycle in the body. The pain can trigger other muscle problems, which in turn aggravates muscle tightness, causing more pain. In addition, the stress of this type of problem can wear down a person—energy is reduced leading to fatigue, stress hormones are elevated disturbing digestion, blood sugar, and sleep, with overall quality of life greatly diminished. This also can lead to significant mental and emotional disturbances. This was Fran's current condition.

My therapy was directed at balancing the abnormal muscles using various biofeedback techniques—the weak muscles were treated by physically stimulating them to contract better, and the tight muscles were left alone.

271

In addition, I asked Fran to stop all stretching. At first she was alarmed by what I said. So I explained that she was maintaining a vicious cycle and that by stretching her muscles, they would not return to optimal balance. Fortunately, within the first week of no stretching and after her first treatment, she began noticing reduction in pain, giving her hope that these procedures might resolve her chronic problem.

After three monthly visits, Fran showed about a 50 percent reduction in pain. In addition, her posture and gait were improved, she was sleeping better, her appetite returned, and her mental state appeared improved. This was the start of a positive cycle of benefits—her body was functioning better, which enabled it to self-correct many of its own problems.

At this point I recommended that Fran begin an easy walking routine. She started with twenty minutes each day and gradually progressed to forty-five minutes over the next month.

After another eight weeks and two more of the same types of treatments, Fran was about 80 percent better by her estimation. Oddly enough, she asked if she could start stretching again. The concept and image of stretching was well entrenched in her mind as a positive activity. But I convinced her that walking would provide adequate flexibility and that stretching would risk a return of the kinds of muscle problems that caused her chronic condition.

Eventually, Fran said she was completely better, with no pain, good energy, and regular walking. Several months later I got a call from Fran, who said the pains were returning and could she make an appointment. I asked what she was doing differently. Now back at a new job and busy with many home projects, Fran was taking a yoga class four times a week. She said it was difficult to fit into her schedule, but she was making the time to get to most of the classes. I asked her to stop the classes and avoid performing yoga at home as well and to call back in a week. She did and reported that before the week was up, the pains had disappeared. It was clear that rushing through her yoga routine was triggering muscle imbalance, and by stopping it, the body was able to make the proper corrections.

Another former patient of mine, Randy, in his late thirties, also had chronic back pain. He began each morning with ten minutes of stretching and then hopped on a bike for his daily hour-long outdoor ride. Even on days he didn't exercise, he stretched. Once on his bike, the first fifteen minutes was spent riding up steep hills from his house out of the valley. This usually made his chronic back pain feel better, only to have it return by midday and last until the next ride. This problem is what brought Randy to seek my care.

During our initial consultation, Randy indicated he also had chronic asthma, was tired from midafternoon until bedtime on most days, and over the past few years had gained about ten or twelve pounds. He recently had to buy new pants for the second time during this period, as his belly was getting bigger.

Randy said he always warmed up before exercise. When I asked what he did to warm up, he said stretching.

Among the evaluations I performed was testing Randy's muscles, which showed that the hamstrings were overstretched and weak. I explained that this was most likely a cause of low-back muscle tightness that was secondary, but very painful.

Randy said that must mean "I'm going to suggest strengthening exercises for the hamstrings." Instead, after explaining that the kind of weakness he had was not the lack of power type problem common due to inactivity, my first recommendation was to stop stretching his already-overstretched hamstrings. My next piece of advice was to use a heart rate monitor.

When he first used a heart monitor, his rate surged to 185 within five minutes. Randy couldn't imagine how any of that was related to his chronic low-back pain. As instructed, he now had the difficult task of adjusting his morning ride to include an active aerobic warm-up and to avoid going directly to the hills, with the resultant high heart rate. The solution was for Randy to warm up by riding his indoor bike for about fifteen minutes before going outside and then riding very slowly until getting past the hills. And to avoid stretching.

After the first week, both his back pain and his chronic asthma disappeared. Within a month, his energy was greatly improved, and over the next two months Randy would lose almost two inches on his waist and had to buy new pants.

Most traditions are not easy to break. That's especially true with stretching. By following the common guidelines I've recommended, you'll become sufficiently flexible for your particular physical needs without risking muscle damage or other injuries. Avoid the peer pressure and temptation of joining others who stretch at the health club, group walk, or other places where many people can be found stretching. Just as important is to discipline yourself to perform an easy, active warm-up for at least twelve to fifteen minutes. Those who still don't feel sufficiently loose after this time period usually require more warm-up time. Likewise for a proper cooldown—it will help your muscles recover from the workout and be better prepared for the next exercise routine. In addition, being fit and healthy overall will significantly help your muscles stay balanced while further providing adequate flexibility.

CHAPTER 16

THE FEET ARE YOUR BODY'S FOUNDATION

G alileo was said to have dropped two objects of different weights from the *Torre pendente di Pisa*—the Leaning Tower of Pisa—to prove his new theory that all objects fall at the same rate regardless of how much they weigh. In 1971, Apollo astronaut David Scott retested this theory from the moon's surface by dropping a hammer and a feather at the same time. While the moon's gravity is weaker than that of the earth, the objects still fell about the same rate, albeit slower, hitting the lunar ground together.

While Galileo's use of the Leaning Tower for his research is probably a myth, he did develop the theory of objects falling at the same rate. But the Tower of Pisa is truly leaning because of the weak shifting soil and the building's weak structural foundation; and the Apollo astronaut actually performed the gravity experiment, but mostly for NASA publicity.

The eight-story Pisa Tower, whose initial construction began in the twelfth century, began falling at some point during the building of its third story. This was due to a shallow foundation of only about ten feet of unstable subsoil. For centuries, preventing the building's fall would be a topic of debate, study, and attempts at correcting the cause of the problem—and the focus was directed toward its faulty foundation. By 2008, after hundreds of tons of earth removal and other careful attempts at replacing and reconstructing the groundwork, architects and engineers finally said the tower's unstable foundation was safe for the first time in history, at least for the next two hundred years. But the tower still lists at just under four degrees.

The human body can be a lot like the Leaning Tower: unstable and with a weak foundation. And the body's foundation begins with the feet. This means healthy, fit feet that can tolerate the downward pull of gravity, with muscles that are balanced, strong bones, good circulation, proper nerve activity that communicates with the brain, and other attributes including regular movement.

The feet must last a lifetime. The more you understand about the feet, the better you can care for them and even fix them when their function goes astray. The feet are subjected to more wear and tear than any other body part. Just walking a mile, you generate more than sixty tons—that's over 120,000 pounds—of stress on each foot! Fortunately, and what's even more amazing, our feet are actually made to handle such natural stress. It's only when we interfere with nature that problems arise. Almost all foot problems can be prevented, and those that do arise can most often be treated conservatively through self-care.

From birth until death, your feet have a strategically important role in health and fitness. But too often, they become one of the most neglected parts of the body. If the feet lose their support—poor muscle function affecting the arches is a common affliction—the body can lean just like the Leaning Tower of Pisa, which in turn can lead to knee and hip problems, low-back pain, spinal dysfunc-

tion, and other physical impairments. And an imbalanced body is more prone to tripping and falling down.

Your feet form the base of the body's physical structure, and any departure from optimal balance can have significant adverse effects not only locally in the feet but for the entire body. These problems are often transmitted through the ankle, an extension of the upper part of the foot. Anatomists technically consider the foot and ankle as two separate areas, but I consider the ankle as a vital part of the foot for ease of discussion. The ankle is a vulnerable area; approximately twenty-five thousand Americans sprain their ankle each day. And probably many more develop at least one unstable foot and ankle.

The body's skeleton is a critical element of one's structural integrity because the muscles attach to bones, allowing one to move properly. The same is true with the bones of the foot—muscle function is a key part of its fitness and health. The early stages of most foot problems are usually secondary to muscle imbalance. Trauma can cause injury to any component of the foot, including a muscle, bone, ligament, tendon, or joint.

Another important job of the feet is to help balance the whole body. The feet continuously communicate with the brain to regulate the rest of the body's daily movements, including standing, walking, and running, and even riding a bike. This is accomplished by powerful nerve endings at the bottom of your feet. These nerve endings are developed from infancy, and their function is necessary

275

throughout your life. Disturbances of these nerve endings due to trauma, disease, poor footwear, or neglect can lead to further health concerns.

The nerve endings at the bottoms of your feet also become a potential source of powerful therapy when properly and specifically stimulated. This approach can be used both preventatively and after some injury is realized. For example, a simple foot massage, even by an untrained person, can be great for your feet and brain because these nerve endings—also the reason it feels so good—are gently stimulated.

While many problems in the body are the result of either obvious or hidden foot imbalances, some foot problems themselves are secondary to more primary disorders. When this happens, these secondary foot problems can, in turn, cause other problems with the body—just like tumbling dominoes. Examples of problems that cause secondary foot dysfunction include structural faults in the spine and pelvis, muscle imbalance, trauma, shoes that don't properly fit, oversupported shoes and those with higher heels, and certain diseases such as diabetes, peripheral vascular disease, neuropathy, inflammation, and arthritis.

Foot problems are very common. And the most typical complaint about the foot is pain. When pain presents in specific areas of the foot, it most often indicates the source of the problem. For example, pain at the top of the foot may indicate a midfoot fracture, although there may be other causes of this type of pain, including tying your shoelaces too tight.

Many foot problems lead to inactivity. Reductions in the level of one's activity can make anyone get out of shape fast; it can also lead to changes in metabolism leading to weight gain, circulatory insufficiency, muscle loss, poor coordination, and other more serious disabilities.

In terms of structure and biomechanics, improper shoes of any type—from dress and casual to all sports types—can alter how the muscles and joints function, not only in the foot but in the leg. For example, ill-fitting footwear can affect the muscles around the knee; the knee joint may move improperly. When this irregular movement continues, the result is some type of knee injury, usually associated with pain.

Foot Anatomy Made Simple

In order to truly understand your feet, it's important to be familiar with the basic aspects of the foot's anatomy—bones, muscles, ligaments, tendons, and other physical aspects. There's really nothing simple about the human foot. It's one of the most incredible and complex bioengineered parts of your anatomy. It combines power and speed with delicate movement and balance, solid stability with acute sensitivity, and the foot has sufficient endurance to take you almost anywhere you want to go throughout your entire lifetime.

The growth of the human foot comes in spurts. During your first ten years, foot growth

276

ARE YOUR FOOT SENSE AND K SENSE BOTH OKAY?

We're all familiar with the sense of smell, taste, and sight. Foot sense is not as well-known but is equally important. If you step on a small sharp object—a rock, acorn, or piece of glass—while barefoot, the body reacts immediately by contracting certain muscles that lift the foot off the ground. Likewise, a painful tiny blister is easily noticed, more so each time you take a step on that foot. Each time the foot strikes the ground, the force of impact through the joints (in the feet, knees, hips, and spine) can be many times greater than the body weight. Usually, this is not a problem because the body is made for this activity, through several million years of evolutionary adaptation, thanks in part to foot sense. Instead of walking on all fours, man became bipedal.

Foot sense is the result of millions of nerve endings at work throughout your feet. They're found mostly in muscles, with the skin, ligaments, and joints containing some. These nerves sense tension, movement, force, pressure, and even temperature. The foot is one of the most nerve-active areas of the body. If you happened to study the structure and function of the foot, such as in an anatomy and physiology class, you would know that the precise scientific word for "foot sense" is "proprioception," which comes from the Latin *proprius*, meaning "one's own" and "perception." Proprioception refers to the sense of the relative position of neighboring parts of the whole body. It's proprioception that allows the brain to adjust the posture and gait to uneven ground, or limp when the big toe hurts.

The foot automatically senses information about ground contact with each and every step. With this data, your brain responds accordingly. That blister might force you to adjust your gait to a limp to alleviate the foot pain. It's also why the tiniest pebble lodged inside a shoe or sock will cause discomfort until you stop, remove the shoe or sock, and get rid of the nuisance once and for all.

As the feet's nerve endings send important information—regarding the foot's movement, tension, pressure—to the spinal cord and brain, it allows the whole body to respond to foot sense. This bodywide activity is called kinesthetic or K sense. "Kinesthetic" comes from Greek *kinein*, or "motion," and *aisthēsis*, or "perception," and refers to any of the body's physical processes by which stimuli are received, transmitted, and interpreted to the brain.

Because of K sense, you don't have to look down to see the position of your foot because your brain automatically "senses" its location. The same is true with the sense of movement—one doesn't have to look at each and every footstep one takes or watch every arm and leg movement in order to walk or run effectively. The brain already knows what's going on because sensations from the feet (and actually, throughout the body) tell it so.

K sense can also be observed while balancing on one foot. The brain interprets incoming messages from the foot one's balancing on and sends back messages to muscles throughout the body to continuously adjust the posture to keep from falling. These movements may include tilting the head, moving the arms up and down, or whatever is necessary to keep balanced. In fact, every step you take relies on K sense.

Muscle imbalance is a common occurrence and a frequent cause of poor foot sense, leading to distorted K sense and increased vulnerability to injury, poor posture, and irregular gait. So are diseases and infections that affect the muscles and skin. The resulting irregular running or even walking gait from a distorted K sense requires expending significantly more energy, which leads to increased fatigue and slowing down.

Hard exercise that results in muscle fatigue—a common outcome of anaerobic training including weight lifting—also can disturb K sense. The result is distorted posture and gait until recovery occurs. During this time, one is more vulnerable to injury.

You can use foot sense and K sense to your advantage as daily therapy. Because the nerves in the feet dramatically affect foot muscles and balance, and communicate with the brain, stimulating them during normal foot movement can excite and improve foot sense. This can be extremely helpful for the whole body, even when performed for relatively short periods. This is a key benefit of being barefoot—the most natural of all positions for the foot. It not only improves foot sense but produces full-body benefits by improving K sense. The result can be better muscle balance, improved posture, and more efficient gait.

Barefoot therapy can be done with almost anyone of any age, and for ten to fifteen minutes per day. You don't need to run a marathon or 10K barefoot. Just walk around the house, yard, or neighborhood to experience the benefits of going unshod.

You can also train and improve K sense by spending a little time each day balancing on one foot, such as when drying your feet after a shower or lacing up your shoes.

The relationship between reduced foot sense and poor K sense is actually nothing new, and its contribution to injury has been understood in scientific circles for decades. While the feet are your body's physical foundation or mobile platform, the more than thirty muscles of each foot provide movement and stability for not only the foot itself but indirectly for the entire body. The muscles give the foot its shape by holding the bones in position. In fact, a foot's various arches are dependent upon muscle function.

Much of the foot support comes from muscles that attach higher up in the leg, with tendons coming down into and attaching on various bones of the foot. Many other muscles are exclusively found within the foot itself.

Equally important is the fact that all these muscles, with their vast networks of nerve endings, provide the primary source of neurological information contributing to foot sense and K sense. "Proprioceptive dysfunction" is a term referring to muscle imbalance that distorts K sense.

Even though the muscles play the primary role in K sense, the skin on the foot provides a critical tactile sensation. Wearing shoes that are too tight that rub the skin in certain areas or otherwise don't fit perfectly can disturb the delicate sense mechanisms in the skin, interfering with normal foot sense and therefore K sense. Even socks that are too tight can cause these problems too. (Many long-distance runners choose not to wear socks—I have avoided them for years most of the time when wearing sports shoes. Because my feet are healthy and my shoes fit well, I don't get blisters or other irritations.

It's easy to see that hiking on a rocky trail requires good K sense. With the uneven terrain, rocks and roots to maneuver over and around, the body should easily and automatically compensate. Yet some people don't, and they tend to trip and stumble more than others who are nimble and sure-footed as they seem to glide over uneven terrain.

Even everyday activity can be an obstacle course for the feet. If you're walking through a crowded restaurant dining room to get to your table, you may have to squeeze past chairs, people, other tables, and perhaps even navigate your way across a wet, slippery floor. You rely on our natural K sense to do this, and the process begins with good foot sense. Those who spend all day in thick-sole shoes or who have worn thick-tread running shoes over the years will have significantly reduced foot sense and therefore K sense, and will need to look down and around to keep from colliding into a chair, table, or person. But with properly functioning K sense, you won't have this problem or most of the other common foot troubles.

Taking care of your feet will keep K sense working at its best throughout the body. This includes spending time barefoot, alternately balancing on one foot, and avoiding shoes and socks that don't optimally match your feet.

averages about one-half inch a year. Between the ages of ten and twenty, the yearly growth rate slows down considerably, with maturity of growth arriving around age twenty. However, the foot still gets larger with age. Throughout an adult's life, it's not unusual for the foot to increase two or more sizes. This is not true growth but a spreading of the foot—often making it wider and longer—due to physical and metabolic changes. For example, body weight, pregnancy, training, lifestyle, and shoe wear all could influence the foot to increase in size. If you don't keep up with foot changes, your shoes may become too tight, which can cause muscle, joint, ligament, and even circulation problems.

At any stage of one's physical development, incorrect posture, poor walking, running and other exercise habits, and improper footwear can also significantly disturb foot muscle function, joint alignment, and the structure of the bones themselves.

The basic anatomy of the foot, like the rest of the body, often has variations in its structures—we're not all exact replicas. But these variations are well adapted for by the muscles. The same is true between the left and right foot. Variations are common, including foot length, which can differ by a whole shoe size or more.

Bones

At birth, the bones in your feet are undeveloped—there is actually just one bone, with the remainder made up of a softer material called cartilage. By the time you are three years of age, much of the cartilage has become bone, and by age six all twenty-eight bones have taken shape but are still partly composed of cartilage. Even in an adult, some cartilage remains. About a quarter of the body's bones are located in the feet. During the developmental stage, interfering with natural foot development can severely impact foot function later in life. For convenience, anatomists divide the foot into three main parts: the forefoot, midfoot, and hindfoot.

- The forefoot bears about half the body's weight, with the ball of the foot (between the big toe and the rest of the foot) responsible for much of your balance. The four smaller toes are made up of three small bones each, called phalanges. The big toe (the hallux) has only two bones (phalanges). Under the big toe are two very small round sesamoid bones within a tendon. The bones of the toes are connected to the longer metatarsal bones that connect to the rest of the foot.

- The midfoot has five irregularly shaped bones, which, with support from the muscles, form the foot's characteristic arches. It is here that much of the foot's natural ability to absorb shock takes place. The bones that connect to the metatarsals are called the first, second, and third cuneiform bones, and the cuboid bone. Behind these sits the navicular bone.

- The hindfoot contains the talus bone (the ankle), which connects the foot to the two long bones of the leg—the smaller fibula on the outside and the main leg bone, the

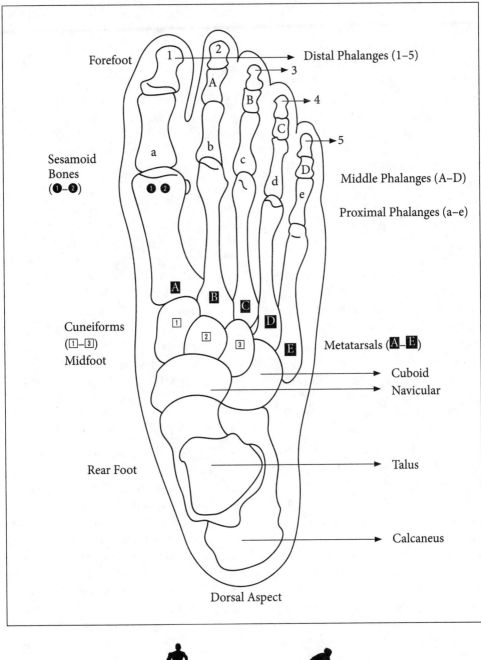

Forefoot

Distal Phalanges (1–5)

Sesamoid
Bones
(❶–❷)

Middle Phalanges (A–D)

Proximal Phalanges (a–e)

Cuneiforms
(▣–▣)
Midfoot

Metatarsals (Ⓐ–Ⓔ)

Cuboid

Navicular

Rear Foot

Talus

Calcaneus

Dorsal Aspect

tibia. The talus bone is also connected to and rests on the calcaneus bone (the heel), the largest bone of the foot, which assists in stability during movement and standing. In the back of the foot, the calcaneus bone is supported by the large Achilles tendon.

In some individuals, small extra bones called accessory ossicles may exist throughout the foot. In addition, there may be extra sesamoid bones, which are also small. When present, these extra bones don't inherently pose any particular problem.

Joints

When two bones come together, they form a joint, which allows smooth movement—flexibility—between the bones. Each bone has a softer articular cartilage at its joint end for protection. Joints are surrounded by a cover, the articular capsule, which contains a thick lubricating liquid called synovial fluid. The joints and cartilage cushion the bones and protect them from making direct contact.

The foot has some thirty-three joints. Coordination occurs with the help of more than one hundred ligaments, which connect bones to bones, tendons, which connect muscles to bones, and muscles. The bones provide a solid foundation and leverage for muscles to move the body. Perhaps most joint problems are due to muscle dysfunction associated with the joint. For example, muscle imbalance typically causes poor joint movement leading to joint dysfunction and pain. While reading about the muscles below, note that the bones and joints are supported by these muscles.

Muscles

The foot relies on more than thirty muscles and tendons for motion and stability—not only in the foot itself but indirectly in areas above the foot. The muscles give the foot its shape by holding the bones in position. Without muscle support, the skeleton and all its bones would collapse. Much of the foot support comes from muscles that attach higher up in the leg, with tendons coming down into and attaching to bones of the foot. Many other important muscles are exclusively found within the foot itself.

All the muscles of the foot, ankle, and leg play a vital role in foot movements. Because of the extensive nature of the structure and function of all these muscles, this discussion will be limited to only the most important muscles and muscle groups.

Tibialis Posterior Muscle

This long muscle attaches to the two leg bones—the tibia and fibula—in the middle of the back calf under the large gastrocnemius and soleus muscles (just below the knee). The tibialis posterior muscle runs down the back of the leg around the inside of the ankle (the medial side) and into the bottom of the foot, inserting into different bones. Contracting this muscle allows you to point your foot down (an action called plantar flexion). It also turns the foot inward. The ability to rise on your toes also requires the function of the tibialis posterior muscle.

The tibialis posterior is one of the most important muscles associated with many foot, ankle, and knee problems. It's a key stabilizing muscle for the fore-, mid-, and hindfoot. When this muscle does not work properly, it can cause a variety of nonspecific symptoms, which can be difficult to diagnose unless the muscle is properly evaluated.

Because of its importance in supporting the medial arch, abnormal inhibition or "weakness" of this muscle, perhaps its most common problem, causes poor arch support that can lead to excess pronation and other problems. Secondary to tibialis posterior inhibition is often tightness of the gastrocnemius and/or soleus muscles, and sometimes pain in the Achilles tendon.

Tibialis Anterior Muscle

The tibialis anterior is also a long muscle and attaches predominantly on the upper half of the tibia on the front of the leg (and slightly to the outside) just below the knee, where it is easily felt as a relatively large mass. It runs downward and becomes a large tendon crossing the ankle, easily visible when lifting the foot. It continues below the ankle and attaches into the first metatarsal bone and the first cuneiform bone.

The tibialis anterior muscle raises the foot upward (an action called dorsal flexion) and assists in turning the foot inward. Like the tibialis posterior, when inhibited (weak), it can cause instability of the ankle and may

be responsible for problems in the first metatarsal joint. It may also be a common cause of so-called shin splints, although the posterior tibialis is also commonly involved.

Peroneus Muscles

The peroneus longus and brevis muscles attach mostly on the fibula on the outside, or lateral side, of the leg, with some parts attached to the tibia. These muscles become a tendon just above the ankle and can be seen just behind the bony end of the fibula (called the lateral malleolus)—the bony protuberance of the outside ankle—where it attaches to the ankle. The longus portion of the peroneus attaches into the cuneiform bone and the first metatarsal bone, with the brevis attaching to the fifth metatarsal bone.

The peroneus longus and brevis muscles stabilize the outside of the ankle, allowing the outer foot to elevate or evert while the ankle is plantar flexed (foot pointed down). If you try to contract this muscle by pointing your foot down and out, you can easily see and feel it on the outside of the leg.

The peroneus tertius muscle is a much shorter but important muscle that also stabilizes the outside of the ankle. This muscle attaches on the lower portion of the fibula bone on the outside of the ankle and inserts into the fifth metatarsal bone. It allows the outside of the foot to turn upward with the ankle. This muscle is often involved in common ankle sprains and, if it does not heal properly after trauma, can help maintain a chronic ankle problem.

Gastrocnemius and Soleus Muscles

The bulk of calf muscle on the back of the leg is made up of the gastrocnemius and soleus muscles. Together, these two muscles are sometimes referred to as the triceps surae. They attach into the upper leg bones and, in part, above the knee into the back of the thigh bone, the femur. These muscles are important for rising on our toes during any movement. These two muscles form the Achilles tendon beginning at about the middle of the calf. This tendon runs downward and attaches into the back of the calcaneus bone. Both the muscles and the Achilles tendon provide great support for the foot through stability of the heel.

Plantar Muscles

There are four layers of muscles on the bottom of the foot consisting of a dozen separate muscles. Overall, these have grabbing actions important for walking, running, foot coordination, and balance. These actions are best observed when barefoot. Wearing shoes can render these and other foot muscles less active and could lead to chronic foot problems. Walking and moving while barefoot improves these and other foot and leg muscle functions.

Foot Arches

As a means of supporting the weight of the body, for shock absorption and propulsion, and adapting to uneven surfaces and other functions, the bottom of the foot is constructed of a series of arches. Muscles are the key factor in supporting these arches, and maintaining them is vital for normal foot function. Interfering with the normal function of the arches, such as by wearing shoes that don't fit or properly match your feet, especially those with so-called arch supports, can often interfere with and disturb the natural action of the muscles that support them.

The medial arch is one of the two large arches and is the one familiar to most people. It runs along the inner aspect of the bottom of the foot. A side view of the bones of the foot (without supporting muscles) clearly shows the magnitude of the medial arch. This arch is maintained by the action of the muscles, especially the tibialis posterior.

The lateral longitudinal arch is the second largest arch and runs along the outside of the bottom of the foot. The transverse or metatarsal arches are in the midfoot across the ball of the foot, and the short longitudinal arches are in the hindfoot. The peroneus longus and brevis and plantar muscles on the bottom of the foot support these arches.

Other Foot Structures

Many other structures in the foot support its actions and maintain foot health. These include fascia, nerves, skin, and blood vessels.

Fascia

Throughout the foot (as throughout the body) are thin yet strong fibrous sheaths called fascia that assists in stabilizing the foot, especially in areas of the joints, and act to bind the tendons, helping the muscles in

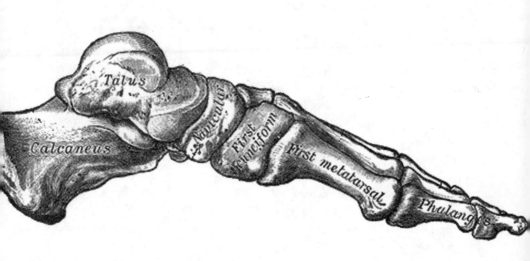

their supporting efforts. The fascia blends with many other soft tissues of the foot and ankle. Important fascia is found on the top of the foot (the dorsal fascia), on the bottom of the foot (the plantar fascia), and around the ankle.

NERVES

Within the muscles, tendons, ligaments, joints, and other soft tissues of the foot are important nerve endings that sense all movement, pressure, and body position. This information is sent along the central nervous system (up the spinal cord and all the way to the brain), so one can respond appropriately to activity affecting the foot. Pain fibers are located in most structures of the foot, including the covering of the bones. Pain is also relayed from the feet to the brain through the nerves. During injury, the intensity of the pain does not necessarily relate to the severity of injury, as sometimes a relatively minor injury can elicit great pain because of the foot's high level of sensitivity.

SKIN, NAILS, AND BLOOD VESSELS

In many ways, the quality of the skin, nails, and blood vessels in and on the foot is a general reflection of an individual's overall health. These areas, like all others within the foot that are not as noticeable, are greatly influenced by diet and nutrition, stress, the brain, and level of exercise.

The skin is obviously important for normal foot function. It protects the structures inside the foot, is an important site for nerve endings, and cushions the foot with the help of a fat pad under the calcaneal (heel) bone.

The skin contains many nerve endings for foot sense, especially on the bottom of the foot. The sole is very durable and can withstand many more pounds of force compared to the hand and fingers before it is cut open. When the skin is subject to chronic stress, such as excessive wear and tear, calluses develop due to a thickening of the skin.

Calluses are almost always caused by shoes that don't perfectly match the needs of your feet. They typically occur over a bony prominence. A callus that forms on a toe is called a corn. Calluses are usually not painful except certain types that are usually on the bottom of the foot. These may be plantar keratoses, or seed calluses, and are quite small. Some calluses put enough pressure on the metatarsal joints to cause pain in the joint. Calluses can usually be differentiated from warts by pinching both sides together—warts are generally tender and calluses are usually not, with the rare exception noted above.

Toe deformities are also indications of poor foot health, typically from wearing ill-fitting shoes for months and years. A hammertoe is a deformity of the joints and bone, typically of the second, third, or fourth toe, causing it to be permanently bent like a hammer. A bunion, also called hallux valgus, is a chronic swelling and enlargement of the first metatarsal joint of the big toe, which can be painful, and makes finding the best-fitting shoes more difficult.

Toenails are adversely affected by trauma, most often by tight shoes. An ingrown toenail usually occurs in the big toe due to either poor-fitting shoes or improper nail trimming, or both. This problem can lead to fungal or bacterial infections.

Another problem found in toenails is the so-called blackened nail. This problem is common in runners and cyclists but those who wear shoes that are too snug. A blackened toenail is usually due to trauma directly on the nail, which darkens from bruising (from breaking of the small blood vessels under the nail). The nail may ultimately fall off. Some dark toenails are also due to chronic fungal infections.

Blood vessels are critical for good foot health. The arteries bring nutrient-rich blood into the foot in the form of glucose, fat, protein, vitamins, minerals, and oxygen. The veins carry blood back to the heart and remove carbon dioxide, excess water, and waste products from the foot. Poor blood flow can be due to poor muscle function or abnormally narrowed or closed blood vessels, often seen in early disease conditions. This can cause or aggravate existing foot problems from within. Improper, restricted blood flow can also cause skin ulceration, which is common in diabetics.

Foot Posture and Movement

When your feet are healthy and fit—with balanced muscles, good circulation, and no distortions—your movement, whether walking, jogging, running, is accomplished most efficiently. This means wear and tear is minimal, as is the energy requirement to keep the feet moving. Any deviation from normal posture and movement causes more wear and tear not only in the foot but also in the ankle, knee, hip, pelvis, and spine. It also causes you to expend more energy on movement—in some cases significantly a lot more. Abnormal foot movement can cause a variety of muscles to overcompensate, adapting in the ankle and knee and resulting in off-balance movement of both joints and related muscles. Foot imbalance can have a negative impact on the knees, hips, pelvis, and spine, and even areas such as the shoulders and all the way to the head.

NORMAL FOOT MOTIONS

The foot has a variety of normal movements. The toes can flex, which curls them downward, and extend, bringing them upward. They have slight movement from side to side—seen in spreading the toes and squeezing them together. These actions can make excellent exercises for those who need to rehabilitate their foot muscles. If you're unable to squeeze or spread your toes, it may indicate poor muscle function and only rarely more serious problems.

INVERSION AND EVERSION

The foot can rotate inward and outward. The inward rotation is called inversion and results in the sole of the foot turning inward. The muscles that accomplish this are the tibialis posterior and anterior. The outward rotation is called eversion, and the sole of the foot is turned out. The peroneus muscles are important for eversion.

The movement of inversion and eversion takes place in the joints between the talus and the calcaneus bones. Pain during these specific movements may indicate a problem with the talus and the muscles that support it, typically the tibialis posterior and sometimes tibialis anterior.

GAIT

The act of moving, such as walking or running, is termed "gait." While the stress on feet can vary, healthy bare feet are made to endure this stress. A full phase of a normal walking gait includes the point your heel strikes the ground, through rolling your foot forward, to lifting and pushing off your toes, to swinging your foot forward to strike the ground again. During this normal gait, the foot makes many adaptations. It can effectively adjust to any uneven surface, become rigid enough to propel itself and roll over the big toe, go through various ranges of motion, and effectively absorb shock. This is accomplished by the actions of muscles, with support from ligaments, tendons, fascia, and bones.

A running gait is similar to walking with some exceptions—especially in the heel. Running should not include landing on your heel but rather farther forward such as midfoot. Runners who land on their heel often do so because of poor foot sense due to the types of shoes worn. To experience a normal running gait, take off your shoes and jog across the room or down the hall. This will usually cause you to land not on your heels but midfoot (or forefoot)—runners who land on their heels often create muscle and joint stress often leading to an injury. See chapter 18 for a full discussion on gait.

PRONATION AND SUPINATION

During walking and running, pronation and supination normally occur in the foot. Pronation is important for optimal movement and shock absorption. During foot strike, many changes take place—the foot begins to roll inward, everting slightly, and the arch flattens. This is called pronation. It is a normal action—one that occurs in every step in every healthy foot. The purpose of this is to loosen the foot so it can adapt to the surface, especially on uneven terrain.

Following pronation, as the foot continues through its gait, supination occurs. This results in the foot turning slightly outward then changing from a flexible foot to becoming rigid so it can propel the foot and push off from the ground. During this phase, the foot inverts slightly, and the arches become higher, thus enabling the foot to properly roll over the big toe.

A number of factors can disrupt a person's normal gait. The two most common reasons are muscle imbalance and wearing stiff, oversupported shoes. Sometimes, areas above the foot, such as the pelvis or spine, can abnormally influence foot function. For example, too little or too much hip rotation can cause the foot to land in an abnormal position. In addition, injury, pain, and other problems that affect blood flow cause inflammation, or disturb muscle function in the foot, which can abnormally alter the gait.

Most shoes change the gait by causing the stride length to become abnormally longer.

This causes an abnormal heel strike—hitting the ground farther back on the heel. It's especially a problem during running, as the longer stride places more shock through the foot and into the knee, and occurs despite shoe cushioning or what is commonly called a "heel crash pad." Barefoot movement does not cause the same stress.

The notion that some people are "pronators" while others are "supinators" is a gross oversimplification that fitness magazines, shoe stores, and footwear manufacturers foist upon the public in an attempt to sell shoes. It's mostly all marketing hype. Everyone pronates and supinates. The reason some people excessively pronate or supinate is more often from wearing oversupported shoes, which causes muscle imbalance. This is especially a problem in children whose feet need to properly develop without shoes.

More importantly, an attempt to "help" a poorly functioning foot with a particular type of shoe or orthotic insert is an example of treating symptoms; most cases of foot dysfunction are usually due to muscle imbalance. Keeping the foot in a rigid, immobile position can actually promote foot imbalance by not allowing the body to naturally correct the problem.

Your feet were made for walking, running, hopping, jumping, and all other natural movements. When you interfere with the movement, such as when you wear shoes, problems can arise. Humans evolved barefoot. For several million years, human feet were free. The first shoes are only about ten thousand years old and were made from cured animal skins. While sandals have been around for at least half that time, only in the past few hundred years have we seen the modern shoe come into its own: stiff soles and uppers that force the foot into an unnatural position. Fashion trends, not comfort, dictate what is popularly worn. How else can we explain why high heels for women continue to be so trendy; yet a shoe with a four-inch narrow heel is forcing the body to put all its weight on a small, concentrated area of the foot, and which can contribute to a series of cascading problems, ranging from bunions to lower-back pain.

Two Types of Foot Problems

Broadly speaking, there are just two types of foot problems. The first, asymptomatic ones, don't elicit pain but are silent in their impairment. Most are due to subtle muscle imbalance in the foot, although muscle dysfunction in the leg, pelvis, or spine can also be a factor. Virtually everyone has subtle muscle imbalance due to normal wear and tear from movement, inactivity, and wearing shoes that don't properly match the needs of the foot. Normally, the stress from exercise and a nine-to-five daily lifestyle is easily corrected by a healthy body with recovery—rest allows the correction of these problems quickly and naturally.

However, sometimes the body does not correct these problems, and they become chronic. This could be due to insufficient rest but more often is caused by poor shoe fit or oversupported shoes. When this happens, a significant imbalance can occur, leading to symptomatic foot problems, such as pain and localized tenderness, to numbness or tingling, weakness, and reduced range of motion in the form of stiffness or limitation in movement. These symptoms indicate that some aspect of the foot or ankle is not working properly and may even lead to further imbalances. Symptomatic problems are usually obvious and may be due to a variety of causes, including three common ones: chronic muscle inhibition, trauma, and disease.

Trauma

More serious trauma can cause fracture, serious laceration, or crushing injury. Ankle sprains, for example, are sometimes due to a preexisting foot dysfunction, typically aggravated by improper footwear such as thick-soled sports shoes or high-top sneakers. The most popular shoe in this category is the basketball sneaker. Plain high-top sneakers were popular for many years, but today they have become fancy oversupported, overpriced shoes. Many nonathletes wear them too. Supposedly, the additional ankle support, which is one of the shoe's main selling features, is thought to protect against ankle sprain. But studies don't verify this. Actually, these shoes can do just the opposite, as basketball players may have the highest rates of ankle sprains of any sport. When the ankle or any area of the body is supported, you run the risk of weakening that area. This is the result of muscles, tendons, and ligaments that sense the support and no longer have to work as much; the result is loss of some of their strength. An ankle sprain typically includes damage to the lateral collateral ligaments on the outside of the foot, but at other times different structures may be damaged such as the tendon, local joints or bones, or even nerves. But in almost all cases, muscle imbalance occurs as well, and many of these muscles stay chronically inhibited, slowing recovery time, maintaining pain, and often allowing a recurrence of ankle sprain. In fact, the majority of athletes who sprain their ankle will do so again.

If you sprain your ankle and rule out serious injury, such as fracture, the area should heal relatively fast. Pain that does not diminish or is almost eliminated within a few days or a week of injury may also be associated with muscle inhibition that has not been corrected or compensated for by the body. Many traumatic injuries will recover significantly faster when normal muscle function is restored as quickly as possible.

THE FEAR OF TRIPPING AND FALLING

Many people, including seniors, are not the same after a bad fall. It's often the start of a downward spiral set of related problems—the fall causes a knee bruise and pain, which produces weakness in the leg, and eventually, low-back pain shows up and then spinal discomfort in the middle and upper back. It can be exhausting—physically, mentally, and emotionally. Too often, a bone fracture because bone density was poor or preexisting muscle imbalance was significant.

Poor function in the feet is one of the common causes of falling at any age. When the feet don't work well, there's usually associated muscle imbalance, poor posture, and distorted gait—all of which further the risk of a fall. You don't have to be a daredevil like a rock climber or downhill speed skier to fall. You can trip over a curb that is only several inches high and still get badly injured.

Reduced brain function also predisposes one to the likelihood of someday falling, even in people without severe cognitive or other physical problems. Those most vulnerable are people who have difficulty multitasking. For the distracted brain, the competing chores of thinking about sending an e-mail to a friend, whether one has enough spinach for that favorite fish dinner tonight, and walking down to the basement freezer sometimes is too much to handle, and the risk of stumbling or falling down increases.

Each year, millions of people fall. The problem is worse in those ages sixty-five and older, where about a third fall at least once. While about 80 percent of falls occur in this age-group, 20 percent occur in those under age sixty-five. About half of those with a history of falling at least once will fall again in the near future. The Centers for Disease Control (CDC) recently reported that "falls can lead to moderate to severe injuries, such as hip fractures and head traumas, and can even increase the risk of early death. Fortunately, falls are a public health problem that is largely preventable."

Prevention of falls is the best treatment. This starts with improved foot function. Exercise also helps prevent falls because it improves aerobic muscle function, gait, and overall balance.

Music can also help the brain with better balance and gait, lowering the risk of falls. In a recent study, Dr. Andrea Trombetti and colleagues of University Hospitals and Faculty of Medicine of Geneva, Switzerland, demonstrated that listening to music as a therapy improved the brain's ability for a better gait and balance, significantly reducing the number of falls. Listening to music stimulates the rhythm centers of the brain, which impact physical movements.

The CDC also notes the following:

- Among those age sixty-five and older, falls are the leading cause of injury death. They are also the most common cause of nonfatal injuries and hospital admissions for trauma.
- In 2007, over 18,000 older adults died from unintentional fall injuries.
- The death rates from falls among older men and women have risen sharply over the past decade.
- In 2009, 2.2 million nonfatal fall injuries among older adults were treated in emergency departments and more than 581,000 of these patients were hospitalized.
- In 2000, direct medical costs of falls totaled a little over $19 billion—$179 million for fatal falls and $19 billion for nonfatal fall injuries.
- Most fractures among older adults are caused by falls—the most common are fractures of the spine, hip, forearm, leg, ankle, pelvis, upper arm, and hand.
- Many people who fall, even if they are not injured, develop a fear of falling. This fear may cause them to limit their activities, leading to reduced mobility and loss of physical fitness, which in turn increases their actual risk of falling.
- Statistically, men are about 50 percent more likely than women to die from a fall, and women about 50 percent more likely than men to break a hip.

While the CDC and other health care establishments focus on recommendations such as getting an annual eye exam, making the home environment safer by reducing tripping hazards, adding grab bars and railings, and improving lighting, the feet are often responsible for falls. Poor foot sense and balance, which are intricately linked, can significantly increase the risk of falling at any age.

Fixing Your Feet

Before continuing my discussion about foot assessment and treatment, there's an important question I am often asked: can age-related problems associated with neglected, abused feet really be fixed? The short answer is yes. Even those with significant debilitating foot dysfunction caused by disease or illness can improve their damaged nerves and blood vessels, severe muscle imbalance, poor balance, and irregular gait.

Let's consider a patient with type 2 diabetes who typically has nerve and muscle dysfunction in his or her feet, and which results in a much slower gait and poor balance, along with an increased risk of falling, weakness in foot, ankle, and leg muscles, and significantly reduced sensation of the ground by the foot. In addition, diabetics often have poor postural stability from toe to head due to foot dysfunction. (Many of these same problems are also found in nondiabetic people as a result of aging in an unhealthy and unfit body.)

A recent study by Lara Allet and colleagues at the Geneva University Hospital, Geneva, Switzerland, that was published in *Diabetologia*, measured gait, balance, muscle strength, and joint mobility in diabetic patients before and after very simple physical activities performed twice weekly for sixty minutes for a total of twelve weeks. It included walking up and down a slope and stairs, standing on toes and heels, one-leg stance, and included interactive games for ten minutes, such as badminton. The result of this study showed significant improvement in the patient's gait speed, balance, muscle strength, joint mobility, and foot sensation. Even upper-body muscle strength was improved.

These are all activities that minimally can improve foot function—even with these short-term basic activities, significant improvements in foot function occurred in a relatively brief time. In my own clinical experience, working with all types of people with foot dysfunction, just by incorporating more physical activity along with improvements in diet and nutrition, and the regulation of stress, dramatic improvements can be made in foot function that contributes to increased health and fitness of the entire body.

292

Self-Assessment of Your Own Feet

If your feet are bothering you, even for only a short time, the first step in correcting the problem is self-assessment. This means asking yourself certain questions. If the problem began soon after you started wearing a new pair of shoes, it may mean the obvious: that those shoes may not properly match your foot. Here are some other factors to consider:

If your aching foot feels better with movement, it's generally a good indication that it's a less serious impairment. As you move the muscles, they get warmed up and are able to function better. Sometimes an adequate warm-up takes twenty minutes, and some problems may feel better only after this period of time. But don't push yourself if the pain persists.

- If a problem worsens during activity, especially after you've had time to warm up, it usually means you should be resting to give the body a chance to heal. Pushing yourself in this situation often makes the problem worse and could lead to a chronic, recurring type of problem.
- If your problem feels worse at the end of the day, activity and weight bearing made it worse. Your foot may need more rest. In some cases, you may have accumulated fluid in your foot, ankle, and lower leg. This may be caused by ongoing inflammation, or because you're not able to circulate this fluid back through the veins. The

retention of fluid is called edema and is often associated with a bodywide problem.
- After being off your feet all night, most mechanical problems will feel better because your foot has had time to recover without mechanical stress. Certain problems may not follow this pattern. Plantar pain and the joint pain of arthritis may feel worse as soon as you start walking and gradually feel better after some movement. This may indicate a dietary or nutritional issue or a metabolic problem that causes too much calcium to deposit in that area during the night.

The wear pattern on your shoes can depict an accurate picture regarding foot balance. Shoe wear on the back of the heels, along the outside of the shoe, and near the ball of the foot should be similar in both shoes. If it's not, there may be muscle imbalance not allowing normal foot movement.

Another clue that the feet are not balanced is your footprints. If you walk in the sand, dirt, or other area where you can see your footprints, they should show very similar patterns. The same is true for your shoe prints. Look for the prints to be facing slightly outward rather than straight. Prints that are facing straight forward or are pointed outward too much may indicate a muscle imbalance in the pelvis that effects how the feet hit the ground. If you use this assessment, be sure the ground is relatively flat; otherwise, you will see a normal deviation in prints.

Finally, most foot problems occur on one side or the other, and rarely are there problems with identical patterns in both feet. When this does happen, it may be a simple muscle imbalance but could point to a more serious systemic condition, such as a spinal or circulatory problem, or possibly arthritis.

In many situations, however, general foot discomfort at the end of the day is simply due to wearing shoes not meant for your feet. This becomes obvious when you take your shoes off and move around a bit, only to find significant relief.

An acute foot problem, one involving trauma that does not start to feel better within twenty-four to forty-eight hours, may require some assistance. For more chronic problems, such as the nontraumatic type, one or two weeks should be sufficient time for at least some improvement to be seen. In allowing your body to fix itself, rest may be the key. One of the most powerful therapies, rest can be a double-edged sword if overused. The key with rest is knowing when and when not to use it.

Improving Foot Function

Without exaggeration, I've spent most of my life barefoot—and I'm not counting the time spent sleeping. Though I never knew it until I studied the merits of foot muscles and biomechanics, I was performing the oldest natural remedy for my whole body—being barefoot. Looking back, I attribute my almost lack of physical injuries, despite being physi-cally active, to staying out of shoes. (There were the rare exceptions of a twisted ankle while running on a rough trail in shoes or calf pain following a hard race.)

Being barefoot is perhaps the most potent treatment that helps the whole body maintain—or regain—the vigor and spring in its step. And it's free. The best time to do it is right now.

Bad shoes of all types have infiltrated our closets, and wearing them has shamed our bodies into making irregular and erratic movements, increasing wear and tear on muscles, joints, ligaments, and bones. It usually happens over a longer period of time, so it's not as noticeable. The results are poorly functioning feet and an unhappy gait that creates back pain, knee and hip problems, spinal distortions, and even shoulder and neck dysfunction. It also reduces our balance, increasing the risk of falls.

The barefoot and minimalist running shoe movements are getting a foothold in mainstream articles and fitness blogs of late, with entire books on the subject filling up Amazon's virtual shelves. While much of this is just the latest trend, many people are realizing that being barefoot is quite healthy for the feet. The 2009 and 2010 national best seller *Born to Run* by Chris McDougall, which focused on the Tarahumara Indians in northern Mexico who can run all day in sandals fashioned from discarded tires and leather straps, brought a surge of acceptance to natural running, either as barefoot or in low-profile flat running shoes. When

PROBLEM AREAS ON THE FOOT

First Metatarsal Jam

Excess pressure and stress through the big toe into the first metatarsal joint behind it is a common problem. It's almost always due to wearing shoes that are too small, which binds the toes. This injury involves the bone of the big toe, the phalanx, jamming back into the first metatarsal bone. The first metatarsal joint, between the two bones—the ball of the foot—becomes inflamed and painful. In some situations, when the onset of the problem is slow, the joint does not elicit pain, but rather the foot adapts, resulting in another problem, one that's symptomatic, elsewhere secondary to the first metatarsal. In a real sense, other parts of the foot are sacrificed to take away some of the stress of the first metatarsal. This is not an uncommon way for the body to adapt when an important structure, such as the first metatarsal joint, has excessive stress placed upon it. Many ankle, heel, knee, and other problems may be caused by a first metatarsal jam.

This first metatarsal jam can be assessed using two key indicators: the toe itself and the shoe:

- In the toe, pain and swelling in the area of the first metatarsal joint are common. Even a relatively minor jamming of the metatarsal joint over a long period will cause swelling of the joint. This is evident by a slight enlargement of the joint, with a warm feeling to the touch due to inflammation. Sometimes a discolored toenail due to the constant pressure from a shoe that's too tight is obvious. This is especially common in people who wear tight shoes. The toenail's discoloration is caused by tiny hemorrhages underneath the nail, similar to other bruises.
- The shoes can also give clues to a first metatarsal jam. Because the foot is wedged forward into the shoe, many toenails can jam into the front of the shoe. Over time, the toenail can bore a hole into the shoe, but more often shoes are discarded before this happens. Even a toenail that is not very long can do this if the shoe is sufficiently tight. This wear pattern can usually be felt inside the shoe. With your fingers, feel inside the shoe in the area where your toenail would rub. You may feel a roughened spot, and in some cases, a layer of material may have worn off the inside of the shoe. This means the shoe is too small—specifically, too short. Keeping the toenail carefully trimmed can be helpful, but wearing the right shoe

size is necessary to prevent a return of the problem. Proper shoe fit is addressed in the next chapter.

If you have a removable insole, take it out and study it. Look at the wear pattern, especially the indentation made from the toes. Observe any areas compressed by the toes that are not completely on the insert, like they should be. Toes that overlap the top of the insert obviously indicate a too-small shoe.

In athletes of any age, "turf toe" is basically the same condition as described here. The toe is injured during forced metatarsal movements, such as a push-off injury or other trauma. It usually includes the sesamoid bones under the first metatarsal joint. They may become inflamed and sometimes fractured. This is evident from local tenderness or pain on the bottom of the foot under the first metatarsal joint.

ANKLE SPRAIN

Many health and medical experts recommend that anyone who sprains an ankle have an X-ray, since it's the only way to determine if a fracture is present. But others say this leads to many unnecessary X-rays and expenses when other options can help rule out fracture. One issue is clear: Every person with a sprained ankle should be treated as an individual. A professional consensus known as the Ottawa ankle rules uses specific questions and examination of key areas to help determine the risk of bone fracture and if an X-ray is necessary.

Immediately after spraining your ankle, a question that should be asked is whether you can bear weight on that foot and ankle, even if it's painful. A second question is whether you can walk four steps, unaided, even with severe pain or a limp, right after your injury. A health professional may also ask you to do this if you go to the emergency room. If you're able to accomplish these tasks, an X-ray may not be recommended because the chances of a fracture are extremely low.

However, despite your ability to bear weight or walk, certain pain patterns may still indicate a potential fracture leading a doctor to X-ray your ankle. The risk of fracture is higher if there is pain in either bone of the inner or outer ankle, along with tenderness in any of the following bone areas:

- The back edge or tip of the lateral (outside) ankle bone
- The back edge or tip of the medial (inside) ankle bone

- The base of the fifth metatarsal (the little toe)
- The navicular bone in the middle of the foot

It should be noted that an X-ray does not always show a fracture. Some fractures are missed because of technically inadequate X-rays, and even good-quality X-rays may not demonstrate the fracture due to its size or swelling of surrounding tissues.

BONE INJURIES OF THE FEET

Bone injuries are relatively common, with a spectrum of three specific problems:

- A stress reaction is the least subtle bone injury, microscopic in nature. It produces vague discomfort following activity. It can't be seen on X-ray or CAT scan.
- Continued pressure on a bone can progress to a stress fracture, which is more painful and usually restricts activity. It can often, but not always, be diagnosed with an X-ray. It is also an example of a microscopic bone injury.
- A fracture is a more serious bone injury, and the damage is more obvious on X-ray.

Stress fractures are common in the foot (and lower leg). Studies show that up to 50 percent of runners have histories of stress fractures. Most importantly, getting a stress fracture means something is wrong—with exercise, diet and nutrition (including vitamin D), hormones, body mechanics (especially muscle balance), shoes, and low bone density. Low vitamin D levels are often associated with stress fractures.

Pain from a stress fracture typically improves with rest and worsens with activity. There is often some swelling in the area, but sometimes it's not noticeable. The swelling around the bone may prevent a proper diagnosis by X-ray within the first two weeks of injury. Only after some healing has taken place will the X-ray show the problem. In these situations, a bone scan may indicate the physical location of the stress fracture.

Most stress fractures will heal quickly when you're healthy and fit, without major therapy. Rest, cooling the site of fracture, cessation of weight-bearing exercise, and hard-soled flat shoes are often sufficient, but each case must be treated individually. Aspirin and other NSAIDs must be avoided as they can delay bone healing.

PLANTAR PAIN

Pain in the bottom of the foot, generally referred to as plantar pain, can come from a variety of sources. Almost all plantar pain is functional, and therefore X-rays will be negative, and the problem can usually be corrected conservatively. If you have plantar pain, first carefully check the skin since a small cut, splinter, piece of glass, wart, or other similar problem can be the cause.

Plantar pain inside the foot, especially in the mid- or hindfoot, frequently comes from tight plantar muscles. This tightness is most often secondary to other muscle weakness. A "diagnosis" of plantar fasciitis is not indicative of the cause of the problem, and no single remedy for this named condition has proven successful. Two people with the same plantar pain due to tight plantar muscles may have very different causes.

A so-called bone spur may be present in some chronic cases of plantar pain. This is usually associated with long-term plantar muscle tightness (often secondary to other muscle weakness). In this case, the tendon of the plantar muscles that attaches to the calcaneus (heel) bone may contain calcium deposits. On an X-ray, this gives the appearance of a pointed "spur," which can give a false impression of a pointed sharp object in your foot. This is another example of the body compensating for a problem: In order to further support the area, the body deposits calcium in the tendon.

Correction of plantar pain usually occurs with improvement of muscle function. A foot with chronic muscle imbalance may need rehabilitation, sometimes best accomplished by spending more time barefoot. In addition, improvements to the body chemistry through better diet and nutrition can also be helpful.

INGROWN TOENAIL

An ingrown toenail usually occurs in the big toe due to either poor-fitting shoes, improper nail trimming, or both. The area becomes inflamed and painful and can lead to secondary fungal or bacterial infections.

Conservative treatment is usually effective, including accommodative shoes. Warm foot soaks and proper nail trimming are also effective. Trimming the nail is best accomplished by cutting it straight across rather than at a curve.

McDougall, a formerly injured runner, swapped out his traditional oversupported shoes for minimalist or barefoot running shoes, and even going barefoot, he stopped getting injured.

But is this just another footwear fad? Because some of the more important, serious issues tend to be left right out of the discussions. The most important one of all is the fact that being barefoot is therapeutic no matter who you are, and not just for the feet, but the whole body.

Of the dozens of therapies I used throughout my thirty-five-plus-year career of treating physical injuries, from acupuncture and biofeedback to manipulation and exercise, being barefoot is one of the most powerful, easiest to apply and quickest to get results.

Barefoot therapy has helped many people rehabilitate their feet—it's necessary because wearing almost all shoes, whether for sports, leisure, work, or night on the town, can damage a foot's delicate muscles, nerves, and bones. But being barefoot allows the most natural of foot movements; it trains the feet to function better and helps support the ankle, calf, knee, hip, back, and all structures up to the head. The result is that many aches and pains—including what some would consider chronic injuries like that bad hip or shoulder—get better.

But one cannot abruptly make the change to being barefoot after years of wearing dangerous footwear: those thick, oversupported shoes that ruin your feet have also weakened your foot muscles. Whether you're wearing common running shoes with thick soles, high heels, or most other footwear, weaning off them must be done at a pace that pleases your muscles—the weakest part of the average foot and the area most in need of rehabilitation.

Here are ten barefoot steps you can take to dramatically change your ailing physical body:

- Take off your shoes. Don't put them on in the morning, unless you're going right outdoors; and when coming home, taken them off before walking into your house. Spend more time standing, walking, and otherwise being barefoot at home, in your office, and in other indoor locations. It's best without socks, but a thin pair would be acceptable. Walk on the bare floor, carpeted areas, and wherever your feet take you. This provides different types of foot stimulation to help muscles work better— the first step in rehabilitating your feet. And it's significant for the many people whose addiction to shoes is damaging the body. Do this for a couple of weeks before the next step, spending as much time as is comfortable each day.
- Now, take the plunge and venture outdoors in your bare feet. This will provide additional foot stimulation over the comforts of home. Stick with smooth surfaces— your driveway, sidewalk, and porch. Do this for at least ten minutes. The different environment—the feel of new materials by your bare feet, including temperature

changes—provides added foot stimulation. Do this in conjunction with the first step. A week or so of this additional activity and you're ready to move on.

- Now venture off to uneven natural ground. Walking on grass, dirt, and sand will provide greater motivation for your feet to function better, helping the structures above be more stable. Start with just a few minutes if you're sensitive, but with three weeks of barefoot training, you'll be ready for this big step: Work up to a short walk of about ten to fifteen minutes.

- Most people will have to wear shoes for various activities—work, running, shopping, social occasions. During this rehab period, there are two important things to do with your shoes. First, start wearing thinner, simple footwear and avoid using orthotic or insole liners.

- Almost everyone can take these first four steps. It will help improve the body's mechanics from toe to head. But many people need more foot stimulus for additional rehabilitation. Being barefoot will do this eventually, but you can speed the process. Here's one way: a foot massage. A professional massage is always great, but you can treat your own feet daily at home, either by yourself or by trading treatments with others. Even a five-minute massage for each foot can work wonders. Start with the feet relaxed, clean, and dry. A small amount of organic coconut oil is a nice option. Slowly and gently rub the foot all over using both hands, working up the leg where key foot muscles originate. Use firm pressure, but it should not be painful. Do this daily or as often as possible.

- A key feature of optimal foot function is that it helps balance the whole body during walking, climbing stairs, jogging or running, and all other movements. Over time, wearing shoes can significantly diminish this balance mechanism. Being barefoot is helpful, but here's a way to speed the process. You should be able to easily balance on one bare foot for thirty seconds or more. If you can't perform this action, it's probably due to foot dysfunction, typically associated with muscle imbalance. Start with attempting to balance on one foot for as long as you can, even if just for a few seconds; next, try the other foot. Balancing on each foot can gradually improve the communication between feet and brain, promoting better balance throughout the body. Here's a way to incorporate this therapeutic activity into a regular routine: After a shower or bath—hold one foot up to dry it while standing on the other. Be sure to get each of your toes and keep your foot relaxed. Then switch feet. Here's another good routine: Each day when putting on your shoes, do it standing, holding your foot above your knee to put on the shoe and tie it, and then do the same with the other.

- If you spend a lot of time on your feet during the day, especially if you must wear shoes, you often get home with tired, sore, sweaty, and warm feet. Cool them. A cold footbath can work wonders, even after a hot shower. It improves circulation, tones muscles and overall improves foot function, and helps them recover from the day. Use a large -enough bucket or foot tub that fits your feet without jamming your toes. Place your feet in cold water so they are completely submerged above the ankle. Add a small amount of ice to prevent the water from getting warm, but do not fill the tub with ice, as this can freeze the foot, risking damage to nerves, blood vessels, and muscles. Keep your foot immersed for five to twenty minutes. A deeper bath can also cool the leg muscles. A cold footbath can do much more than an ice pack placed only on the area of discomfort. Take a footbath while answering an e-mail, catching up on phone calls, or use it as a time to relax and listen to music.

- Sometimes, the use of a hot footbath can be therapeutic, not to mention comforting. Moist heat works better than a heating pad because it penetrates into the foot better. Use the same-size footbath as mentioned above and fill with hot water—not scalding—but most people can tolerate temperatures of around 90 to 100°F. Adding Epsom salt (magnesium salt) is also soothing. Beware: Heat can have unwanted side effects. Do not use heat if you have an acute injury, especially one that's inflamed, swollen, or bruised,

and avoid heat with any skin disorder, diabetes, circulatory problem, or an open wound. When in doubt about using heat, avoid it.

- For many people, here's one more step: turn your outdoor barefoot walk into an easy jog or run, expanding your walk as described in the third step. There are many ways to describe this process, but like other natural activities, your body already knows how to do it. Whether you begin on blacktop, smooth dirt, or other areas that are comfortable, as you naturally thicken the skin on the bottoms of your feet, you may be able to run anywhere barefoot. Use this barefoot time as a warm-up for your longer run in flat shoes, a cooldown, or keep it as a separate therapy. Many people take this as a launching pad for regular barefoot running, whether as a thirty- to forty-five-minute workout or even running in races.

- This final step is most important and for everyone. Once you've weaned off bad shoes, rehabed your feet, and restored good foot function, be careful to avoid returning to old unhealthy habits by wearing bad shoes. It's that simple.

Rehabilitating your feet with barefoot therapy and ridding your body of improper footwear will bring renewed physical function. It can quickly bring back the spring and vigor in your step, prevent injuries, and help maintain overall physical activity for years to come.

301

CHAPTER 17

FOOTWEAR MADE SIMPLE
Finding the Right Pair of Shoes Is a Key Step to Better Health

The human foot evolved over several million years, enabling early man to walk long distances and not stay close to heavily forested areas like his arboreal ancestors. Our closest living relatives—the chimpanzee—use their feet mainly for climbing and scampering short distances. The shoe is a recent development, just over ten thousand years old. Man went either barefoot or covered the bottom of the foot with bark or animal skins for protection from sharp rocks, thorns, and rough terrain. Shoes didn't interfere with natural foot function. Sandals were common in warmer climates, with moccasin-type shoes used in colder environments. Today, simple sandals and moccasins are still the most common footwear worldwide.

But with the advent of today's modern shoes came a whole array of foot problems as well as the growth of a new footwear industry that also made therapeutic devices and professionals to treat such conditions. The running shoe industry has benefited the most; annual revenues now approach $20 billion. And it's not just runners who are buying shoes.

A 1997 *British Journal of Sports Medicine* paper by Steven Robbins, PhD, described the hazards of deceptive advertising of athletic footwear. Writing about modern athletic shoes, Robbins stated, "Deceptive advertising of protective devices [in shoes] may represent a public health hazard and may have to be eliminated presumably through regulation."

For most of history, shoes were made straight with left and right being identical. Records show that between the fourteenth century BC in Egypt and the mid-1800s, shoes were essentially produced the same way—by hand. For centuries, shoemakers kept secret the measurements of their clients' feet to help assure continued business.

In 1845, the rolling machine, followed by the invention of the sewing machine a year later, dramatically changed the shoe industry. By 1860, other more effective shoe-making machines were developed. The next manufacturing breakthrough came in 1875, when Charles Goodyear Jr. developed a machine that made shoes using a new material called rubber, previously invented by his father.

Today, most shoes are made on machines, but they also require manual assembling. The manufacturing of many shoes, especially athletic shoes produced by big companies, is accomplished in third world countries because it's very cheap, often a dollar per pair or less.

How Shoes Can Harm Your Feet

When was the very first time the human foot was injured by a shoe? Probably the first time one was worn. Nothing is more stable, supportive, shock protective, and efficient than bare feet. As soon as a shoe is placed on the foot, there is a loss of mechanical stability and the potential for injury. Perhaps the very first shoe-related injury was a twisted ankle due to surprise instability. Or worse, being overtaken by a lion due to slower running speed or poor maneuverability in shoes. While most of us don't have to run from wild animals, our shoes can still be dangerous.

One of the earliest published studies describing the harm from shoes came in the early 1950s when Canadian scientist Dr. John Basmajian showed that wearing shoes affected foot function through impairment of muscle activity. Known for his work in the area of electromyography (EMG) and biofeedback, Basmajian's work played a key role in other studies, which continues today, demonstrating that shoes, especially most running ones, have a negative impact on feet and legs. These findings are readily available to read in online medical libraries, whereas the running magazines, which depend on advertising support from footwear companies, stay clear of the topic.

There are a variety of specific problems associated with wearing shoes. I've broken these subjects down to four general categories:

Shoe Stress

Many types of ill-fitting running shoes, and those that are oversupported, too much cushioning, and rigid tread and heel can put stress on the foot's delicate structures, including muscles, bones, ligaments, joints, and even the skin. In addition, shoes that produce a noticeable height difference between the heel and front of the foot can be an unnatural stressor, especially on the knees. Going barefoot means that there is the same height front and back, or "zero drop," but a shoe with a thicker heel causes the front of the foot to drop farther down. Many conventional running shoes have a drop over twelve millimeters, or half inch to an inch. Some have much more.

Don't be seduced by the shock-absorbing material of the shoe's sole. The thicker the tread, the harder it is for the brain and foot to properly communicate with the body. In other words, the soles of the feet can't stay in "contact" with the ground. You want that earth-to-foot rapport. While an overdeveloped shoe bottom might be protecting your foot from rocks and tree roots if you are running on a trail, there's still a lack of foot sense, which, in turn, restricts if not allows optimal bodywide kinesthetic or K sense. This can throw off a stride and cause further biomechanical stress, because the brain is also less aware of where the foot is landing—and how to make minute adjustments.

With poor K sense comes a response from the brain to the muscles that may be disrupted or altered. As a result, the body does not properly compensate for a minor foot problem, or even normal wear and tear, ultimately leading to a more serious injury such as Achilles tendonitis or inflammation in the metatarsal area of the foot, stress fractures, or other problems in the knee, hip, and even lower back.

weight bearing, foot sense and orientation, muscle and bone, and gait.

Weight Bearing

Your feet support the entire body's weight. Normally, this weight is distributed through specific areas of the feet in order to handle the weight most efficiently. During standing, walking, and running, this efficient weight-bearing distribution can significantly reduce the risk of injury. High heels and a small toe box, for example, concentrate all the weight onto a smaller area. But when you wear a flat shoe or are barefoot, the distribution of weight is over a larger area. While casual, sports, or running shoes are not in the same category as high heels, they also cause weight-bearing distortions due to the exaggerated heel support. This can be seen with the following experiment. Get your feet wet. Now stand on a flat dry paper towel. Step off the towel and observe your footprints. Drawing an outline around the print may help you see it better. Next, take a pair of flat shoes that you have worn for a while and observe the area of wear—this will be mostly the back outer corner of your heel and the ball of the foot and sometimes along the outer edge of the shoe. Now compare the size of your footprint with the area of wear pattern on your shoes. In most cases, your footprint area will be larger, sometimes a lot larger. This is because your contact to the ground is greater when barefoot than in shoes.

The surface area that makes contact with the ground is a significant factor associated with many types of foot problems. If the weight of your body is forced through a smaller area of your foot—meaning less surface area—more stress is induced in your foot. Instead, your foot is supposed to disperse the weight-bearing stress through a greater surface area. In addition, with less surface area making contact with the ground, the body has a lessened ability to maintain proper overall balance.

The flatter and thinner the sole of your shoe, the more your weight bearing is likely to be more natural as in a barefoot state. Changing to this type of shoe could have significant benefits for your feet, but you must do this carefully if you're used to thick-sole shoes, those with high heels, or those with a lot of cushioning and support.

Impact

Your weight-bearing contact with the ground is intimately connected to foot sense. For many years, sport shoe manufacturers focused on impact, promoting shoes with shock-absorbing materials to protect us from the impact forces that supposedly caused injury. But after decades of scientific research, experts are unable to demonstrate that our feet are vulnerable to injury from the result of impact, whether from standing, walking, running, or jumping. In fact, what the studies show is that there's no difference in injury rates between running on hard surfaces and on soft surfaces, or between runners who have heavy or light impact on the ground.

Certainly, excessive impact can injure our feet and other parts of the leg. And any impact can cause injury when muscle imbalance is present. However, the action of standing, walking, running, and performing other common types of physical activity is quite natural—your feet are made for these activities and the normal impact associated with it. The forces of impact are a natural phenomenon that your feet were made to deal with. Actually, your feet use the impact on the ground to decide how much muscle work is needed to move most efficiently. This action is mediated through the nerves and muscles in the feet.

The muscle response to impact also affects comfort. For this reason, all shoes, from the moment you put on a new pair to those that appear too old and worn out, should be completely comfortable. Otherwise, the shoe should not be worn because of the risk of foot damage. So-called worn-out shoes may be just fine as long as they are comfortable and not falling apart.

Still other benefits are obtained from your constant impact on the ground. Bone strength can be improved in those who perform activities that result in harder impact, such as dancing, running, and even walking especially when compared to activities that have low or almost no impact such as swimming.

More on Shock Absorption

Shock absorption is another popular selling point used by running and walking shoe companies. But just because a sneaker has plenty of shock-absorbing ability, that does not mean it can accomplish much cushioning. In fact, shoe materials with good shock absorbency properties are not effective enough to reduce stress in the foot during physical activity. This is because shock absorption in the feet occurs at the same level of intensity whether you wear shoes or not.

The notion that shock and repetitive impact are harmful over time has caused footwear companies to heavily base their marketing on the notion that one needs extra cushion while walking, jogging, or running. It's easy to understand why cushioning is a concept most people relate to in terms of comfort and safety. Cushioning can protect your feet against bruising if you should step on a hard object like a sharp stone. However, cushioning can have drawbacks. Shoes that are too cushioned can give your brain the

improper perception that the impact is much less than it actually is, which can result in inadequate or improper response by the foot (and rest of the body) to the actual impact. In a December 1997 issue of the *British Journal of Sports Medicine*, researchers Robbins and Waked wrote that "expensive athletic shoes are deceptively advertised to safeguard well through cushioning impact yet account for 123 percent greater injury frequency than the cheapest ones."

Support

Many shoes have a "support system" built into them. This may be a simple insert or a complex arrangement of built-up stabilizing structures with fancy technical names. Most of these exist for marketing reasons and serve no real important function. When you artificially support the feet when they don't need it, you're asking for trouble. And for most individuals, this need usually does not exist. Some people, however, may need extra support because they have stayed in shoes with too much support for too long, thereby weakening the natural support mechanisms within the foot. For these individuals, their feet don't feel right without the added support. This vicious cycle can only be broken by weaning off oversupported shoes and strengthening the muscles of the feet. Going barefoot, even for only several minutes per day at the beginning, is a good start.

Support systems in many shoes contribute to a thicker heel area. When barefoot, your heel and forefoot are about the same level, but

306

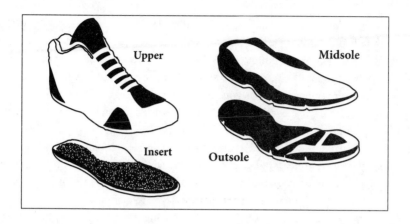

most shoes are made so that your heel is higher than the rest of the foot. This unnatural state can ultimately result in reduced muscle function in the gastrocnemius, soleus, and tibialis posterior muscles in the back of the calf, and tibialis anterior on the front of the leg.

Recall the importance of foot sense. Within the foot are important nerve endings that sense foot contact with the ground. This information is sent to the brain and spinal cord so you can respond appropriately to activities of the feet and help regulate all movement and body position. In effect, you orient yourself—and the whole body—as a result of foot sense.

The primary reason for many common foot injuries is the lack of feedback from the foot despite the same level of shock absorption. This can be the result of increased thickness of the sole or the types of synthetic materials used in many shoes. In other words, the soles of our feet are not able to properly communicate with the ground. The

relationship between reduced foot sense and its contribution to injury has been understood in scientific circles for over forty years.

Those who wear popular running shoes must contract their tibialis anterior more than normal during each step in order to land on their heels. During natural running, with a very flat shoe or when barefoot, this constant high level of tibialis anterior contraction does not have to take place. This excessive muscle contraction could trigger tightness, followed by weakness of the tibialis posterior muscle or other patterns of imbalance. In addition, gastrocnemius and soleus muscle tightness can also be a secondary problem, with increased tension in the Achilles tendon. In any of these situations, the resulting muscle imbalance can lead to common injuries. The exact area of injury can vary from person to person.

Buying the Right Pair of Shoes

Not all shoes are harmful. The best shoes are those with little or no support, such as moccasins, sandals, flat sneakers, and running shoes with thin and hard rather than soft soles. The correct shoe should feel almost perfect, whether it's used for walking, running, or other sports. This also applies to shoes you may wear much of the day or even just on special occasions, from casual work shoes to a black-tie affair. The right shoes should wear well, keep their shape over time, tread safely, allow for sufficient foot freedom, minimally distort the foot, if at all, and hold together for years. These characteristics depend on the quality of materials, the manufacturing process, including how the shoe was put together, and how well each shoe matches the structure of your foot. In general, the best shoes are those that are flattest, and ones made specifically for your feet. Unfortunately, most people buy off-the-shelf shoes, so it's important to follow strict guidelines for optimal fit.

Considering that your feet are probably two different sizes, shoe-size numbers (for example, size 10 or size 7) have no real meaning, and most companies don't have consistent sizes, which makes finding the optimal shoe a difficult challenge. However, there are a number of things you can do to eliminate common dangers and find the best match for your feet. The most important factor is fit.

Finding Your Proper Fit

Optimal shoe fit may be difficult for some people, while others have an easier time. While there's a subjective component to shoe fit, other factors are more concrete. You can't predict your size based on previous shoes with specific sizes as shoes between companies can be different, and even the same shoe in one company can vary in size. This means it's difficult to get the proper fit without actually trying them on and walking or running in them.

The Battelle Memorial Institute, a non-profit scientific research and development facility in Columbus, Ohio, shows there are at least thirty-eight factors that influence shoe fit, ranging from length, width, and height to feel. This makes most shoes difficult to fit properly. The subjective opinions and attitudes come from both the consumer and the salesperson, but ultimately you determine if the shoe fits.

Sizing Your Foot

The majority of people in the Western world probably wear shoes that are too small. Certainly in my own private practice, where for over thirty years I studied the shoes and feet of my patients, that was the case. In many situations, I would measure both the feet and shoes of the patient—and show how off they were.

Some patients I have seen bought larger shoes after discovering their initial problem of a tight fit, only to find that their feet kept getting larger. At some point in time, they ended up with an increase of a whole size or more. I have even seen increases of 2.5 U.S. sizes over a two-year period in adults!

Today's shoe sizes include three popular but different length-sizing systems depending on where the shoes were made. These systems include sizes for shoes made in the United Kingdom (U.K.), which originated in the late 1600s; the United States, originating in the late 1800s; and the Continental or Paris point metric method, originating in the late 1600s. Other sizing systems also exist. More recently, the Mondopoint system was proposed to replace all other systems. This is based on a simple length and width measurement in millimeters. It would be a great benefit to consumers, but it will probably never be accepted by the shoe industry since it would put all shoe sizes on the same playing field, making marketing—and deception—more difficult.

Measuring Your Feet

Most adults don't measure their feet when buying new shoes, especially considering that many shoe purchases today are online. As a result, many people squeeze into the same shoe size for years or even decades. As I have discussed in the previous chapter, while adult feet stop growing by age twenty, they still get larger through the years—sometimes more than two U.S. sizes. They also get larger within a twenty-four-hour period, typically as the day goes on, returning to "normal" by the next morning, so always measure your feet and try on new shoes at the end of the day. Combine this with the fact that units of measure for shoes are not consistent, you can easily get frustrated and not want to take the time needed to find the best fit.

Consider shoes sold in the United States. A shoe marked size 10 may be made differently than another shoe from the same footwear manufacturer that's also marked size 10. Both will measure different lengths. Still another pair of size 10 shoes made with a different manufacturing method can measure differently than the other two size 10s. Actually, it's possible that a shoe marked size 10 could be one of five different sizes. So much for those silver gadgets, also called the Brannock device, that shoe stores used to measure your feet. In addition, shoes for men, women, and children have different size units—a size 8 men's is much different in length from a size 8 women's.

The three popular size systems don't have much in common either. In the United States, a men's size 10 is the same in Canada, but in the U.K. it's a size 9. The same size in Japan is 27.5, and the Continental (Paris point metric) equivalent size is 43.

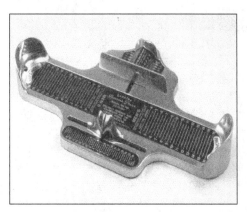

The Brannock device

In addition to length, width is an important dimension. The width is measured across the ball of the foot. Add height to the foot and you have volume as another important measurement that is usually neglected. An example of the complexity of shoe fit is with volume, which is best assessed by foot comfort when trying on shoes on a hard floor. By now you may be thinking that this is complicated. It is. But since there's no standard for size, none of these numbers should really mean anything to you, with one exception.

Measuring Devices

One benefit of measuring your feet is keeping track of their relative size. This may not relate to shoe size. The Brannock device was introduced in 1927 with the purpose of providing a starting point for shoe fitting, not to dictate the best shoe size. The Brannock device is standardized within itself—they all have the same standard measurements—but these don't precisely match any one kind of shoe size made by any of the companies.

By either using the Brannock device in a shoe store or doing the measuring yourself as described below, you could, and should, keep track of your foot size just like you would keep track of your weight with a scale or overall health with a regular blood test. Like most health-related tests, measuring your feet is an important general guide.

Any measurement of your feet should be done in a standing position on a hard floor.

Do this at the end of the day. Any meaningful daily size fluctuations must be differentiated from serious health problems, such as edema, certain pathological changes as seen in arthritis, or side effects of drugs.

For an accurate measurement, make a footprint on a piece of paper. Use a damp foot on a paper towel or draw the outline of your foot with a pencil. Measure the back of the heel to the end of the big toe in each foot. The purpose would be to see how much your feet change from year to year, and not related to any shoe's size.

High-Tech Shoe "Systems"

In the past twenty years, almost all athletic shoes, including tennis, golf, and even walking, have become more specialized. This makes finding the optimal one more difficult. For example, there are several different pedaling systems available for cyclists, with different ones for road or mountain bikers. The different pedal systems provide increased efficiency during pedaling, but the shoe still must fit or foot stress will follow. Finding the shoe and system that best matches your need, like a running shoe, is a matter of trying them on; but this can't be done as easily as trying a few running shoes in the store—it's a more difficult feat since you need to try the whole system on your bike. Once again, comfort is key. Unfortunately, comfort in a shoe can change after thirty minutes of easy riding. Pay particular attention to comfort in the front of the foot, where most wear and tear occurs.

TEN STEPS TO A BETTER SHOE FIT

You can get the best fit by following some key points:

- Never assume you'll take the same size as your previous shoe, even if it's the same type or model.
- Rely on fit and comfort rather than on any particular size.
- Always plan on spending adequate time when shopping for shoes. Don't rush—if you're short on time, postpone it and set time aside for this important event. You may not find the right shoe in the first store you visit. Most outlets carry only a few of the many shoes on the marketplace.
- Always try on both shoes. First, try on the size you think would fit best, then walk on a hard floor (not carpeted). Even if that size feels fine, try on a half-size larger. If that one feels the same, or even better, try on another half size larger. Many people don't realize that a larger shoe may actually feel and fit better.
- Continue trying on larger half-sizes until you find the shoes that are obviously too large. You know especially by the heel—it will start coming off when you walk. Then go back to the previous half size—more often that's the pair that best matches your feet. There should be at least a half inch between your longest toe and the front of the shoe for most shoes.
- Each time you try on a pair of shoes, find a hard surface to walk on rather than the thick soft carpet in shoe stores, where almost any shoe will feel good. If there's no sturdy floor to walk on, ask if you can walk outside (if you're not allowed, shop elsewhere).
- You may also need to try different widths to get the best fit, although many shoes don't come in different widths. The ball of your foot should fit comfortably into the widest part of the shoe without causing the shoe to bulge.
- Use comfort as the main criterion. Don't let anyone say you have to break them in before they feel good. The best shoes for you are the ones that feel good right away. While many sales clerks are aware of how to find the right shoe size, many are not. Often shoes from mail-order outlets cost less. But be prepared to ship them back if they don't fit just right.

- If the difference between your two feet is less than a half size, fit the larger foot. If you have a significant difference of more than a half size between your two feet, it may be best to wear two different-size shoes. How you accomplish this is up to you.
- For sports shoes, many women fit better in men's shoes than in women's. The first rule, though, is that the shoe must fit properly. Some women don't fit into men's shoes, and some stores don't carry or companies don't make men's shoes in sizes that are small enough for many women.

One problem with cycling shoes is that the tighter they are, the more efficient they may be, because there's less energy lost in foot movement. This makes the need for a "perfect fit" even more important. Just don't sacrifice comfort for the notion that a bit more efficiency will make a dramatic difference in performance—it won't. One option over off-the-shelf shoes is to get them custom-made; it might be well worth the effort and cost. Just have both feet measured at the end of the day when they may be slightly larger.

Remember, the manufacturer makes new shoes based on trends of style, color, and fancy gimmicks to market the shoe. That's why shoe styles come and go. If you find the shoe that fits perfectly, buy more than one pair. Just be sure to try them all on, since the same shoe may also vary in size.

Or take the example of a golf shoe. If ill-fitting shoes can disrupt normal foot function, golf shoes can adversely affect your game. Legendary golf instructor David Leadbetter once told me, "With all activities, especially golf, balance is of the utmost importance. Understanding your feet and how they interact with the ground is the main ingredient in balance." This is the reason that companies are starting to make a new type of golf shoe—a minimalist, flat-sole shoe to simulate being barefoot.

Traditional golf shoes are even more rigid and unforgiving than running shoes, and while golfers don't run, except for the few who play speed golf, they can walk up to five or six miles during a full round. So many of the same biomechanical principles apply to those who run or walk. The University of Calgary's Human Performance Laboratory conducted a study (published in the November 2009 *Journal of Clinical Sports Medicine*) on golfers and their shoes. The study looked at how sandals would fare compared to golf shoes on low back pain in forty golfers. After six weeks there was a significant reduction in low-back pain in the test group wearing sandals and without any loss of balance or performance.

Weaning Off Bad Shoes

If you feel it's time to make a healthy change for your feet, you may have to go

Socks

When trying on shoes, wear the socks you would normally wear in them. Socks are not necessary but are mainly for added comfort, especially in avoiding blisters. Like shoes, socks can be too tight, contributing to foot irritation and stress. For most situations, socks should be thin and not tight. Thicker socks may require a half-size larger shoe.

Which style of socks you wear (low-cut or above the ankle) and what they're made of (natural fibers such as wool or cotton—my preference—or synthetics) is up to you. But like shoes, make sure they fit well; and be careful to avoid the sock interfering with shoe fit.

through a "withdrawal" from bad shoes to good ones. It might be impossible to stop wearing bad shoes one day and start with good ones the next. The reason has to do with the posture of your foot, specifically the function of your muscles.

Let's take the case of a person wearing thick-sole running shoes for everyday use and walking. If he's been wearing this type of shoe for several years, his foot muscles, along with tendons and even ligaments, have changed in length to adjust to the shoe. When he suddenly starts wearing a flatter shoe, his

muscles, tendons, and ligaments will have to readapt. This process may be uncomfortable, and even painful, if he tries to do it all at once. In making this change, he may feel discomfort right away or it could take a day or two. If his feet have more significant unnatural changes in the joints, such as hammer toes or a bunion, the problem could be worse and take much longer.

For many individuals, these changes need to take place slowly if they're going to make the transition without much discomfort. In many cases, the muscles have become weak and will require a period of strengthening, which could happen during normal movement in good shoes. For some, rehabilitating the feet may be necessary, which can be accomplished by being barefoot. It's not necessary to be barefoot all day to accomplish this, but just spending time on your feet—around the house or office—will help balance and strengthen foot muscles.

For these and other shoe problems, making the change to flat shoes or even being barefoot, as natural as that is makes your foot feel rather odd and may sometimes be uncomfortable. After all, your feet have been addicted to being coddled and oversupported and have become weak. This does not mean that flatter shoes or being barefoot is a stressful state because you don't feel as good; rather, your feet are changing back to their more natural state.

For many people, weaning off bad shoes may take at least one extra measure. First, look at the highest heel height of a current shoe. Compare this to a lower heel or a flat shoe. Your first step in weaning off bad shoes may be to wear a shoe that's about half to three quarters less in height than the height of the one you currently wear. Try wearing a shoe with this height heel for a few days to make sure your feet don't become painful. If there is pain, you'll require two extra steps and have to wean slower by wearing a shoe whose heel is only one-quarter to half the height of what you're used to wearing before going to one that is half- to three-quarters. In some cases, just removing the insert in your current shoe is a good first step to better feet.

With running shoes, there is also the need to potentially make a slow transition. Don't immediately go from conventional shoes with large heel crash pad for cushioning support to barefoot running shoes in which the heel and toe box are on the same plane. In this case, use a shoe that's about half the size of the original sole's thickness.

Whether you need to take one or two intermediary steps in making the transition from bad to good shoes, it may only take a month or two to make the appropriate adaptations to the new foot position. For others, it may take longer, especially with running shoes. Be patient and prudent. Rushing things will only lead to possible injury. Still others may need assistance from an appropriate health care professional. Rely on the feet feeling good for at least a week or two before progressing to the next step. Once you've weaned down to a more flat shoe, you'll wonder how you survived all the others.

Old Shoes

It's been said that old, worn shoes can cause foot or leg injuries. This may be true if your old shoes were bad to start with. Sports shoe companies want people to get rid of their shoes sooner to buy new ones more often. But a good shoe that has a lot of wear may still be good. Properly made sports shoes that match your feet could last years depending on your habits. Marketing has made many people believe that we have to replace our shoes frequently. This may be true when the shoes are poorly made, but even cheap shoes can last a long time.

A number of factors may cause you to either repair or replace your current shoes:

- First and foremost, they should remain comfortable. As soon as they cease being comfortable, they need to be repaired or replaced.
- Another factor is wear. The two heaviest areas of wear are the heel and under the ball of the foot. If you're a runner, there should be less wear on the heel. If your shoes wear very unevenly, this could be a problem. For example, if one heel is worn a quarter inch more than the other, this can cause a significant muscle imbalance (which may be the cause of this excess wear to start with). If one heel is worn down much more than the other, repair both heels if possible, or buy new shoes. If the area under the ball of the foot is worn through the sole, sometimes due to an

imbalanced gait while running, this is also a reason to repair or replace the shoe.

- A common problem in some shoes is the breakdown of the stiffener in the heel area. This is especially troublesome when the heel height is more than about an inch thick. This can create instability in the feet and lead to balance problems.

Arch Supports, Orthotics, Shoe Lacing, and Other Foot Support

Many shoes have built-in or removable supports, which supposedly help your foot function better. Various types of supports are made for the heel, sole, arch, and ankle and include soft and hard materials comprised of cotton, leather, synthetics, plastic, wood, and metal. They come in the form of heel and sole supports, ankle braces, a variety of inserts, and arch supports, including orthotics and others.

In addition to conventional supports, some health care professionals use taping methods to help support the foot and ankle. In my clinical experience of using conservative treatments for many types of foot problems in athletes, successful outcome does not require any type of support in the vast majority of cases. Instead, correcting the cause of foot problems such as muscle imbalance is usually what is necessary. Only on occasion would additional foot support be required and almost always for a short period during

which time the foot can heal. In rare situations, support would be necessary long term.

Stabilizing or immobilizing the foot or ankle may be necessary in the case of an emergency when the risk of serious damage is suspected and until such time that a proper assessment can be made.

Unfortunately, the long-term use of foot supports by both active and inactive people is all too common. Despite the potential risk of further weakening the foot and not treating the cause of the problem, orthotics and other foot supports are heavily marketed and readily available in many retail outlets and online sites. While these supports come in different sizes and shapes, these are essentially "one size fits all" products since they usually don't specifically match the needs of the individual foot, despite what the manufacturer says.

Some people use these devices for short period without seeing any real change, only to try one brand after another with many different kinds of supports ending up in the drawer. If you don't specifically match a particular support to your precise needs, it could lead to long-term worsening of the condition, making proper treatment much more difficult.

In most cases, the use of shoe supports should be considered only after more conservative therapy has been tried without success and before more radical treatment is considered, such as surgery.

How Supports Can Weaken the Foot

The greatest harm caused by the use of foot supports is the failure to address the cause of the problem. This is especially true when supports provide temporary symptomatic relief, giving the false impression that it's cured. In some cases, a support will provide symptomatic relief in the area of pain, only to trigger an imbalance or discomfort in another area that's previously not a problem. For example, you may start using a particular support that provides relief for your foot pain. A week later, your knee may begin to hurt. This can occur due to the initial change made in the structure of your foot by the support, causing other structural changes and possible injury—sometimes up the leg into the knee, hip, or even lower back. This is due to muscle imbalance. With the additional artificial support, the foot's natural internal support is relaxed. In other words, the foot muscles have less reason to work as much since something else (the added support) is doing the job for them. And no support can ever take the place of proper muscle function.

In certain instances, a reduced range of motion may be necessary to assist in healing, such as after an ankle sprain. However, it's important to remove the support of the body as soon as possible to complete the healing process in order to prevent a continuation of a reduced range of motion. This in turn will allow the foot's muscle function to return to normal.

Even when a support is necessary, a softer or semirigid support such as leather, rather than a hard or rigid support like hard plastic, may work best for most individuals and may even quicken the healing process. This may also apply to the case of a foot fracture, where a semirigid rather than a rigid support is usually best. However, these more serious conditions must be treated individually.

Arch Supports

The notion that our arches always need support is incorrect. They work just fine in their own natural state, as evident from our evolution, where humans have been mostly barefoot. Today, the foot naturally has a higher arch when not bearing weight, and it flattens out considerably with weight bearing. This is especially true in those who spend a lot of time barefoot and have maintained healthy arch function. Some people confuse this normal flattening with "flatfeet" or a pronation problem.

As discussed earlier, the arches of the foot are supported and maintained by muscles. The medial arch is very important, with the tibialis posterior muscle being a key support. Disturbance of muscle function due to shoe problems can lead to muscle imbalance with resulting medial arch dysfunction. In this common situation, addressing the cause of the muscle problem should be the primary treatment rather than using an arch support to take the place of the muscle's normal activity.

Many shoes come with generic supports or insoles that can be removed. Some can be easily taken out while others may require a little pulling. These are very general supports that usually don't match the specific needs of your foot. In most cases, you're better off removing as much as possible from inside the shoe. In addition to allowing your foot to function more freely, the shoe will become thinner and more firm, both healthy attributes. Some of these inserts are meant to cover poor manufacturing work underneath, which can be very rough—in this case it may be uncomfortable to be in this type of shoe without the insert. If the insert is thick, you can replace it with a thinner one.

Orthotics

The use of an orthotic device should not be a first line of therapy for most foot problems. Orthotics are often prescribed to patients with knee pain. However, many studies have not shown this to be effective. In addition, EMG (electromyographic) studies fail to show any significant differences in the average muscle activity of the tibialis anterior, peroneus longus, and gastrocnemius muscles when orthotics are used.

Placing orthotics in your shoes most often results in the shoe fitting differently, usually too tightly. In this instance, the shoe must either be modified or a different shoe used. Unfortunately, this is not usually done and many people with added support now have worse ill-fitting shoes.

Most orthotics are not custom-made to your foot but adhere to a general model of an average foot. They are often made from hard materials—plastic and sometimes even metal. I could never understand these materials for use in a person without a serious permanent condition as these materials are often used for people who have functional problems. Your foot moves through many ranges of motion during the course of standing, walking, or running. The best material to use is leather since it will move with the foot.

Heel Lifts

The use of heel lifts has been popular for many years. These are often recommended for plantar fasciitis, Achilles tendon pain, or the so-called short-leg syndrome, said to contribute to low-back and other pains. Just because they may provide some symptomatic relief, however, does not mean they address the cause of the problem.

Heel lifts can make structural changes in the feet, ankle, legs, pelvis, and spine. Yet studies show that the use of heel lifts can also result in increased impact and increased instability of the foot. The result can be higher weight-bearing stress on the joints in the foot and ankle and possibly the knees, hips, and pelvis. Like other supports, even if you feel better with lifts, the cause of the problem is usually not addressed.

- Heel lifts may provide relief of symptoms in a variety of problems.

 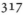

- Heel lifts may temporarily improve symptoms of plantar pain. However, in the process, other areas of the foot and ankle may become physically stressed.

- Some people use heel lifts to attempt to improve low-back pain. It's clear that heel lifts can change the posture of the pelvis and low back. However, whether this change makes a real improvement of the problem, no change, or a worsening of the problem is left to chance.

- For those with so-called short-leg syndrome, heel lifts are sometimes recommended. However, if the "short leg" is functional, which is almost always the case, and due to muscle imbalance and not a true shortening of one leg compared to the other, heel lifts are not the best remedy since they do not address the problem. For those with a history of a broken bone in the leg or thigh or other causes of a true or anatomical short leg, a heel lift may be helpful since one leg is actually shorter. (Although even in these situations, muscles should compensate for a short leg, and using a heel lift may interfere with normal compensation.)

- Heel lifts are sometimes used for those with Achilles tendon pain. This is due to the elevated heel reducing the activity of the gastrocnemius muscle, thereby reducing tension in the Achilles tendon. However, the cause of this tension may be due to other more important muscle imbalance that requires treatment, such as the weakness of the tibialis posterior.

- The temporary use of heel lifts may be important in certain surgical conditions, such as postoperative management of a ruptured Achilles tendon.

Elastic Support

The popular use of elastic support, such as an ACE bandage, is different from taping. These supports don't have much effect on foot sense, presumably because they don't "stick" to the skin like tape and have much less of an effect on the nerves within. Studies have shown that compared to other devices, elastic supports are much less effective in treating various foot and ankle conditions. Like other supports, elastic devices may cause muscle dysfunction if worn for too long.

Shoe Lacing

Some shoe problems are not due to fit but poor lacing technique. How difficult can it be to tie your shoes? After all, we learned that a long time ago as children. Well, the fact is, many people don't lace their shoes correctly, and sometimes it can make a significant difference in how the shoe fits. In addition, many people don't tie the laces of their casual shoes, making them too loose. This creates a very unstable stress in the feet.

Sometimes lacing too tight is a sufficient-enough stress to cause problems. Lacing should be snug—not too loose but not tight. There should never be discomfort associated with lacing, or any discomfort under the area of the laces. The most important aspect of lacing is that, after tying your shoes, they should be completely comfortable, and after they've been on for a while, they should be just as comfortable. This should be true for not only the laces but the whole shoe.

There are many different types of lacing used for many different types of shoes by different types of shoe wearers. Using comfort as your guide, you'll always get the best fit. Here are some general tips to lace more effectively:

- Always lace from the toes upward, beginning with the holes or eyelets farthest down.
- Each set of eyelets you go through with the lace, pull the laces snug, but not tight, so the same amount of tension is evenly distributed through the lace.
- Use a crisscross or zigzag pattern—most people and most shoes function best with this approach.
- When you finish lacing, all areas of the lace should have the same tension.

Crisscross style of lacing is the most common way to tie shoes in the United States. In Europe, it's more common to use straight lacing, where instead of all the laces going up the shoe in a diagonal pattern, some go from hole to hole straight across.

It's been shown that both the crisscross and European pattern is equally effective. If you find either of these patterns of lacing not comfortable, most likely your shoe does not fit correctly. In addition, the crisscross

pattern requires the least amount of lace, so you'll always have sufficient lace for tying. The European style is the second most efficient approach for lace use.

If you have a very irregular foot, you may require any number of different types of lacing, one that matches your particular needs. In this case you may also be wearing special shoes and a specialist should be able to help with lacing. In any situation, don't be afraid to experiment. But always use the comfort factor as the ultimate index.

It is easy to get seduced by the marketing hype associated with the latest footwear fads. But your most prudent path is to steer clear of the bold, extravagant claims offered by the shoe companies. Overall, those who wear shoes less often have healthier feet. You need to experiment with different shoes and styles, while continuing to make adjustments and self-assessments. Your feet are quite adaptive.

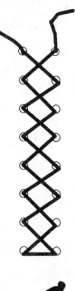

Humans, to a great extent, owe their survival as a species to their feet. Forty thousand years ago, we left Africa by foot and have been moving ever since.

CHAPTER 18

EVERY RUNNER IS DIFFERENT

The Intimate Relationship Between Footwear and Gait, and What You Can Do to Improve Both

The numbers speak for themselves. Running events like the marathon have been steadily rising every year. In 2009, 468,000 people completed a marathon, which was almost a 10 percent increase from 2008. Another 10 percent increase occurred in 2010. Many are first-time runners whose goal is simply to finish, usually several hours after the winners, and even if it requires a bit of walking. The number of participants is even greater for 10Ks and half marathons.

The national organization Running USA estimates that over ten million Americans completed a road race in 2009. Aging baby boomers are fueling this interest; the average age of a male runner is forty-four; for female runners it's thirty-eight. They want to stay fit and active, and running is an easy way to get in a high-quality aerobic workout, whether on a treadmill in the guest bedroom or by simply stepping out the front door and trotting down the road. Running requires little in the way of equipment—some clothing and a pair of shoes (for most) are all that are really needed.

Compared to other sports, running can be done on the cheap, which is an appealing quality in difficult economic times. Given that a pair of shoes is the only real investment required, runners tend to be obsessive about what they put on their feet. The average runner purchases three pairs of running shoes each year. Understandably, runners develop deep and lasting relationships with brands and models, and they rely on their footwear to protect them and carry them to new heights of achievement.

But there are other important considerations that often come into play when it comes to running, especially for those who would like to go faster, longer, or more efficiently. Long before I entered private practice, I was a competitive runner who specialized in short distances on indoor wooden and outdoor cinder tracks. But like so many others who caught the jogging bug in the '70s, I, too, became a runner who liked seeing how far he could run. That was a primary reason I ran in the 1980 New York City Marathon.

Around this time, I also began treating and training runners as well as top-ranked endurance athletes. And as word got out of what I did, I began to receive invitations to speak at running clubs, cycling clubs, and even aerobic classes. I'd be lecturing to a group of, say, fifty runners about the importance of running technique, and on the hour, like clockwork, nearly everyone's digital wristwatch would beep almost in unison. Except for me, I didn't wear one. But I did talk about heart rate monitors, although they were bulky and didn't come with a watch back then.

Understanding Gait

Beginning runners often just run because they enjoy it. They care little about the nuances regarding form, technique, or proper gait. But at the elite level of running, gait takes on an entirely new dimension of complexity, research, and questioning.

But first, what is precisely meant by the term "gait"? It is typically defined as moving posture—in running, it's the whole body's forward progress, including the foot strike and pelvic position, to arm swing, head and knee movement. It's not unusual for coaches, kinesiologists and other biomechanics experts, and elite runners to dissect each component of one's gait. From this assessment, each element of the gait that's viewed as "flawed" is "corrected"—the runner is told to lift the knee to this position, swing the arms that way, or hold the elbows this way.

Yet nothing is more natural than the biomechanics of human running. Or should be. With every step a runner takes, the limbs, trunk, head, and spine participate in various combinations of movement, ranging from flexion, extension, and rotation, to abduction and adduction, along with the feet, which pronate, supinate, invert, and evert. Only by understanding the normal range of motion can one detect "abnormal" movements so as to help assess an injured athlete or observe for the potential of future injury.

This is what I like doing as a coach, trainer, and also in private practice—applying what I learned about biomechanics as a student and using that knowledge to help patients correct their painful injuries and hidden imbalances. But before I became adept at treating common athletic injuries, I had to learn the biggest lesson yet: Understanding the details of each of the body's movements—some are so subtle that most runners don't even notice them—had to be put aside, almost forgotten. Instead, I had to look at the big picture. In other words, when it comes to gait, the whole person moves better than the sum of each of his or her parts. This is what makes the running gait uniquely individual.

More importantly, there's no ideal running form. While all humans have the same basic running patters—just like other animals—your gait is yours alone. In fact, it's easy to recognize your running partner from a distance, even before the face comes into focus, because you know his or her unique running fingerprint.

Even looking at the best athletes in professional sports, there's one common feature—everyone's movements are slightly different. Each golfer follows the basic swing, while at the same time each has a swing all his

own; the same for every pole vaulter, baseball pitcher, tennis player, or marathoner.

That is, unless something interferes with movement. When something causes the gait to go astray, two things happen. First, there is the risk of getting injured because it meant something went wrong, and it will be reflected in running form in a subtle—or sometimes more obvious—way. There might be irregular movement in the hip joint causing the pelvis to tilt more to one side than the other, more flexion of one knee than the other stressing the hamstring muscles, too much rotation of the leg causing the foot to flair outward excessively, and erratic arm movements. The most common reason for this is muscle imbalance, and it forces the body to compensate by contracting certain muscles to keep the imbalance from worsening.

The second problem is that the body's energy is being used inefficiently. It will raise the heart rate more than usual, making one fatigue quicker, and resulting in a slower pace. There are several common abnormalities that could interfere with the brain's ability to let the body run free and efficiently.

Physical interference is most often the result of bad shoes or muscle imbalance, sometimes both. Stretching can disturb the gait too—by making a muscle longer with a loss of power. By stretching muscles before running, it's very possible to cause muscle imbalance.

Mental-emotional interference is most typically the result of misinformation, usually from bad advice. The images seen on TV, of lead runners in the marathon traveling at sub-five-minute paces, remain in the brains of millions of people who jog along at a ten-minute pace in the same race. We all want to run that way, but we can't. And we should not pretend either.

Another mental-emotional factor is a bad habit. It's easy in our society to develop bad postural habits. A lot of energy is devoted to some movements, like running or lifting weights, but we neglect other activities like healthy posture. The result is that we slump at our desks, stand with poor posture, and even walk with a bad gait—all because somewhere along the way we allowed our bodies to get lazy. For many, these bad habits carry over to running.

What Is the Best Running Gait?

Over the years, I was often asked about the best way to run. Faster leg turnover? Lean forward with the body? Keep your arms by your side? Push off with your feet? I wish there was a simple answer. But there's not. What is best to tell a runner, however, is the notion that if your feet hit the ground properly, the rest of the body tends to follow, resulting in your natural gait. While this is the most important place to start improving your gait—and if there's a problem—here's the one to fix first. But this is easier done than said. Most running shoes interfere with the feet doing their job, which could cause the whole body to have a poor gait, inducing stress into muscles, bones, and joints. By wearing the wrong shoes, you'll never find your natural effective gait.

A specific problem that's most common is that many running shoes cause you to land on your heel instead of farther forward on your foot. This is because they are built with large oversupported heels and are marketed as providing as a "smoother, more cushioned ride." But over time, the repetitive action of landing on the heel causes foot dysfunction as well as the potential for an ankle, knee, and hip injury. Now your body's foundation is cracking at the most vulnerable areas.

The arches in your feet, supported by muscles and many tendons, especially the large Achilles, work in such a way that when unimpeded, their built-in springlike action makes running a perfectly natural activity. Not only can your foot take the pounding force with each step without damage, but it also takes that energy—from the gravitation force—and recycles it back to the foot to spring forward instead of falling back. But by wearing shoes with built-up heels, you are virtually falling backward with each step.

Try running barefoot even for a few yards to feel the difference. You can't land on your heel. Being barefoot will change all that. It will allow you to run free, natural, and efficient. Generally, by running barefoot, you'll tend not to slump. It will be easier to keep an upright posture. This is because you'll land on your mid- to forefoot, not your heel. And

WALKING VERSUS RUNNING

Walking is associated with first striking the heel, whereas a running gait involves landing farther forward on the foot—a midfoot strike in most cases with more forefoot landing as running speed increases.

Making contact with the ground imparts impact forces—the foot literally collides with the earth on each step. While impact is often seen as a negative aspect of running, equating to trauma and injury, a proper gait is potentially associated with better bone density and improved muscle and tendon function, better circulation, and other healthy benefits associated with exercise. With proper gait, colliding with the ground is well compensated for—humans have evolved an effective gait mechanism.

Impact forces during walking are relatively minor. But heel striking while running can be a significant loss of energy, a common example of an improper gait producing stress from impact. The overall mechanics of the foot, ankle and leg, and many body areas above are stressed with abnormal heel striking compared to the runner who lands farther forward. Mid- or forefoot running is associated with a more optimal gait that's usually not impact impaired. Let's consider these two gaits.

A key difference between walking and proper (mid- and forefoot) running is how the foot muscles work and, in particular, the energy used for propulsion. The walking body acts more like an inverted pendulum, swinging along step by step, literally vaulting over stiff legs with locked knees. Muscles use the body's metabolic energy created by the conversion of carbohydrates and fat.

Things are quite different with running. This action is sometimes referred to as an "impulsive" and "springy" gait, rebounding along on compliant legs and unlocked knees. Instead of using all the body's energy, the leg and foot have a built-in "return energy" system for a significant amount of energy. This relies on the Achilles and other tendons to recycle impact energy. (Don't confuse this with claims made that some running shoes have a "return energy" system, they don't—it's simply marketing hype.)

In running, the body has an effective muscle work-minimizing strategy—many of the foot muscles don't technically push you off the ground like during walking. Instead, the muscles provide an isometric-type tension to stabilize the tendons and help in the function of the unique mechanism that takes impact energy, sometimes referred to as "elastic energy" associated with gravity and impact, and uses it for propelling the body forward. In particular, the large springy Achilles tendon on the back of the heel that runs up the leg and attaches into the large calf muscles (the gastrocnemius and soleus) plays a key role in recycling energy for propulsion. This tendon must function with sufficient tension to help in the return energy process, and the muscles it attaches to, also important postural supports, require a certain level of tautness, even at rest. (Trying to "loosen" these muscles and tendons through stretching, aggressive massage, or other therapy may be counterproductive, impairing the natural springy gait. Excessive tightness of the Achilles certainly can induce poor function as well—think balance.)

Those with shorter, more compact Achilles tendons, unlike taller runners who also have longer heel bones attached to the Achilles, generally have a more efficient spring mechanism—one reason why shorter runners typically can run faster, especially in sprinting, although there are exceptions. Carl Lewis and Usain Bolt, past and present Olympic champions, respectively, are taller than average. Bolt's height advantage worked against him in the start, but then he would later cover more ground using fewer strides than his competitors.

Here's how the body's natural gait uses recycled energy for propulsion. As a runner's foot hits the ground, impact energy is stored in the muscles and tendons, and 95 percent of this energy is then used to spring the body forward like a pogo stick. This mechanism provides about 50 percent of the leg and foot energy for propulsion (the other 50 percent comes from muscle contraction). If this process isn't working well, such as if you land on your heels, are wearing bad shoes, or have muscle imbalance, the impact energy is dissipated or lost, and you must make up for the problem by contracting more muscles for propulsion, which requires the use of more energy. Not only is this mechanically inefficient but it will also slow you down, due to the higher cost of energy. This can be further compounded if you burn less fat for energy, thereby relying more on sugar that's associated with the more rapid onset of fatigue. And the impact energy that's not recycled often places a strain on muscles and tendons (and ultimately, ligaments and bones) and can contribute to an injury.

In addition, movements above the ankle, especially in the knees, hips, and low back can help—or hurt—the natural spring-ahead mechanism. Too much motion in these joints can reduce the body's ability to recycle impact energy. By running more upright—you should be running tall—rather than adopting a lazy, slumped-over position, you'll minimize knee, hip, and low-back movements, and thus helping to utilize the foot's spring mechanism. This involves using muscles similar to when you have to stand up straight—they include the abdominals, gluteus maximus, and even the neck flexors that prevent the head from tilting back.

Other movements are different between walking and running. Most notably in the knee, which is locked during a walking gait but not while running. The slightly flexed knee is more active during running and requires much more effort by muscles to support the joint while the foot is on the ground. This is a key reason why many runners with improper gait have knee injuries.

Those who run slowly often wonder if it's better to sometimes just walk fast as the pace can be the same. This is especially true on hills. Deciding on which option is best is the job of the brain, which will naturally tend to make the right decision about making the transition from walking to running.

The energy cost of walking and running not only varies with speed but with the type of ground surface and other environmental factors such as temperature, humidity, and wind. But when the gait is irregular, both walking and running share a common feature: Both movements will cost more in energy. The worse or more inefficient the gait, the greater will be the energy expenditure.

with each step your foot will spring your body up and forward.

This natural gait will help you sense your feet springing off the ground, almost as if they have more energy. In fact, they do. That's the energy return that occurs naturally in a healthy stride. Focus on the feet springing off the ground. When you feel it, your body will actually be moving more quickly. If you're wearing a heart monitor, you'll see that your pace can be faster without a rise in heart rate. (I have witnessed, on many occasions, a difference ranging between ten and twelve beats—with higher rates associated with an improper running gait.)

Need more help? Think of running on hot coals—if you were going to do that, your feet need to stay off the red-hot coals as much as possible. So from the instant each foot touches the ground, quickly pick it up. I've used this "hot coal" technique to help runners be more efficient with their gait. The longer your foot stays on the ground, the more energy you waste, the more vulnerable you are to injury, and the less likely you will use that energy for better running. Instead, think about your feet coming off the ground after each step. All while you're relaxed. Look at photos of the great runners; they are actually airborne much of the time because they spend much less time with each foot on the ground.

In the unlikely event that your body is being particularly stubborn and you can't relate to what I've just explained, it could be that your feet are so used to working improperly that they need more time to learn natural movements. They may require additional retraining or rehabilitation. If this is the case, keep forging ahead with barefoot activity, slowly increasing the time spent unshod. This process is particularly difficult and challenging for those who have already developed poor running habits or for those with a long history of wearing improper shoes.

Interference from Muscle Imbalance

Even if you're doing all the right things—performing your brief barefoot jog, using the correct flat-sole shoes during the rest of your workout and throughout the day—muscle imbalance can interfere with a more efficient gait. One of the most common problems people develop in their feet is muscle imbalance. This can become a vicious cycle—you can't walk or jog without your shoes because your muscle imbalance prevents proper support, but the shoes continue maintaining muscle imbalance.

But for some people with muscle imbalance, going without shoes often doesn't feel right, or in some cases it's painful. In both cases, the shoes have literally become a crutch—you're addicted to the artificial support. It's like being in a wheelchair all day—getting up after ten hours will make you feel

stiff and achy—being in the wheelchair for months will render you unable to even walk!

By gradually weaning yourself off over-supported shoes—and this means going barefoot whenever you can or when it's convenient—you can often fix the muscle imbalance in your feet by stimulating them in such a way as to enlist proper function of all the muscles, ligaments, tendons, and even the skin.

This can take time for some people. It might first be necessary to wear slightly thinner-soled shoes and gradually work down to those that are half or more in thickness from your usually shoe. Only then, as your feet start to work and feel better, will barefoot walking finally achieve that wonderful natural sensation that was originally hardwired into your body as a youth. Then only after a couple of weeks of just walking more naturally, you will be able to jog barefoot.

In stubborn cases, or to speed the process, it may be necessary to find a health care professional who can determine which muscles are not functioning correctly and fix them.

You don't have to become a barefoot runner. For those who want to progress from walking to running, even professional athletes, many choose to run barefoot for the whole workout. But for others, just spending time at home or work without shoes is the start of a great therapy. Then add a walk on the grass barefoot, even for ten minutes a day. The more time barefoot, the more your feet will work better in a proper shoe. Jogging or running short distances barefoot to retrain your body's natural gait is the quickest, most powerful, and most effective way to accomplish this task. It helps if you have a great location for barefoot running—a grassy park, a hard-sand beach, or a track.

By taking off your shoes and jogging or running barefoot—even for fifty or one hundred yards—you'll eliminate interference between your feet and ground and quickly have better form. Among other things, this will improve your foot strike—from a heel striker to landing more forward—produce better pelvic movement and arm swing, and allow your head to better control eye-and-body coordination (a very complex but important part of running efficiency). But because of bad habits, some people need more than just taking off their shoes—this behavior is unfortunately well ingrained into the processes of the brain, nervous system, and muscles. Perhaps this programming first began at an early age in gym class, at summer camp, or from watching a video, reading a running magazine, or from a well-meaning coach.

Once your gait is more natural, shoes will interfere much less. In fact, as your feet function better, you'll feel more sensitive to shoes that are not a perfect match—you'll focus on finding the ones that fit just right on each foot, are flat, and don't disturb your normal foot mechanics. Once your feet are happy, you have the best chance of finding your ideal running form. In the process of finding the perfect shoe, you'll become a "pain" for those

salespeople in places like Foot Locker. That's okay.

A Quick Primer on Running Right

The notion of barefoot running to improve your form and gait is fine and good, but what if you've trained your body to bend forward too much, can't get the image of a world-class marathoner-type stride out of your head, or have learned other bad running habits such as landing on your heels. What then? So here are some additional recommendations that can help you get out of the rut:

1. Avoid Trying to Emulate the "Perfect" Gait

You can't fool Mother Nature, so don't mess with gait. Trying to run with some "perfect" running form is a quick way to get hurt. It's been tried over and over, without long-term success. In fact, it was a common history I heard from runners coming to my clinic with an injury. The sad story was a common one—many of the comments went something like this:

- I started running strides on the track to improve my form . . .
- I was watching the New York City Marathon on TV and couldn't help notice the running style of the leader and thought I should run the same way . . .
- I began training with my friends who were running four-hundred-meter sprints . . .

328

THE PROS AND CONS OF VIDEO GAIT ANALYSIS

For the past several decades, video analysis of human movement has been used in virtually all sports by coaches, athletes, and health care professionals. Because of the relative ease of combining video and treadmill activity, this approach is now common in the evaluation of running gait. Properly applied, video analysis can be an important assessment tool, helping reveal gait abnormalities and add to our knowledge and research of body mechanics.

In isolation of other factors, however, video gait analysis has limited value. An abnormal irregular gait pattern is most often the end result of some imbalance in the body or wearing improper shoes and rarely due to just bad running posture. The ideal use of video analysis of gait combines it with a complete assessment, including a health and fitness history, a thorough physical examination, and others such as blood and urine tests or X-rays that may be necessary to uncover a problem that influences gait, for a comprehensive evaluation of an individual.

Even to the untrained eye, it's not difficult to observe an asymmetrical or awkward gait, even without a video—just watch other runners on the roads, track, or in parks. Fatigue can worsen most gait problems, so at the end of a 10K race or during the second half of a marathon, irregular gaits are more common and most obvious.

One must differentiate an abnormal, irregular-looking gait from one that is an individual's normal running pattern. Regardless of one's speed, running incorporates the use of more muscle mass than virtually all other regular activities. As such, one's gait reflects individuality because the muscles (and their tendons) and bones (and associated ligaments) are not perfectly symmetrical between the left and right side and also vary from one person to the next. Like a unique "fingerprint," this contributes to each person's particular gait.

Other than the effect of wearing ill-fitting shoes or those that have too much heel or are overly rigid, muscle imbalance may be one of the most common causes for an abnormal, irregular gait because the body's neuromuscular system (including the brain and nerves connected to the muscles) is responsible for all movement. For example, let's say you pulled your right hamstring a few months ago, which caused weakness. A secondary problem might have developed as compensation—tightness in the right quadriceps. One possible end result of this muscle imbalance is that the pelvis tilts downward on the same side and rotates forward, triggering tightness in the low-back muscles. The result is an irregular gait—the right leg may stride slightly longer than the left, and the tension in the low back increases extension in the spine, distorting it all the way up to the head. (In addition to slowing you down at the same heart rate—the energy cost of running increases—you'll fatigue easier and be at risk for an injury, typically one associated with inflammation in the hip, knee, or spine.)

Video analysis won't necessarily tell you which specific problem or imbalance exists, but rather, it provides images of how your body moves as a result of these particular imbalances. A common example of gait irregularity is associated with dysfunction of the tibialis posterior muscle, which is a frequent cause of foot, leg, and knee injury. One end of this muscle attaches on the bones in the back of the leg and the other end in numerous locations of the bottom of the foot. The tibialis posterior supports the medial arch and significantly controls ankle and foot movements. Specifically, it stabilizes the back, middle, and front of the foot while it's on the ground during the run. A video analysis may demonstrate the abnormal gait associated with this muscle problem. The atypical foot mechanics associated with tibialis posterior muscle dysfunction may include excessive dropping of the medial arch—abnormal pronation—or other erratic motions observed when the foot hits the ground. After observing these movements on video, a follow-up assessment involves a precise evaluation of the tibialis posterior muscle (and perhaps other potential causes of the irregular gait) followed by an appropriate therapy that restores normal muscle function (such as the various techniques used in rehabilitation, physical therapy, or massage). In many cases, positive gait changes can be observed once the tibialis posterior muscle (in this case) is corrected, which can sometimes be in one or two treatments. In other cases requiring more therapy, a slower improvement in gait would follow.

But not everyone who pronates has this particular problem. Consider another runner with the same excessive pronation when the foot strikes the ground. In this case the cause of pronation may be dysfunction of the psoas muscle in the pelvis. The psoas attaches to the front of the lower spine, going through the pelvis and hooking on to the upper part of the inner thigh bone (the femur); and though it's a primary flexor of the hip, it also affects leg rotation. Psoas dysfunction can result in the lower limb rotating outward too much, causing the medial arch of the foot to fall excessively inward on impact—abnormal pronation. As often occurs after video analysis, encouraging a runner to keep the leg from rotating too much or point the toes more forward rather than too far out may seem logical, but this can put significant stress

330

on other muscles, potentially triggering an injury in a different location, such as a muscle strain that affects the knee joint. Just as important, if this is the only recommendation, the psoas dysfunction remains untreated.

A video analysis of your gait can have the greatest value if a trained professional performs the test and interprets the images. There are individuals with diverse educational and professional backgrounds who are experts in this field, including kinesiologists, physical therapists, medical doctors, chiropractors, and others engaged in sports medicine. But the video is only part of what is often a complex process—a full evaluation might include postural analysis, physical examination, blood tests, and assessment of other aspects of your life that could directly or indirectly impact on gait. This might also include exercise schedules, diet, nutritional status, and the types of shoes you wear during sport, leisure, and work.

Physical therapist Jay Dicharry, director of the SPEED Performance Clinic and the Motion Analysis Lab coordinator at the University of Virginia, uses three-dimensional motion analysis systems in his state-of-the-art facility to digitally reconstruct the individual's body as a multisegment system. In a recently published paper in the journal *Clinics in Sports Medicine* (2010), he describes part of this assessment procedure: "After infrared markers are placed at specific anatomic landmarks, their position is triangulated by cameras to calibrate the individual into the system. Construction of the coordinates and orientation of the rigid body segments allow calculation of joint angles of the proximal and distal segment, joint angular velocity, and joint acceleration. Measurements are collected for each joint in all three cardinal planes of motion." The 3-D gait analysis then produces graphs for each plane of motion of each specific joint. Dicharry also states that "in a clinical setting, barefoot gait evaluation can yield a plethora of information about the foot, but clinicians must be aware of the complex foot mechanics."

Just as important as a complete gait assessment is an athlete's follow-up. After a video analysis and following any therapy or exercise recommendations that are made to improve your gait, another assessment should be made to observe whether improvements in gait have indeed occurred. How soon this is performed after the first video analysis depends on the individual and his or her particular problems. And most importantly, all this should correlate with any previous signs or symptoms—a prior injury should be completely gone if the process has been successful.

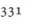

Video analysis of gait is too often used to help an athlete run more "efficiently." In this case, the runner's gait is compared with some textbook or "ideal" style, and the recommendations might include lifting the knees higher, swinging the arms differently, bending forward more, or, as mentioned above, preventing the lower limb from rotating outward too much. Put into practice by the runner under the watchful eye of his or her coach, it can be counterproductive and can even lead to further dysfunction. I've seen too many athletes, even elite runners and professional triathletes, who tried to mimic a so-called perfect running gait—one that uses a world-class marathoner's gait as a model—only to get injured, along with worsening performance. One reason is that the causes of an irregular gait—such as muscle imbalance—are never evaluated and corrected. Instead, the person consciously runs with a different gait, which can further add stress to an coach, it can body. Correcting abnormalities must be done first. This will allow the brain to better regulate muscle, joint, and other mechanical function to provide the most efficient gait for that particular individual. (Another problem with trying to copy the fluid form of a world-class marathoner is that most people simply can't run that fast.)

Other key factors in video analysis of gait are cost and availability. The equipment in a modern gait laboratory might include a three-dimensional motion analysis camera system, a high-tech treadmill with special force platforms and pressure mats, and video-editing software necessary to compile the images. But this type of facility is less available to the average runner, who more often is evaluated with a simple camera on a basic treadmill, which has its limitations. However, in many cases, a proper gait analysis using modern high-tech equipment can cost significantly more than visiting the right therapist who may be able to effectively assess and treat the causes of irregular gait without the need for video analysis.

Here are some other thoughts if you're ready to have your gait analyzed. In quantum physics it's been said that the mere act of observing an atomic particle changes its state—in video analysis, when someone is watching you run, you will usually, perhaps subconsciously, change your gait. Furthermore, when running on a treadmill, the "ground" is moving, and this can create a slightly different gait than on a track.

Like most assessment tools for use on humans, video analysis of gait is not perfect. But the science of observation—a key part of my work with athletes since the 1970s—would not be the same without the large volume of important research that has been performed, often by assessing the running gait.

This is not to say there aren't ways to make the running gait more mechanically and metabolically efficient. Physical strain and wasted energy can come from excessive arm movement, overstriding, and improper footwear.

Despite the many possible benefits of video, the simplest, least expensive, and most effective approach for most runners to experience a better gait is to just take off their shoes and run a short distance slowly while barefoot. (A barefoot video analysis of gait is the "raw data" that's vital before seeing the body while wearing shoes.) Just jogging barefoot down the hall in your home is a start. Doing this on a smooth surface, such as an outdoor track or grass for a couple of hundred meters is helpful. A daily "therapy" of jogging barefoot—even working up to a quarter mile—can be great for the feet and overall body mechanics. In addition to this routine having the potential to correct muscle imbalance, it enables one to immediately experience how natural running truly feels—something a video analysis usually won't accomplish. There's nothing high-tech about going barefoot, and yet it can do wonders in improving a runner's gait.

One elite runner, Dr. Mark Cucuzzella, forty-five, is a highly accomplished marathoner (2:24 PR), race director, family physician, associate professor at West Virginia University School of Medicine, lieutenant colonel in the Air Force Reserve, and owner of Two Rivers Treads, a center for natural running and walking, in Sheperdstown, West Virginia. He is a big believer in video analysis and barefoot running. "I have been enlightened in how not just my own body works and how to correct it, but also in how I can assist others, by participating in gait evaluation and the corrective prescriptions with Jay Dicharry at his SPEED Performance Clinic. Jay has taught me to see and understand what I could not see. The analysis which involved motion and joint forces helped me identify asymmetries, joint mobility and stability deficits, and stride patterns, which were suboptimal for efficiency. By cueing certain movements and muscles I made immediate corrections in form and through proper rehabilitation of weaknesses made long-term stability corrections. Retesting proved in the lab what I was feeling in my body—a more relaxed, stable, and efficient stride. That being said, I continue to learn and am doing a lot of true barefoot running now, and it's really impossible to overstride barefoot. The lower leg never gets out beyond perpendicular to ground."

We too often forget that the human body, when given the opportunity and in the proper environment, is the best teacher and coach. We just need to be more attentive students.

- I read an article on form in the running magazine . . .

All these statements ended with . . . soon afterward I started feeling this pain . . .

What's particularly typical is that a coach or runner himself will attempt to break down the gait into separate components—arms should be horizontal, knees should come up high, thigh horizontal, heels should almost hit your butt, and so on. When all these aspects are performed "correctly," you supposedly have the perfect gait and can move at a faster running pace. But in reality, most runners revert back to their old habits, physically unable to make these dramatic changes. And what often happens next is a muscle twinge here, a joint ache there, and soon a run-stopping injury. That's because the runner is often starting with an already-improper gait, especially if he or she is a heel striker wearing the wrong oversupported shoes. The fact is that there are actually dozens of interrelated components regarding gait—and even if you make them picture-perfect, it doesn't mean your body works better that way. Additionally, consciously making a lot of gait changes can raise your heart rate significantly— a sign of increased stress. And if you only change some of the individual pieces of your gait, you just end up with another form of improper gait that can cause physical stress elsewhere in your body.

2. Don't Lean Forward

It seems obvious. If you lean forward, you'll fall forward and propel your body in the direction it's going, so it must be a good way to run. It's not. The problem with leaning forward is that most people do it by bending at the waist; that's unnatural. Bending forward forces your lower and upper spine to extend back more and, in fact, the whole body to adapt to a potentially worsening posture. The result will be added stress on your muscles, tendons, joints, ligaments, and bones anywhere in the body.

Instead of bending at your waist, which flexes the pelvis and triggers a whole serious of abnormal changes in posture leading to a more irregular gait, think about the whole pelvis being slightly more forward instead of tilting forward. Properly done, this will make you run in a more upright posture. Think about being taller when you run, which technically you are when your posture is right. As the spine is straighter (it has normal curves), you will also want to make sure your head is in a natural position. Do this with your eyes and your head will follow: Look slightly below the horizon—not gazing straight ahead, not looking up, and not with your head looking down at the ground.

By unnaturally bending or tilting forward, you could cause the powerful gluteus maximus muscles in the area of your butt to gradually lose power because they contract much less (which causes the quadriceps on the front of the thigh and possibly the psoas muscles in the front of the pelvis to tighten too much). And both the lumbar (low back) and cervical (neck) spine can extend too much, producing an exaggerated curve along with extensor muscle tightness in the back of the neck and the low back. This could also cause weakness in the neck flexor muscles, making the head less stable, which can further worsen your form. All this makes the body use more energy to accomplish the same task of moving forward.

When running, think about a forward pelvis and you'll feel your quadriceps contract as you hit the ground with your foot. If you do this correctly, you'll feel your butt tighten and even produce slight muscle soreness between workouts if you have chronic gluteus maximus weakness. Doing this will also allow your abdominal muscles to contract more, and become firm, further helping you run with a better upright posture.

All this may be difficult if not impossible to do if you wear oversupported or thick-soled running shoes because you'll land on your heel, which forces your pelvis back instead of forward. By wearing proper shoes and landing mid- or forefoot, your gait is more likely to be optimal.

Even better is this idea: Instead of trying to lean forward, focus on the "hot coal" technique mentioned earlier. By getting your foot off the ground quicker (which is a process of bending and lifting the knee), you'll

encourage the foot and ankle spring-forward mechanism, which will propel you most efficiently.

3. Pushing Off

If you follow the actions noted above, pushing off from the ground with your foot is not something you need to consciously do with each step. Your brain will take care of that action (along with the hundreds of others your body undergoes during running). Pushing off should be natural and occur without you doing anything if your gait is right. As noted above, the body has an incredible spring mechanism, an important job of the tendons attaching to foot muscles that make up the arches of the feet, and especially the Achilles tendon supported by the calf muscles. As you hit the ground, you recycle that pounding energy to spring forward. In other words, you will be naturally using the force in your favor for a better gait. If you have to force your push-off, you're probably doing something wrong, such as wearing the wrong shoes. In that case, the pounding becomes a negative effect and ultimately can contribute to an injury.

4. Fast Leg Turnover

A fast leg turnover is fine, but can you mimic a world-class runner stride for stride? For most, the answer is no. Just as you can't shorten your stride too much to get a faster turnover. Too long or too short a stride is

 335

unnatural and stressful, but finding your most relaxed gait will produce the lowest heart rate, all while maintaining the same pace. (Or a faster pace with the same heart rate.)

You can run within the natural boundaries of your own biomechanics and still increase leg turnover by incorporating downhill runs into your training. By running down a slight or moderate grade (not too steep), you can maintain the same heart rate and run at a much faster pace and without overstriding, thereby having a faster turnover. This is a great workout for those who compete, and performing it once or twice a week (not back-to-back days) is not excessive for most runners. You can do this with several downhill repeats if you have a long grade of a half mile or more (with an easy jog up the hill to start your downhill run again) or just run a hilly course with adequate downhills.

5. Cadence

Humans move in an incredibly similar fashion regarding cadence or tempo. It may be hard to believe, but most of us all run about 180 steps per minute. Anyone who is healthy normally walks at a basic pace of about 120 steps per minute. Even our daily activity has been shown to have a "pace" of 120 steps or moves per minute. (The exception is walking or running on a treadmill, which poses a particular stress due to its unnatural circumstance—the brain senses the body movement but the body remains in one place. In this case, there's a wider variation in tempo.)

These numbers—180 and 120—are approximate and are typical. Virtually all runners have a range of tempo between about 150 and 190 steps a minute whether jogging, running a marathon, or sprinting. This allows one's brain some leeway to adjust one's pace and body mechanics as necessary. Muscle imbalance, fatigue, caffeine, time of day, the weather, and other factors can affect one's running efficiency for a given workout, and the brain will sense these factors and make appropriate changes such as slightly slowing our tempo or speeding it up.

It's more than the brain, the rest of our head is important too, not only influencing tempo but also gait. The eyes (a part of the brain) play a role, as does the inner ear, which contains a tiny otolith on each side. These contribute to collecting information about body movement and balance. In addition, various muscles around the neck and those of the jaw joint (which connect directly to the brain as opposed to all other muscles which first connect to the spinal cord) continually send messages to the brain about body movement and help the eyes and ears do their work. All this feedback, combined with the sensory input coming from the feet, spine, pelvis, and elsewhere helps the brain better adapt to changes during a run. Most of these adjustments are subtle and barely noticeable. The result is the most efficient run possible. In order to do this, the brain may decide 176 is a good tempo, at least for the first twenty or so minutes, then it may change to 182, and so on.

RUNNING WITH PHIL

Coralee Thompson, MD, writes about natural running in her new "toe-finger" shoes:

I've been working out for much of my adult life, and since first meeting Dr. Phil Maffetone in 1997, running always included wearing very flat shoes. The past few years while living in the mountains of Southern Arizona, we sometimes combine three daily activities that might include hiking, running, walking, biking, and swimming. In addition, moving heavy mounds of soil for the garden, lifting large rocks, and other chores more than satisfy the anaerobic aspects of the neuromuscular system.

Recently, I noticed my cheap $20 running shoes, about four or five years old, were ready for retirement. They served me well. Phil helped me find a good stride and cadence and maintain a good posture while running. But even though I'm ten years younger than him, my heart rate was always ten beats higher.

We often discussed barefoot biomechanics, not to mention many other aspects of health and fitness—we live it. Luckily, if anything ever goes wrong with my muscles or joints, he's quick to fix it. But I miss not being barefoot outdoors more. The Arizona desert, with its windblown thorns everywhere, especially on the seemingly smooth trails and dirt roads, is not the place to be barefoot, especially for running of any significant duration even though we're that way much of the day inside and near the house.

The other day I went into Tucson for gardening supplies and succumbed to my intrigue of owning a pair of Vibram FiveFingers, which have tiny sleeves for each toe and a thin bottom rubber tread. It was not an impulsive decision, but it was just time. Before doling out $100-plus for a cute light gray and green pair called Bikila and in a size 42 men's, I made sure that Summit Hut sports store offered a return policy. It did.

Phil and I talked about the potential issue of having to get used to this type of footwear. "Your muscles are very well balanced, and your feet quite healthy, so in your case, making the change should not be difficult or require a period of breaking them in," Phil told me.

Apparently, a lot of runners are having trouble making the transition. We've read and heard about runners having to wean into using these glovelike shoes, sometimes taking weeks to get used to them or not able to run in them without causing blisters or pain.

Just to be sure, I wore them when I left the store and kept them on until I got home—making about a dozen quick stops at various stores along the way. So far they felt great.

When I wore them for my first morning run, the shoes felt even better. In fact, I felt like a great runner—like those photos of lead-pack marathoners. Well, almost.

Phil did say my gait, stride, and cadence were even better than usual, and the time my foot stayed on the ground appeared to be much less. I was running with grace and ease that I have never felt in my life in all the years I've run.

Phil also noticed that my improved mechanics seemed like it would reduce the cost of running. Daniel Lieberman, PhD, was recently quoted in *Harvard Magazine* that running barefoot is about 5 percent more efficient than wearing shoes. But that's an estimate, and he's not taking into account people whose feet fall apart when they take off their shoes. Since their feet are full of distortions, due to daily trauma, such as bone injuries often disguised as a "normal" ache or pain, muscle dysfunction, and toe damage that creates an adequate-enough nervous system injury so that the whole body will twist, bend, warp, and otherwise need much more energy to do the same work. Likewise, a person with near-perfect feet would take their shoes off to run and feel, well, aaaahh—balance, comfort, freedom, and the need for less energy. That's the difference.

I had never felt that elusive spring-forward effect that kinesiologists and Phil often talked and wrote about. But there it was, a sensory sensation, with every step I took.

I have also read about people who buy the Vibrams, then run too fast or too far, and develop pain. Some even keep running after the pain comes on—this is the ultimate no-pain, no-gain blooper. Others develop bone fractures in the toes, apparently not an uncommon complaint. Now it's quite obvious—it's not the shoes, it's the feet!

But all this really didn't hit me until halfway through our short forty-minute trail run—my heart rate was about ten beats lower than usual. This was evident because I felt myself going faster—much faster.

I thought Phil was behind me all that time to analyze my gait, but now it was evident that not only did I make up the difference of ten beats between Phil's heart rate and mine, but it was also lower by a couple more beats. I need to get him a pair of these (well, even if it made him run faster).

All these new albeit relatively minimal but noticeable changes in my gait translated to almost a minute a mile faster at the same heart rate! We also run by time, not sure of the exact distance, and don't have mile splits, so this was not a scientific study.

But the following days and weeks, we ran again—same course, same time of day, same result. I love running fast! The human body never ceases to amaze me.

6. Got Rhythm?

It so happens that humans have a rhythmic brain, and the walking tempo of 120 and 180 for running are examples of this pattern. Ask anyone to tap out a rhythm with his or her fingers and the tempo will usually be around 120 beats a minute. Even listening to music at this tempo is preferable. Scientists have evaluated over seventy-four thousand pieces of modern music between 1960 and 1990 and found that the average rhythm was around 120 beats per minute.

It's no wonder music can help one's running, like all other sports. Music can promote the activity of the cerebellum, that "little brain" at the base of one's brain that controls tempo and rhythm. People who can't maintain a smooth gait while running may benefit from listening to music—not in the background and not necessarily while running, but focused listening to music as therapy any time of day even if it's only for a few minutes; it helps the brain regulate the rhythm of the gait.

Another way to help your gait is by using a metronome. A small handheld digital metronome, available in most music stores or online websites, is easy to carry and adjust throughout your workout. This simple therapy can help you learn to run more smoothly by following the beats of the metronome adjusted to your pace. It's best to do this on an easy running surface such as a paved road or track rather than a rough trail. Start with a proper warm-up, adjusting the metronome to your slower pace—the metronome should beep in conjunction with each footstep. As you increase your speed, adjust the metronome again. With each new tempo, make sure your feet are hitting the ground in step with the metronome's beat. It may seem difficult at first to maintain the right rhythm—syncing the brain's coordination of beats with your feet hitting the ground. You may find your mind drifting away at times, causing a brief loss of beat-step coordination. But as your cerebellum gets the idea, as the therapy succeeds, your gait will become smoother and the run will feel easier and more relaxed. For some people, just a few training sessions with a metronome can work wonders. Others may require a few weeks.

Section
THREE

Self-care

CHAPTER 19

STRESS AND HORMONES
How They Affect Your Overall Health and Fitness

O f all the problems I've seen in patients throughout my career, excess stress is the most common one. It typically triggers a multitude of signs and symptoms but at the same time is very elusive to detect and control. In our current health care environment, the focus on end-result complaints usually means the cause—some particular stress or combinations—remains untreated. As a consequence, most people are left unaware of the underlying stresses.

Stress is such an incredibly powerful influence on health and fitness that even if you are doing everything right in terms of exercise, diet, and nutrition, too much stress can make you feel old and run-down. Enough stress can contribute significantly and directly to inadequate fat burning, physical injury, aerobic deficiency, and poor brain function. And it can directly affect many health conditions, both as a cause and an aggravating factor, including cancer, heart disease, Alzheimer's; and it can also contribute to fatigue, bacterial and viral infections, chronic inflammation, blood sugar problems, weight gain, intestinal distress, and headaches. Stress-related problems account for more than 75 percent of all visits to primary care physicians and are responsible each day for millions of people needing to take time off from work. So stress comes with a monetary price tag as well that far exceeds the cost of antianxiety drugs or antidepressants, which are readily prescribed and yet don't address the causes of the problems.

Proper adaptation to stress first involves being as healthy and fit as possible and reducing unnecessary stresses—those that can be eliminated. This allows your body to better cope with the reality of life—that a certain amount of stress will always exist.

Adaptation is not always a conscious choice one makes. It involves the relationship between the brain and body and the specific hormones that help regulate stress. However, choosing to eat and exercise properly and deciding to better control stress is the major step in effectively adapting.

The mechanism by which you adapt to stress involves activity of the brain and nervous system with actions carried out by hormones. But dysfunction of the immune system, the balance of fats, blood sugar regulation, aerobic fitness, and all the health factors discussed in this book so far can lead to a maladaptive response to stress. In other words, you won't easily cope with relatively minor stresses unless you're healthy and fit. But as you can see, stress can easily become a vicious cycle in itself.

Stress is not without a remedy. In fact, you have a great coping mechanism for stress—it includes the brain and adrenal glands, important parts of what's called the hypothalamic-pituitary-adrenal axis. However, when part or all of this mechanism is functioning poorly, bodywide problems can result.

There are effective ways to help protect oneself from harmful stress, and the first step is to better understand it. So let's begin by addressing the three main types of stress: physical, chemical, and mental-emotional. These stresses can generate many different effects throughout the brain and body. Moreover, each person responds differently to various combinations of these stresses.

Physical Stress

Physical stresses are strains or exertions on the body, something many people take for granted. Overworking your muscles is an example of physical stress. Slight physical stress is what makes exercise beneficial and is an example of good stress. However, too much physical stress, or that same good stress without adequate rest or recovery, can potentially result in a variety of problems. A common example of physical stress is exercising too much or too hard—beyond your body's ability or threshold. This may result in sore muscles or joint inflammation that can then affect your lower back, knee, or hip, causing pain.

Likewise, dental problems can be a physical stress. It can affect more than your mouth, often causing stomach dysfunction, shoulder, neck, or head pain. Other physical

343

THE HYPOTHALAMIC-PITUITARY-ADRENAL AXIS

The brain plays a major role in regulating hormones throughout the body. This impacts muscle function, energy production, water and mineral balance, as well as the glands that produce the hormones. In a small region of the brain called the hypothalamus, the important link between the nervous system and hormone control takes place. This part of the brain can provide information to the pituitary gland, housed in the middle of the brain, to produce a variety of hormones sent to the body. The pituitary is also influenced by memories and emotions stored in nearby regions of the brain.

The pituitary releases hormones that stimulate the body's other glands, in particular those of the adrenal and thyroid, to control metabolism, muscle function, and sex hormones. Often referred to as the "master gland" of the body, the pituitary has significant control over one's entire hormonal system and helps funnel information to it from the brain.

The pituitary also secretes growth hormone, which stimulates muscle development in men and women. Its production occurs during sleep. While the amount of growth hormone made is higher in childhood and is reduced as one ages, sufficient amounts are still secreted even in older, healthy individuals. Like other hormones naturally produced in the body, poor health may reduce the level of growth hormone. In rare cases, pituitary problems at any age, such as a tumor, might require the necessity of a patient to take a synthesized form of human growth hormone—HGH.

Unfortunately, it's become too common for those seeking to restore youth, control weight, or enhance sports performance to also take HGH. However, the use of HGH does not actually guarantee more muscles or improved performance. It's a banned substance in sports and its use is dangerous. Taking HGH can reduce the pituitary's ability to produce growth hormone, creating an even more serious problem when HGH ingestion is stopped. Side effects of HGH include fatigue, muscle weakness, reduced sex hormones and sexual function, and blood-sugar irregularities. Don't believe the extravagant claims by so-called anti-aging clinics that want you to believe that HGH is the "new fountain of youth" drug.

stresses include irregular gait, poor posture, eyestrain, and even bad shoes.

Chemical Stress

Many chemicals from our environment can adversely affect the body's metabolism and cause stress. This can adversely affect your immune system, intestines, breathing, heart rate, and other areas. Dietary and nutritional imbalances such as too much sugar or too little vitamin D are examples of chemical stresses. In addition, drugs obviously influence body chemistry; examples of bad stress include excess caffeine or the side effects of prescription or over-the-counter drugs—virtually all have the potential for harm. Other sources of chemical stress include air pollution—secondhand smoke, indoor and outdoor toxins in the air. Reducing harmful chemicals from air, water, and food, and improving diet quality are key ways to reducing stress. Chemical stresses can also affect physical and mental-emotional problems.

Mental and Emotional Stress

The mental and emotional state includes the behavioral aspects of health. The mental state may be referred to as cognition—sensation, perception, learning, concept formation, and decision making. The emotional state typically describes pain, moods of anxiety or depression, and loss of enthusiasm or motivation. It's usually difficult for most people to separate the two, and so I prefer to combine both.

A multitude of physical, chemical, and mental-emotional stresses can come from your job, family, strangers, infections, allergic reactions, and even the weather. Most people are affected by more than one form of stress and frequently by all three types. And, stress is cumulative; the response to a physical stress from the weekend's 10K run may be amplified by Monday's chemically related stress of too much coffee and poor eating, further compounded with a family-related mental stress on Tuesday and another with the boss on Wednesday. All of this may affect your brain and body by Saturday with symptoms of fatigue, headache, or intestinal distress.

The weather is a potential stressor too and can affect us physically, chemically, or mentally. Seasonal affective disorder (SAD) is a good example of how the weather at certain times of year, typically in the fall and winter in the Northern Hemisphere, can have a dramatic adverse effect on people. Cold temperatures, low barometric pressure, and reduced daylight can increase feelings of depression and trigger low metabolism, which causes weight and body fat gain.

Some people accumulate so much stress that they lose track of it. When I ask a patient to list their stresses, for example, they may recall three or four—but if I ask, "What about this or that?" they say, "Oh yes, that too." When you're ready to deal with stress, the first thing to do is make yourself aware of it. The best way to do this is write it all down as a stress list.

Stress List

Reducing or eliminating individual stresses is easier if you write them down on paper. Here's an example:

- On a page, make three columns, one each for physical, chemical, and mental-emotional stresses.
- In each category, write down what you think are your stresses. This may take several days to complete since you probably won't think of all your different stresses right away.
- When you're done, prioritize by placing the biggest stress of each category on top.
- Then work on reducing or eliminating one stress at a time. Or, if you can handle it, work on one stress at a time from each category.

Reducing or eliminating unnecessary stress from your life will give your body a better chance to cope with other stresses you may not be able to change right now.

As you make your list, put a check mark by the stresses over which you have some control. This may include unhealthy eating habits such as rushing or skipping your meals,

drinking too much coffee, or not taking time to warm up or cool down properly during exercise.

Simply draw a line through those stresses that you can't control. If there's nothing you can do about them anyway, don't worry about them for now. Many people expend lots of energy on stresses they can't—or in most cases won't—do anything about. This may include job stress or the weather, though in reality almost any stress can be modified or eliminated—it's just a question of how far you're willing to go for optimal health and fitness. As time goes on, you may want to reconsider some of the items you've crossed off. You'll realize, for example, that changing jobs is a must, or moving to a more compatible climate will significantly improve your health.

Once you can "see" your stress listed on paper, it will be easier to manage. Start with your checkmarked stresses first, because you have more control over them—not that it's always easy. Circle the three biggest stresses from this list and begin to work on them. You may be able to improve on some and totally eliminate others. Some will require habit changes. It's a big task, but one that will return great benefits. When you've succeeded in eliminating or modifying each one, remove it from your list and circle the three next most stressful ones, so you always have three to work on.

What's most important about stress is that too much of it interferes with rest. Or

Stress—Just Say No!

In addition to self-managing your stress list, here's some other strategies for dealing with stress:

- Learn to say no when asked to do something you really don't want to do.
- Decide not to waste your time worrying about the past or the future. That's not to say you should ignore the past or not plan for the future, but live in the present.
- Learn some relaxation techniques, and perform them regularly. This also includes listening to or even playing music.
- When you're concerned about something, talk it over with someone you trust.
- Simplify your life. Start by eliminating trivia. Ask yourself, "Is this really important?"
- Prioritize your busy schedule: Do the most important things first, but don't neglect the enjoyable things. Before getting out of bed in the morning, ask yourself, "What fun things do I have planned for today?"
- Know your passion and pursue it.

more accurately, recovering from excess stress requires more downtime. If you don't get enough rest, usually in the form of sleep, the effects of stress will continue to accumu-late. One of the questions to ask yourself is whether you're getting enough sleep, considering the amount of stress you have. As you will see, one of the symptoms of excess stress is insomnia. In fact, too much of the stress hormone cortisol can interfere with sleep, waking you in the middle of the night and causing difficulty returning to sleep. A disturbed night's sleep is not only a stress but also reduces recovery for everyday activities.

By learning to take control of the various types of stress in your life, you can literally improve the quality of your life. This will also help your brain and adrenal glands regulate other stresses better.

Stress and the Adrenal Glands

No matter what type of stress you encounter—whether it's physical, chemical, or mental and emotional—your body has an efficient mechanism for coping. This is the important job of the adrenal glands. On the top of each kidney, these small glands work with the brain and nervous system to regulate important coping mechanisms, including the fight-or-flight reaction. The adrenal glands accomplish their work through the production of certain hormones, making them not only essential for stress coping but also for life itself. In addition to the regulation of stress, these hormones also help with sexual activity and reproduction, growth, aging, cellular repair, electrolyte balance, muscle function, and blood sugar control. This is why stress can affect so many different aspects of health

347

THE "RUNNER'S" HIGH—NOT JUST FOR RUNNERS

Many people believe that working out is one of the best ways to reduce stress. The so-called runner's high—a feeling of euphoria during or right after exercise—is often perceived as a way for a runner, hiker, cyclist, or other active person to feel great. But what really is this "high"?

We don't really know exactly what the runner's high is or why it occurs. In past decades, research has associated this state with natural opiates in the brain, or a cognitive state of dissociation. This usually centers on a discussion of endorphins—different types of hormonelike chemicals produced in the brain; some may even be produced in the skin, associated with sun exposure and vitamin D.

More recently, the so-called runner's high has been associated with the same brain receptors for substances like marijuana. While these receptors in the brain are still being studied in the lab, and undoubtedly other chemicals will be discovered that might better explain that elusive feeling gained from working out, the brain is far too complex to pinpoint just one cause for an "elevated state."

I believe the runner's high phenomenon is an important state of consciousness. Normally, when one is sleeping, in a business meeting, or in the middle of a good workout, the brain produces certain brain waves. When you're mentally relaxed, unstressed, and doing something that takes you into your own private world, the brain produces alpha waves. This state also can be promoted by listening to music, mediating, prayer, and other activities. Unfortunately, not all people experience the high because, for some, stress can overpower the enjoyment of the workout, impairing the ability to produce alpha waves.

and fitness—when the adrenals become overwhelmed with stress regulation, they may have to reduce their work with all other tasks.

Cortisol is a key adrenal stress hormone and commonly measured by simple blood or saliva tests that can be performed like other tests from your health care practitioner. Saliva is a better way to measure cortisol in most instances because having a needle thrust into a vein in your arm evokes stress—and cortisol production—sometimes making the blood test quite inaccurate. A saliva test only requires a small sample of your saliva in a little test tube during the normal course of your day. And since cortisol fluctuates throughout the day and night, a saliva test can easily be taken four different times throughout the day for a more accurate evaluation. (Most research studies on stress also rely on measurements of salivary cortisol rather than blood tests.)

When your body is under high stress, cortisol level can increase dramatically, and when the stress passes, the level returns to normal. In chronic stress states—the continuation of stress without relief—high cortisol levels can become prolonged and dangerous. This can adversely affect the brain, including the pituitary gland, and especially reduce memory, impair aerobic function, create blood sugar problems, reduce fat burning, suppress immune function, lower the body's defense against not just cold and flu but any infection, and cause intestinal distress. Long-standing stress can result in the "burning out" of adrenal function, with a serious loss of normal hormone production. In this state, cortisol levels become dangerously low, along with other hormones made by the adrenals.

Sex hormones, including estrogens and testosterone, are also important adrenal hormones that help both males and females to maintain proper sexual function and reproductive health and strong muscles and bones. In addition to production of both estrogens and testosterone by the testicles in men and ovaries in women, significant amounts of these sex hormones come from another important adrenal hormone, DHEA. When stress raises cortisol, DHEA is often reduced. The end result may be lowered sex hormones, which cause poor sexual function and loss of desire.

The Physiology of Stress

Our knowledge about stress and adrenal function began in the 1920s, when famous stress-research pioneer Hans Selye began to piece together the common problems resulting from excessive adrenal output. These include poor immunity and intestinal dysfunction, which in turn can trigger many other problems—like a domino effect. Selye developed what is called the general adaptation syndrome, which has three distinct stages:

- Stage 1: The first stage begins with the alarm reaction, when you're initially hit with stress. This could be job or family related. This increases the adrenal hormone production of cortisol to help the body cope. The purpose of this first stage by the adrenal glands is an attempt to battle and adapt to the increased stress. If it is successful, and the stress is reduced, you recover; adrenal function returns to normal, especially with sufficient rest. If this stage takes a bit longer to complete, a variety of mild symptoms may occur: noticeable tiredness during the day, mild allergies, or even some nagging back, knee, or foot pain. If over time—a few weeks or months—the adrenals fail to meet the needs of the body to combat the stress, they enter the second stage.

- Stage 2: During this period, also called the resistance stage, the adrenal glands themselves get larger through a process called hypertrophy. Since the increased hor-

349

mone production of the first stage couldn't counter the stress, the glands enlarge in an attempt make even more cortisol to do the same. During this stage, more advanced symptoms may occur, including fatigue, insomnia, and more serious back, knee, or foot pain, or poor recovery. Many people with chronic stress problems are stuck in this stage, often for months or years. They usually no longer function at their best—physically or mentally, are frequently ill, injured, or have other chronic health problems. If people in this stage continue to push themselves, thereby maintaining high levels of stress, the adrenals eventually can enter the third stage, called exhaustion.

- Stage 3: People who enter this stage are exhausted, often with chronic illness, and most likely are not able to function in life near the same level of effectiveness. Getting through the day—and night—is usually difficult. The adrenal glands are unable to adapt to any stress and are unable to produce adequate levels of hormones, including cortisol. The person is usually more seriously ill—physically, chemically, or mentally.

This discussion is not about adrenal disease; rather, it concerns the gray area between normal adrenal function and disease. Addison's disease occurs when the adrenal glands are unable to produce sufficient cortisol to sustain life. It can occur in men and women of all age-groups; symptoms include severe weight loss, muscle weakness, fatigue, low blood pressure, and sometimes darkening of the skin. The disease is also called adrenal insufficiency or hypocortisolism.

Diet and Adrenal Function

Adrenal stress can be caused or aggravated by the consumption of refined carbohydrates and sugar. This includes hidden sugars in many foods. How much is too much? Less is best.

Caffeine is a common source of adrenal stimulation, and one of the main reasons people depend on it to get through the day. Coffee, tea, and cola are the main sources. If you have an adrenal problem, assess your caffeine intake. For many, no caffeine is best; for others, a single cup or two of coffee or tea may be tolerable. You must determine this, as objectively as possible, by listening to your body to see how much caffeine you can tolerate. Feeling jittery and high-strung, a rapidly rising heart rate, or queasiness in your stomach may indicate you've consumed too much caffeine.

Breakfast is always the most important meal of the day, but most especially for those with adrenal dysfunction. A healthy breakfast includes protein but is void of refined carbohydrates. An egg-based meal can be the cornerstone of an ideal breakfast.

People with adrenal stress often need to snack between the three main meals, as much as every two hours, in the early stages of recovery. Healthy snacking means eating healthy food in small portions.

ADRENAL STRESS CHECKLIST

Ten common symptoms of adrenal dysfunction are listed below. Note those that pertain to you. While any of these can be caused by other imbalances in the body, together they make up the most common complaints experienced by those with adrenal dysfunction:

- *Low energy.* This is common especially in the afternoon, but could happen anytime or all the time. The fatigue can be physical, mental, or both. When the adrenals are too stressed, the body uses more sugar for energy but can't access fat very well for energy use. This can significantly limit one's energy for daily activities and even sleep.

- *Dizziness upon standing.* Standing up from a seated or lying position, or just bending over to pick up something from the floor, can make you dizzy because not enough blood is getting to the head quickly enough. Check your blood pressure while lying down and then immediately after you stand. If you suffer from adrenal dysfunction, you will often notice the systolic blood pressure (the first number) doesn't rise normally—it should be higher when you're standing by about six to eight millimeters.

- *Eyes sensitive to bright light.* Adrenal stress often causes light sensitivity in your eyes. You may feel the need to wear sunglasses even on cloudy days or have difficulty with night driving because of the oncoming headlights (often misinterpreted as bad night vision). Some people find that their nearsightedness (ability to see distances) worsens with adrenal stress.

- *Asthma and allergies.* Whether you call it exercise-induced asthma, food allergies, or seasonal allergies, they are all similar symptoms of adrenal dysfunction.

- *Physical imbalance.* Problems in the low back, knee, foot, and ankle are particularly associated with adrenal problems. They can produce symptoms such as low-back pain, sciatica, and excess pronation in the foot, leading to foot and ankle problems.

- *Stress-related syndromes.* Emotional despair and depression can often be the result of adrenal exhaustion. While both these problems can become serious enough to warrant medication or hospitalization, adrenal dysfunction occurs long before this point.

- *Blood sugar stress.* With adrenal dysfunction, the body is unable to properly regulate blood sugar. Symptoms include constantly feeling hungry, being irritable before meals, especially if meals are delayed, and having strong cravings for sweets or caffeine.

- *Insomnia.* Many people with adrenal dysfunction fall asleep easily (from fatigue) but wake in the middle of the night with difficulty getting back to sleep. This may be due to high levels of cortisol occurring at the wrong time (levels should be low during sleeping hours). Many people say they wake up in the night to urinate, but it's usually the adrenal problem that awakens them, and then they get the urge to urinate. Rest is a key factor in recovering from adrenal dysfunction. Are you getting at least seven to eight hours each night? If not, you may need more sleep. Adrenal stress increases the need for recovery.

- *Diminished sex drive.* This is a common symptom of adrenal dysfunction due to low levels of the hormone DHEA, which makes estrogen and testosterone.

- *Seasonal affective disorder (SAD).* This usually occurs during the colder months. As the hours of daylight lessen and the temperature drops, many people go into a mild state of hibernation. The metabolism slows and the body and mind become sluggish, sometimes resulting in a mild or moderate depression. (This corresponds with a combination of stresses: the weather, lack of sunlight and vitamin D, and even the start of the holiday season—people don't eat well, are less active, and weight gain is typical.)

In addition to these signs and symptoms, excess abdominal fat is common in those with high levels of stress. Because high cortisol level encourages sugar burning and reduces fat burning, belly fat tends to accumulate for many stressed-out people.

Recognizing the symptoms of adrenal dysfunction can be useful in your own self-assessment. You may also want to test some of your adrenal-hormone levels with the help of a health care professional. The best initial test for adrenal function measures cortisol and DHEA in saliva and is performed with four samples of saliva over the course of a typical day and evening, rather than just a single test.

Nutrients and Adrenal Function

Your nutritional needs may vary with adrenal stress. These include factors to help the immune system, intestines, and the adrenal glands themselves. Most, if not all, nutrients should come from an optimal diet. Below are some possible supplemental nutrient needs:

- For many types of adrenal stress, especially those that cause insomnia, additional zinc may be useful. Studies show this important mineral can help lower high cortisol levels that accompany adrenal stress. Taken right before bed, for example, zinc may improve sleep patterns associated with high cortisol.
- Choline is a nutrient commonly needed by some people with adrenal stress, in part due to the relationship of choline with the brain and nervous system. Individuals who are always on the go, overworked, and trying to do too much are examples of those who may benefit from additional choline. A smaller dose several times a day, rather than one or two higher doses, may be most helpful. Those with asthma (exercise-induced or not) may need higher doses. The best source of choline in the diet is egg yolks.

Exercise and Adrenal Function

Building a great aerobic base can be a significant strategy for improving adrenal function. Anaerobic training, including any type of weight lifting, can worsen existing adrenal problems. Once adrenal function is improved, anaerobic exercise can be resumed, though the balance of aerobic and anaerobic exercise must be maintained.

Natural Hormones

All hormones play a major role in one's physical, chemical, and mental well-being. Three important hormones, produced by both men and women, include a group of

---

EXERCISE AND STRESS: WELCOME TO THE RAT RACE

The following is excerpted from my good friend Bill Katovsky's latest book, *Return to Fitness: Getting Back in Shape after Injury, Illness, or Prolonged Inactivity*:

Research scientists love tormenting lab rats. The furry little rodents are starved, shocked, bullied, and even water-boarded. Their torture is encouraged under the rational aegis of science—to find out how stress affects the brain. Because rats provide a fairly reliable indicator of human behavior, scientists use them to examine how stress affects overall health, including blood pressure, immune system, and depression.

In 2009, scientists at the University of Minho in Portugal discovered that chronically stressed rats acted rather un-ratlike. They'd continually press a bar for food pellets even when they had no intention of eating. The rats were stuck in a habit-forming groove of futile, nonproductive behavior. It's as if their stressed brains were unable

---

to make intelligent decisions like, "Hey, no food, so why don't I do something else with my time?"

Speaking with *The New York Times*, Robert Sapolsky, a neurobiologist at Stanford University School of Medicine, called the Portuguese study "a great model for understanding why we end up in a rut, and then dig ourselves deeper and deeper into that rut. We're lousy at recognizing when our normal coping mechanisms aren't working. Our response is usually to do it five times more, instead of thinking, maybe it's time to try something new."

Stress had an important evolutionary role in keeping our ancestors alive. Survival in the forest or on the savanna demanded quick action when danger lurked. Stress hormones like cortisol and adrenaline would suddenly flood into the bloodstream, causing the heart to beat faster, which increased blood flow to the muscles. But after the danger passed, the flight-or-fight hormones would settle down and the body would return to its normal physiological state.

But in today's modern world, stress receptors often get stuck open in a locked position. Since the body can't function all the time like this, stress hormone production is ultimately affected. Natural defense mechanisms weaken. The overloaded brain shuts down critical areas such as the hippocampus and prefrontal cortex, which affect learning, memory, and rational thought. A stressed-out person will end up engaging in harmful, counterproductive behavior, like having three beers after work, or eating junk food when not hungry.

Given identical stressful conditions, such as losing a job or breaking up, some people are better able to cope, while others will emotionally fall apart—and remain depressed for a long time. In a 2009, *Newsweek* cover story titled "Who Says Stress Is Bad for You?" science reporter Mary Carmichael cited several studies that pointed to genetic differences in determining the individual outcome to stressful situations. But which specific genes are responsible? No one knows. "The science is still young," she writes.

Yet there's good news for the stressed-out population. The Portuguese scientists found that stress-caused behavior is indeed reversible. Once removed from a stressful environment, the rats resumed acting like normal rats. No more pressing the food bar when there wasn't any food. Their brain circuitry had somehow rewired itself.

"The brain can grow new cells and reshape itself," says Carmichael. Furthermore, "meditation appears to encourage this process. Monks who have trained for years in

meditation have greater brain activity in regions linked to learning and happiness."
The monks grew new brain cells.

Carmichael brought up another classic rat study: "Something that should lower stress can actually cause stress if it's done in the wrong spirit. Scientists put two rats in a cage, each of them locked inside a running wheel. The first rat could exercise whenever it liked. The second rat was forced to run whenever its counterpart did. Exercise, like meditation, usually tamps down stress and encourages neuron growth. The second rat, however, lost brain cells. It was doing something that should have been good for its brain, but it lacked one crucial factor: control. It could not determine its own 'workout' schedule, so it didn't perceive it as exercise. Instead, it experienced it as a literal rat race."

So even too much of a good thing like exercise can turn harmful if it's controlling you rather than vice versa. It's a primary reason why many athletes get injured or sick if they train or race too hard and don't take time off. The stress switch can't indefinitely remain open.

estrogens, testosterone, and progesterone. As one ages, and with increased stress, the production of these hormones is diminished. This occurs especially when cortisol rises, reducing the production of DHEA, and subsequently diminishing the estrogens and testosterone.

In many, if not most, cases, improving health and fitness will also correct hormone imbalance. This is especially true when adrenal hormone problems exist. In difficult cases, since the hormonal system is complex, it's recommended that you seek the input of a health care professional to assess and treat the problem. In some stubborn cases, natural hormone supplements may be an option.

Estrogen

This most well-known of hormones is actually a group of about twenty compounds. The most important estrogens are estrone, estradiol, and estriol. The different estrogens have unique roles in the body. For example, estradiol is the most stimulating to the breast, potentially increasing the risk of breast cancer. Estriol protects against breast cancer. Normal production of both by the body is the right balance. A variety of benefits are attributed to the effects of natural estrogens, including prevention of hot flashes, better memory and concentration, slowing of the aging process, and reduced depression and anxiety.

BIOIDENTICAL HORMONES

What are bioidentical hormones and are they safe? The answer is not what you'd expect. Any hormone, synthetic or natural, must be identical to the ones your body make; otherwise it would not work (some are only similar and the body may convert them to the identical type). For the past dozen years or so, the FDA literature—those difficult-to-read tiny-print inserts that accompany prescription drugs—have been using the marketing term "bioidentical." While this term sounds safe, it may not be—it's simply a consumer-friendly term. Bioidentical hormones may or may not be natural—some are even synthetic.

But bioidentical hormones can be deadly if taken improperly. Estrogen's commonly known risk of breast cancer is one example. A healthy body normally orchestrates the production of a whole range of hormones that are produced, do their work, then disappear. It's the liver that breaks them down, through a process called detoxification, and eliminates them through the gut. When this does not happen, it may be due to poor liver function or an imbalance in hormone production.

But if you do have an imbalance, hormonal therapy may be an option, but you first need to consider all the potential risks. Before taking any additional hormone, the question about why you're not making enough of your own must be answered. This involves a proper assessment by a health care professional. Good liver and gut function becomes even more important during any hormone therapy. So make sure your liver is working well so it can properly control the hormones. To do this, the body needs the active (natural) B vitamins, listed in chapter 9, and a proper detoxification system discussed in chapter 22.

For most people, hormone therapy is not necessary. Why? Because by being healthy and fit, hormone activity usually remains in balance, at any age. An example is when a woman's ovaries no longer produce adequate amounts of estrogens. After menopause, the adrenals normally adapt by making more of this hormone. But without healthy adrenal function, this may not happen, triggering common menopausal symptoms with health care professionals recommending hormone therapy instead of improving adrenal function.

Bioidentical or not, hormone therapy is tricky as exemplified by the use of estradiol, one of the estrogens. It's the most common hormone prescribed to women and the one that's responsible for the alarming rates of breast and uterine cancer.

Estradiol is normally not produced by itself but with other estrogens and, along with progesterone and other hormones, provides the body's natural "checks and balances" that avoid the increased risk of cancer.

There are times, however, when natural hormone therapy is warranted—this is an individual issue.

Estradiol (Premarin) is a commonly prescribed estrogen that places woman at high risk for breast cancer. This is due to the fact that it's not broken down in the liver as quickly as your own natural estrogens (affecting the cells for a longer time). Premarin, made from the urine of pregnant horses, simply doesn't function exactly like the estrogens made in the human body.

One of the common risks of taking an estrogen replacement drug is the higher dosage compared to what the female body would normally produce. The most common symptom of too much estrogen is water retention. This can lead to breast tenderness and swelling, weight gain, and headaches. Excess estrogen can also lower blood sugar and increase your cravings for sweets. Too much estrogen also increases a woman's risk of uterine cancer and gallbladder disease.

While the idea of estrogen replacement is often "sold" to female patients by touting the benefits of building strong bones, estrogen doesn't actually do this. Rather, it decreases the rate of bone loss that occurs naturally throughout life. The hormones that have the greatest impact on new bone growth—some-

thing the body is always doing—are progesterone and testosterone.

Progesterone

Unlike estrogen, which is a group of hormones, progesterone is the only hormone in its class. It improves sleep, builds bone mass, protects against breast and uterine cancer, improves carbohydrate tolerance, helps burn fat, prevents water retention, increases sex drive, and in many women has a calming effect on the nervous system. (Men also produce progesterone, which has similar health effects.)

Provera is a commonly used synthetic version of progesterone. However, it doesn't have the same functions as the natural hormone your body produces. While natural progesterone acts like a diuretic, Provera can increase salt and water retention and body fat. Too much of this synthetic hormone can cause bloating, depression, fatigue, increased hair growth on the body, and increased weight gain. Provera can also cause your body to diminish its own production of natural progesterone, forcing you to rely more on outside sources. Other synthetics can cause birth defects, epilepsy, asthma, and heart problems.

It's important to note that both estrogen and progesterone work together. In a real sense, they balance each other when in their natural state. Taking one prescription hormone without the balance of the other often creates the side effects noted above.

Testosterone

Testosterone is also a naturally occurring hormone made by both men and women. It's important for healing, helps build and maintain muscles and bones, increases sex drive and overall energy, and is a very important hormone for healthy metabolism. There are a variety of synthetic testosterones, such as fluoxymesterone and methyltestosterone, with side effects including hormonal imbalance, intestinal distress, increased cholesterol, hair loss, depression, and anxiety.

Outside sources of testosterone are sometimes used to enhance strength performance—not just for athletes but those who work out very little. The use of this hormone and its potential to help "restore youth" may go back thousands of years with the consumption of animal parts containing this hormone, namely, the adrenal glands and testicles. Today, it's produced in drug-company labs and is classified as an anabolic steroid and is the most commonly detected drug in athletes who are tested, often causing a fine or banning from competition (depending on the particular sport's rules). Androgen abuse in men is associated with reduced size of the testicles and low sperm counts, and low production of natural testosterone; symptoms can include violent mood swings, acne, and excessive muscularity.

Taking synthetic testosterone can cause the pituitary gland to shut down the supply from the testicles—a chemical castration. The inappropriate and dangerous use of testosterone is not only a problem with some athletes and bodybuilders but is also becoming more popular among older men, with a side effect of increasing the risk of prostate cancer.

Like all hormones made by the body, the sex hormones are important for optimal health and fitness. The ideal scenario is to have your body make the types and amounts of hormones necessary for you. That amount varies from day to day and year to year (even from minute to minute). If reduced health interferes with this delicate mechanism, imbalances can occur.

If you have signs and symptoms related to hormone imbalance, measuring your hormone levels, such as by testing the blood or saliva, is an important part of a complete assessment process. A reevaluation of the same tests will help you know whether improved lifestyle habits or any replacement therapy is successful.

For menopause, premenstrual syndrome, muscle or bone loss, or other hormone-related imbalances, the use of hormones can improve your quality of life. What's most important is to understand that no one has to live with the pain, displeasure, and discomfort that too many doctors (along with the media and pharmaceutical companies) have told us are normal with aging. But I can't emphasize enough that preventing and correcting hormone imbalance by improving adrenal function and overall health and fitness is the most effective and best first option.

CHAPTER 20

GETTING TO KNOW YOUR BRAIN
Diet, Physical Activity, and Lifestyle All Play Important Roles

What is the brain? The simple act of reading those four words requires the work of hundreds of millions of brain cells (called neurons). Though the brain weighs less than 5 percent of total body mass, it controls nearly every bodily function, from holding this book to going up a flight of stairs. The brain uses between 20 and 50 percent of the oxygen one breathes. Your everyday tasks are achieved with the brain's arsenal of more than one hundred billion neurons and one hundred trillion interconnections—greater than the number of stars in the universe—existing between those neurons. The brain is more complex than the greatest supercomputers, and this makes the organ truly magnificent, almost beyond our comprehension.

There are a variety of lifestyle habits that will help you develop and maintain better cognitive function, including proper nutrition and exercise. So let's start with the latter.

Physical activity is intricately related to ongoing brain development. This process begins at the earliest age when a child's first movements stimulate brain growth and continues throughout life unless one stops being active. This activity increases levels of a family of natural protein-based chemicals in the brain called neurotrophins. Perhaps the most researched chemical includes brain-derived neurotrophic factor (BDNF), which promotes cellular growth and repair in the brain and body. BDNF improves brain function by helping cell-to-cell communication, which is important for learning, memory, and overall cognition. BDNF also stimulates the production of new brain cells—a process called neurogenesis—and protects cells from degeneration, associated with a decline in brain function with age. Physical activity also stimulates BDNF to help mobilize gene expression, switching on many of the genetic benefits programmed within the body while turning off the bad genetic profiles. BDNF also affects one's muscles by helping them function more effectively through improving contraction and fat burning for energy production throughout the body. Even an easy workout can benefit the brain in another way by promoting plasticity—the ability to improve overall brain function at any age. Those individuals with depression, Alzheimer's disease, and other brain disorders often have low levels of BDNF. Those with high body fat and diabetes are typically low in BDNF.

Stimulating Brain Health

Which workouts are best for brain health? The answer is any training that promotes overall health, especially those that are aerobic. This can even include an easy walk, regardless of one's level of fitness. Just like with any sensible exercise or workout, when you stress your muscles, you must use the brain by pushing it a bit to reach new limits, but not too much to hurt it. To paraphrase the great singer-songwriter Bob Dylan, if we're not busy being born, we're busy dying. This sums up the remedy for optimal brain function throughout life. This use comes in the form of sending a variety of sensations into the brain from the body. This can be accomplished through various means:

- Physical stimulation. Every step you take, each movement you make influences many different brain areas significantly. Even a physical massage can provide great stimulation for the brain, as can walking barefoot.
- Auditory stimulation. The best example is listening to enjoyable, soothing music, which may stimulate all the brain's areas.
- Visual stimulation. Even taking in the sights during a workout is a great exercise

361

for the brain (not always possible if your running is done indoors on a treadmill).

- Avoid stressful stimulations. Try to keep away from annoying sounds, sights, smells, and environmental factors (such as running or biking in a crowded urban setting, with all that traffic noise and vehicular air pollution).

Diminished brain function can result from either too little or the wrong kind of stimulation. It's estimated that one in four people in the United States suffers from some form of mental or emotional disorder also known as brain injury. (This is similar, but not usually as severe as getting knocked on the head or other trauma.) Many more have diminished brain function or rather stress-caused mental impairment, which is often temporary. These and other brain injuries can be improved, often corrected, by providing the brain with sufficient stimulation, nutrition, and the right environment.

Human error is a common result of diminished brain function leading to forgetfulness, fatigue, or poor decision making and is the cause of the majority of automobile, airplane, rail, boating, and other tragic accidents reported in the media on an almost daily basis. Medical mistakes, which kill and maim millions of people each year in the United States, are also usually due to human error. In most cases, memory-related problems are preventable through proper food and nutrition, stress regulation, and lifestyle. And the idea isn't just to go slack altogether and avoid confronting cognitive challenges—you want your brain to function at a high level until you die! In fact, it's never too late to pick up a new intellectually challenging hobby even in your fifties, sixties, or seventies.

Brain Biofeedback

One way to improve brain function is to stimulate certain levels of consciousness—in particular, those that result in particular brain waves. This is accomplished with an important form of biofeedback that I developed during my years in practice and called it "respiratory biofeedback." The procedure is similar to EEG (electroencephalograph) biofeedback, or neurofeedback, which helps improve brain function by increasing alpha wave production. Increases of this brain wave help overall brain function and reduce unwanted stress hormones.

Before I go into how respiratory biofeedback actually works, allow me to first discuss some of its preliminary aspects. Everyone can benefit from respiratory biofeedback, which helps not only the brain but the body as well. This biofeedback can reduce high levels of stress hormones to improve adrenal function and fat burning, control blood sugar, and other benefits such as correcting and preventing muscle imbalance. You can use it on yourself as a quick, effective daily remedy to improve overall health. Respiratory biofeedback can also be performed before other physical therapies are used to help improve the efficacy of these remedies (and sometimes eliminate their necessity). For example, before getting a hands-on treatment from a chiropractor or osteopath, respiratory therapy can help prepare your body for these other therapies. In fact, some health care professionals use respiratory biofeedback on their patients.

Respiratory biofeedback is associated with a number of significant health benefits that can also improve both health and fitness:

- It can increase oxygen to the brain, potentially improving a variety of neurological imbalances. This is accomplished through more efficient breathing that brings more air into the lungs and more oxygen to the brain.
- Respiratory feedback can help restore and improve normal breathing. Improper breathing is often associated with brain and spinal cord injuries and is sometimes a hidden problem even in relatively healthy people.
- It can help improve the function of the diaphragm and abdominal muscles. In addition to breathing, these muscles play a significant role in physical activity, improving posture and supporting the spine and pelvis.
- Because of its effect on the brain and nervous system, respiratory biofeedback can help improve the function of other muscles in the body as well and help reduce pain—two reasons to perform this procedure before other therapies.

- It can help reduce harmful stress hormones, especially cortisol; balance the autonomic nervous system; and promote muscle relaxation—all critical features for a healthier brain and body.

Respiratory Biofeedback Procedures

Once you have a better understanding of brain waves and normal breathing, you can then perform respiratory biofeedback. While it's important to relax the body as much as possible during this process, if this procedure is new, you may be a little tense as you go through each step. But soon, you'll be able to relax and obtain the maximum benefits of respiratory biofeedback.

While each of the steps below can produce some alpha wave activity, combining all of them can be a very potent five-minute therapy. Here are the five steps for respiratory biofeedback:

- It's best performed relaxed, in a lying position, although slightly reclined while sitting is also effective.
- Place your hands or arms on the middle of the abdomen and keep them relaxed. This sensation and weight provide a biofeedback effect on the diaphragm and abdominal muscles during movement.
- Close your eyes.
- Listen to enjoyable, relaxing music—popular or classical. The tunes that are your favorites work best, especially if head-

363

A QUICK LOOK AT BRAIN WAVES

An important component of respiratory biofeedback is the production of healthy brain waves. The brain produces different frequencies and amplitudes of electrical waves depending upon our levels of consciousness. Sensation, attention (self-awareness), intellectual activity, and the planning of physical movement have distinct electrical correlates in the brain that can be measured using an EEG.

There are four commonly measured waves, and at least two others that have been observed:

- Beta waves (12–32 Hz) are associated with full awareness and high cortical activity—typical of a busy brain, such as during a business meeting, planning a trip, or when mentally doing several things at once.
- Alpha waves (8–12 Hz) are associated with a sense of "relaxed alertness" and high creativity—typical during meditation, listening to music, and when eyes are closed. The ability to generate alpha waves is associated with the self-regulation of stress and may contribute to an expanded state of consciousness.
- Theta waves (4–8 Hz) are associated with an awake but dreamy state common just before the onset of sleep; most prevalent in babies and children because the brain has not yet fully developed, they also occur during deep creativity and meditation in adults at any time.
- Delta waves (0.5–4 Hz) are slow waves occurring during most stages of sleep. It is abnormal for them to occur while one is awake and may indicate a lack of nutrients such as glucose or oxygen, medication effects, or poorly functioning neurons.

Another brain wave type is gamma (30–80 Hz). Much less is known about this type of wave. It may be associated with more complex cortical function and higher levels of consciousness. A sensory motor rhythm (12–15 Hz) above the higher-end alpha and entering beta has been associated with alert but muscle-relaxed states.

Your brain should make specific waves in certain regions at appropriate times. For example, delta waves that occur while driving to the store are abnormal, leading to distraction and increasing the risk of a traffic accident. And the presence of theta waves while listening to someone give you driving directions could result in your mind drifting off and not paying attention, with the result of getting lost.

The ability to produce alpha waves is associated with an overall healthy brain and body, especially in relation to controlling stress. It is one reason people have, for thousands of years, pursued meditation, the use of psychedelic or hallucinogenic drugs, prayer, and other activities that seek to promote the alpha state. Specifically, alpha waves can reduce high levels of the stress hormone cortisol and help balance the autonomic nervous system. These alpha waves can have dramatic effects on the whole body, such as improved memory, learning, and comprehension; better blood sugar regulation; improved gut function; and balanced hormones. When you're relaxed, creative, meditating, or happy, the brain produces large amounts of alpha waves. For these and other reasons, one main focus of respiratory biofeedback is the creation of alpha waves.

The inability to produce alpha waves signifies underlying problems. Inadequate sleep, nutritional imbalances, and very high levels of stress hormones can impair the ability to produce alpha waves. Even certain structural problems, such as those in the jaw joint or neck muscles, can significantly reduce our ability to generate healthy alpha waves.

phones are used, which keep out distracting noise.

- Breathe easy and deep. Most people can comfortably, slowly inhale for about five to seven seconds, then exhale for the same five to seven seconds. If five to seven seconds makes you feel out of breath or dizzy, adjust the time—try three to four seconds during inhalation, for example, and the same for exhalation.

Continue respiratory biofeedback for about five minutes.

Caution: it's important that you do not fall asleep, or even start drifting into sleep, which produces delta waves. If you start getting sleepy after two minutes, perform respiratory biofeedback for just less than that time and gradually work up to five minutes—but always avoid getting sleepy. If you consistently get sleepy during respiratory biofeedback, there may be other sleep-related issues such as sleep deprivation or sleep apnea (often caused by carbohydrate intolerance).

As a powerful self-therapy, respiratory biofeedback can be performed once or twice daily or more if necessary. By correcting muscle imbalance and improving the nervous system, it can also help control pain, correct and prevent injuries, and overall, reduce stress.

Brain and Blood Sugar

Do you remember where you were when President Kennedy was assassinated? Maybe you weren't born yet. How about when the space shuttle *Challenger* exploded? Or when the World Trade Center towers collapsed? Most people have vivid memories of where they were when these historical events occurred. At the same time, many people can't recall a friend's frequently called phone number or the name of someone they just met a half hour ago. The strong memory of traumatic events persists due to the powerful adrenal response—the fight-or-flight mechanism—that raises blood sugar to optimum levels. While the body utilizes both fat and sugar for energy, the brain is primarily dependent upon sugar. If the level of blood sugar rises too much or falls too low, the brain has an immediately reduced capacity. This means you don't remember as well, have a diminished response to external stimuli, and can't learn as easily. Overall mental and physical performance can be affected by the following:

- High-glycemic carbohydrates, especially sugar and processed flour products, can reduce and impair brain function due to the effects of insulin.
- Blood sugar can be controlled exceptionally well by snacking on healthy items. By eating five or six meals daily, you can help stabilize blood sugar, allowing the brain to do its job properly.
- Stress can wreak havoc on blood sugar and reduce overall brain function.

Mental Energy

Diet can have an immediate and profound effect on brain chemistry, often as much as drugs, but is easier to regulate and without unwanted side effects. A meal at dinnertime can influence your sleep, dreams, and how you feel during your morning routine. And what you eat, or don't eat, for breakfast can determine your overall human performance for the rest of the day.

Most of the forty or more types of neurotransmitters are made from amino acids derived from the protein in your diet. Certain vitamins and minerals are also required for their production, including vitamin B_6, folic acid, niacin, iron, and vitamin C. There are many important neurotransmitters related to mental function. They include serotonin and norepinephrine—the two most commonly discussed substances.

The reason many people get sleepy after a big lunch or dinner is usually due to too many carbohydrates, including sugar. In the case of a large meal such as a Thanksgiving dinner, it's not the turkey but the bread (usually high glycemic), potatoes (including sweetened sweet potatoes), gravy (made with flour), cranberries (sweetened with sugar), and of course, those extra servings of pie (there's always more than one type to taste). Throw in some alcohol, and it's no wonder you end craving more than just one cup of coffee afterward just to stay awake.

The carbohydrates cause a rise in the level of the brain neurotransmitter serotonin—this has a calming, relaxing, sedating effect on the brain because the more carbohydrates you eat, the more sedating its action.

Sleepiness after any meal may be indicative of carbohydrate intolerance because of higher levels of insulin. This would also indicate that your body is burning more sugar and less fat, just the opposite state you want for optimal health. So if you often feel sleepy after meals, it's time to evaluate, or reevaluate, your eating habits. While sweets are traditionally thought of as providing energy, they are in actuality mentally sedating. Sometimes sweets may give the feeling of a pickup, but that is short-lived until insulin lowers the blood sugar, resulting in more fatigue.

If you need a mental pickup, try eating some protein. A protein-based meal with little or no carbohydrates causes your body to produce less insulin and provides a higher amount of tyrosine and increased norepinephrine levels. This neurotransmitter has a stimulating effect on the brain.

Drugs and the Brain

A variety of over-the-counter and prescription drugs can impair brain function. Many of these drugs won't signal obvious symptoms that the brain is adversely affected. Alcohol can depress brain function, although in small amounts it can improve social activity by lessening inhibitions. But balance or moderation is key—even if it's only one small alcoholic drink, whether wine, beer, or distilled booze, if you don't feel right drinking or your behavior worsens, or you feel the effects the next morning, avoid alcohol altogether.

Drugs are often prescribed to balance brain chemistry. Depressed patients are given medication to restore balance to the neurotransmitters. Prozac, Elavil, BuSpar, Aventyl, Tofranil, and Zoloft are antidepressants that affect the balance of serotonin and norepinephrine. But these medications have side effects that may initially include headache, nervousness, and upset stomach. Fatigue and drowsiness, weight gain, insomnia, and reduced sexual function, including decreased sex drive and difficulty reaching orgasm, are other common effects. In addition, antidepressants can reduce glutathione, the body's most powerful antioxidant, and which protects the brain from damage.

Brain and Eicosapentaenoic Acid (EPA)

One of the most important brain nutrients is the omega-3 fat EPA (along with its related fat, DHA (docosahexaenoic acid). Most people usually don't get enough of this nutrient from food because of reduced consumption of wild, cold-water fresh fish such as salmon and sardines, so supplementation is often necessary. The omega-3 fats are key ingredients for the development and repair of the brain, especially the eyes. Imbalances in essential fatty acids—particularly deficiencies in omega-3 fats—have been implicated in depressive disorders in adults and behavioral problems in children and adolescents, including attention deficit/hyperactivity disorder, difficulties with learning, impulsivity, hyperactivity, aggression, and anger. I've helped many restore normal brain function and eliminate medication, often with the help of EPA. These brain problems often go hand in hand with chronic inflammation; EPA can not only improve brain function but can also help balance fats so the body can make natural anti-inflammatory chemicals for body repair.

Researchers continue to identify the positive effects of EPA on the brain and also have established a direct link between an imbalance in fatty acids and depressive disorders. In fact, it appears that these fats regulate neurotransmitters in ways that mimic the effect of some antidepressant medications. These fats also coat the brain cell membrane, serving a protective function when neurotransmitters are fired in the synaptic phase.

EPA and DHA have other benefits in brain function as well. They are most vital for the fetus and child during development of the brain. They may also help control the release of the stress hormone cortisol, resulting in improved brain and adrenal gland function. And they may help reduce the severity of degenerative brain diseases that lead to memory loss and dementia, including Alzheimer's disease.

Other Brain Requirements

Any dietary inadequacy can potentially have a dramatic impact on brain function. Numerous studies show that many people with depression also have low levels of the nutrient folate. Consuming foods containing this nutrient can significantly improve depression. For this reason, anyone considering antidepressant medication should first be screened for folate levels through a blood test for homocysteine, the best indicator of folate levels in the body. For depressed individuals who have low folate levels, adequate folate intake and use may be as effective as Prozac or other antidepressant drugs for treating mild, moderate, and severe depression. Folate is contained in green leafy vegetables and fruits; in some cases, fruit, especially citrus (such as oranges and grapefruit) can be a better source than leafy vegetables. For many people, synthetic folate, labeled as "folic acid" and found in most supplements, may not be as effective or as well utilized as folate obtained from real food sources.

Other micronutrients are important for the brain too:

- Sodium, potassium, magnesium, and calcium improve sending messages through the brain.
- Zinc is for the growth and maturation of the brain and is used for many chemical reactions in the brain, especially those related to behavior.
- Copper deficiency has been associated with deterioration of mental function and physical coordination, but too much of this mineral can have the same results.
- Manganese, like copper, facilitates proper brain function and has potential for

adversely affecting the brain if taken in excess.

- Lead, arsenic, and mercury are toxic to the brain and pose real health problems. Lead poisoning has been known about for centuries. For years, scientific literature has described mercury poisoning, which can happen through consumption of fish contaminated with accumulated methylmercury (introduced to the food chain by industrial waste) or consumption of grain treated with mercury fungicide. The debate over dental fillings is still a concern to many in the scientific community.
- Vitamin B_6 is used in the regulation of certain neurotransmitters. Because estrogen can reduce the levels of vitamin B_6, women who are taking birth control pills and estrogen-replacement therapy often need this supplement.

Millions of people consume and even rely on caffeine to help get through the day. Though caffeine isn't considered a nutrient, it is a drug with potentially significant brain effects. This is obvious to those who regularly consume caffeine—in coffee, tea, colas, or even the so-called energy drinks. Don't think so? Try *not* having your daily fix for even one day! A key effect of caffeine is increased mental performance and alertness, though negative brain effects can appear soon afterward when the drug wears off and you crave more, especially if your healthy food intake is inadequate. The physical side effects of caffeine can be unhealthy for some while others can tolerate relatively small amounts of caffeine each day. It's up to you to determine if your brain and body can tolerate caffeine and, if so, how much.

Music and the Brain

Currently, one of the hottest fields in medical science is research into the brain—how it functions, what consciousness and memory are, biofeedback, behavior modification, and biological self-repair. Music plays an especially key role in illness and injury treatment. Being in the right mental state while listening to music can affect one's brain waves, which, in turn, can improve one's overall health and fitness.

In Dr. Oliver Sacks's best-selling book, *Musicophilia*, he investigates the profound relationship between music and the mind. In one passage, the well-known neurologist describes how he hurt his leg while mountain climbing and was able to get down the mountain before nightfall by singing "The Old Volga Boatman." He said that he "musicked along" and the rhythms and melodies made his mind forget the pain. Later, in the hospital, he repeatedly listened to a cassette of a Mendelssohn violin concerto. Then, after weeks of struggling to walk, he stood and found, "The concerto started to play itself with intense vividness in my mind. In this moment, the natural rhythm and melody of walking came back to me . . . and along with this [came] the feeling of my leg as alive, as part of me once again." This example of the healing powers of music is one everybody can benefit from.

Music can help reduce stress hormones, allowing the healing process to proceed more effectively and quickly. Music also helps coordinate the brain and muscle memory. Think about the power of music and muscle memory in complicated dance routines. Visualization is a practical application of this for anyone. I've extensively worked with many people who had serious muscle problems and found that through biofeedback—by improving communication between muscles and brain—normal function can be restored even in those with strokes, spinal problems, and brain injuries.

When you listen to music, the brain focuses on all the sounds, which then affects other brain areas. The more sounds, the more involved the brain becomes. In a piece of music with just a guitar and vocal, like a simple folk song, the brain will "light up" all over, lyrics may trigger all kinds of memories, melodies affect other brain areas, and bass notes can awaken still other brain regions, and so on. A song about social injustice might get the brain working more diligently than simple nonsense or pop lyrics. The act of listening to a full symphony orchestra playing a complex piece of music will let an enormous number of sounds enter the brain. In turn, this can increase blood flow to the brain, bringing in more nutrients to help brain function—including those areas that control our muscles, ranging from relaxation

to power. As a simple experiment, spend a few minutes listening to Vivaldi's *Four Seasons* or Beethoven's Fifth Symphony—not while doing something else or as background music. Close your eyes and let the auditory experience take over your brain. Or go to PhilMaffetone.com and listen to the song "Rosemary" during your five-minute respiratory biofeedback session.

Music "therapy" is similar to using a heart rate monitor, it's just a different form of biofeedback. You listen and your body responds. This approach to brain biofeedback is basic and one I like using because the increased alpha waves can improve brain and body function, improve oxygenation, balance the nervous system, and control stress. With music therapy, there is no need to pay for a series of expensive biofeedback sessions. Using music during respiratory biofeedback helps make this technique even more powerful as a brain therapy.

Music as therapy is thousands of years old. Perhaps the first written therapeutic use came from Chinese medicine about five thousand years ago. About 2500 BC, followers of Pythagoras developed a science of musical psychotherapy. Today, the long, winding road of music includes treatment for many types of patients, including those with depression, autism, learning disabilities, and Alzheimer's. In fact, music therapy has been making substantial inroads into contemporary mainstream health care. Music therapy is used at many medical facilities, including Greenwich

Hospital in Greenwich, Connecticut; Beth Israel Hospital in New York City; and Children's Hospital at Vanderbilt Medical Center in Nashville, Tennessee. The University of Michigan Medical Center is among a growing list of schools that offer programs to certify music practitioners. The American Music Therapy Association has specific curriculum requirements including courses in research analysis, physiology, acoustics, psychology, and music and therapy. There are about six thousand certified music therapists in North America alone.

The musical beat or rhythm can also help improve certain brain areas such as the cerebellum, which acts as one's internal metronome—this part of the brain controls physical coordination and balance. Consider carrying a digital metronome during your walk or run. This can stimulate key communication between at least two brain areas—the cerebellum and motor cortex—to maintain steady, continuous, muscle activity. As I discussed in the chapter on running, these actions can improve the economy or efficiency of your gait and even help posture.

So which song or type of music produces the best training or therapeutic response? That depends on you and your circumstances. Music can rev you up as easily as it can relax you. Thus, one key is picking the songs most appropriate for what you want. Those needing additional help with their rest and recovery, soothing music—like the slower classical pieces—may be best.

Sometimes, it's how you listen as much as what you listen to. When hearing high-energy songs that get you moving, it's often the drums and bass guitar that affect your nervous system and rev you up. The melody (in songs with words, it's the part that's sung) is what most people remember and can be a powerful therapy. Or by listening to things you may not have heard before in a familiar song, such as one of the background instruments like a subtle piano chord or acoustic guitar, the brain responds accordingly

Often, those who normally don't respond to music can't seem to take their mind off everything else around them when the music is playing. They are easily distracted. If this happens to you, try using a good pair of headphones (especially the noise-cancellation types) and close your eyes. In this state, the brain doesn't have to listen to anything except the music, and there are no distractions from visual stimuli, which turn on more of the brain than anything else. This gives the brain more "energy" to focus on the music, and often in this state, you can hear things you may never have heard before in a favorite song.

Which songs do I like listening to? Ask me this question tomorrow and I'll have a different list. Virtually any Beatles song will work well, especially "Hey Jude," "Yesterday," or "Here Comes the Sun." I've used "Day Tripper" in measuring brain waves with patients. I also like "For No One." Most classical music works exceptionally well too. Like many Beatles' songs, Mozart's modal music

371

is great, but experiment—there is almost an endless supply. Some great pop picks include "Chelsea Morning" by Joni Mitchell, "Heart of Gold" by Neil Young, "Hey" by Red Hot Chili Peppers, "Hallelujah" by Leonard Cohen, "San Diego Serenade" by Tom Waits, "Time of No Reply" by Nick Drake, Dylan's "Like a Rolling Stone" or "Desolation Row," James Taylor's "Fire and Rain," John Lennon's "Imagine," Paul Simon's "Graceland," and Tom Petty's "Learning to Fly."

There's nothing like listening to Mozart, the Beatles, or Cat Stevens to reduce stress or meditatively ponder life. There's a place for Chopin and Dylan in your day and evening. Match the music and your mood, and you're on your way. Relaxing and listening to some good music can help the brain and body—both can come together in a healthy way.

Eleven Ways to Building a Better Brain

Who doesn't want to prevent the age-related problems of memory loss, mental fatigue, and trouble concentrating so often seen in the elderly? But the truth of the matter is something that may surprise you: you can not only prevent brain dysfunction but also correct it and actually grow your brain. It's not a fantasy, it's real. The first step is the most difficult—deciding you really want to do it.

Not too long ago, most researchers and health care professionals thought it was impossible to improve the brain once it's damaged or loses function with age. This

not only includes intelligence, but the brain's ability to regulate muscles, hormones, vision, and its many other functions. But scientists now know that stimulating the brain through the five senses—eyes, ears, touch, smell, taste—and just by thinking certain ways, will trigger new connections within the brain and between the brain and body. It's even possible to grow new brain cells through these activities.

With the right mental activity, blood flow to the brain increases, bringing more oxygen and other nutrients to cells—the first step to better brain function. Listed here are some powerful routines to significantly help your brain.

1. *Finger touching.* Learning to type or play the piano are powerful brain exercises. Typing, the real format of touch-typing, not poking at keys with one or two fingers, is relatively easy to learn. There are many Internet sites, programs, and booklets available. It involves using all your fingers. Learning the piano does essentially the same thing—you teach your brain to place your fingers on specific areas of the keyboard, guided by your brain. Both touch-typing and playing the piano work both sides of the brain, with many sensory and motor brain regions stimulated. Too many of our daily activities activate only one part of the brain, leaving the less dominant areas relatively inactive

372

Brain Food

Of course, a great diet is necessary for optimal brain function. In fact, the entire first section of this book has direct and indirect relationships with improving your brain. Here is a review of some of the key items:

- Eat sufficient amounts of healthy fats (60 percent of the brain's volume is fat), preferably organic items: extra-virgin olive and coconut oil, fresh raw nuts and seeds, avocados, wild fish, free-range meats, and eggs (the yolks). Balance fats too—starting with about two-thirds of the diet as monounsaturated fats (especially olive oil). The remainder of diet can be about equal amounts of saturated (coconut oil, meat, and dairy), omega-3 (fish), and omega-6 fats (raw nuts and seeds).
- Control chronic inflammation by balancing fats and avoiding all vegetable oils such as corn, soy, safflower, peanut, etc.
- Avoid high-glycemic foods, eliminate processed carbohydrates. Avoid sugar, white flour, white rice, pasta, crackers, bread, cereals, cookies, and so on. They also contribute significantly to chronic inflammation.
- Drink enough plain water.

- Eat at least ten servings of fresh organic vegetables and fruits a day. This is the foundation of a great diet, providing thousands of nutrients you can't get anywhere else.
- Get adequate high-quality protein each day. The best organic sources include grass-fed animal meats, eggs, and wild fish. Vegetable proteins are found in beans, lentils, and nuts.

2. *Stimulate taste and smell.* These are both very powerful ways to improve brain function. Stimulate your sense of taste and smell daily with different types and textures of food, spices, oils, and other pleasant sensations. Each healthy meal is a great opportunity—something you can't do when you rush your meal. Avoid artificial and chemical tastes and smells. The sense of smell is especially powerful and is associated with the memory centers of the brain, so don't be surprised if certain sensations bring back interesting memories.

3. *Be bilateral.* From an early age, one learns to be unilateral—to do things one-sided. The most common example is using your right hand for most things if you're right-handed. (This is different from being ambidextrous, which refers to the ability to do things equally well on both sides.) Evaluate your habits and start using your opposite hand, and

373

foot, for more activities. It will seem odd at first, but even performing this task once starts improving brain function. Be careful with things that can be potentially dangerous such as shaving or using the opposite foot for the brakes while driving.

4. *Brain routes.* In your mind's eye, take a tour of a common route in your life—your drive to work, a walking trail, or the train to the office. As you go through the chosen path, recall as many objects, smells, sounds, and colors as possible. Visualizing routes pumps blood to the memory centers of the brain, feeding the cells there. Many memory experts use routes to memorize large amounts of data. You could easily memorize something shorter—a poem, song, or list of things—using routes. Here's how. Using a familiar route, attach a key word or phrase of your poem or list you want to memorize to objects you see along the way. Then, when you want to recall your poem or list, think of each point of the route and the key words or phrase will come out of your memory.

5. *Create categories.* Many brain functions are best accomplished by creating categories of information. This can help improve the speed of your thinking. As an example, suppose you had a long list of items to buy in the grocery store: red peppers, lettuce, summer squash, carrots, onions, tomatoes, zucchini, blue-

berries, beets, and eggplant. Instead of writing a list, create a single mental category containing those different items. In this case, the category could be rainbow. Then, further categorize the list of fruits and vegetables into their respective colors: red (peppers, tomatoes, beets); purple (blueberries, eggplant); green (lettuce, zucchini); and yellow (summer squash, onions). Keep the number of items in one category to no more than ten. Once those bits of information are entered into the brain, it can be treated as one chunk. So instead of having to remember ten things, you only have to recall one. Chunking is very effective for helping memory recall and long-term memory. Other categories can be created by asking yourself questions. As an exercise, ask yourself, what are five ways of using a ballpoint pen when the ink is gone? What are five things you can do with a shoe other than wear it? The more fun and challenging you make the questions and answers, the more you stimulate your brain.

6. *Learn a language.* While the optimal window of opportunity to learn language occurs before age seven, adults can still learn other languages. Pick one you've always wanted to speak. There are many booklets, tapes, and other learning tools available, and most likely you know someone who speaks another language who can help. Add one new

word to your vocabulary each day, and use it in your daily life. Listen to "native" speakers through recordings or people you know. If you're learning Japanese, for example, go to your favorite sushi bar and speak with the chef, or if Italian, to your local Italian deli (they will love talking with you). Like everything else, have fun doing it. The non-Latin-based languages may be best, including Japanese and Chinese, but any language works well for the brain.

7. *Storytelling*. At least seven major areas of the brain are activated during the telling of a story. Before the age of printing, people relied upon the oral tradition of storytelling to pass on great works of poetry and sagas (the most famous examples are Homer's *Odyssey* and *Iliad*). While memorizing stories and poems stimulate brain function, storytelling is even more creative and imaginative for brain development. Dream up some exciting stories, or use real-life experiences if you aren't feeling creative, then put "twists" on the truth such that you have created fantasies that may be silly, romantic, or wildly unbelievable. Have a storytelling wine and cheese party, write down your tales, go to an open-microphone gathering at a café and tell stories, or just talk to yourself. Even daydreaming your stories, like during one of those boring business meetings, will be great for your brain.

8. *Love*. Being in love is a powerful stimulus for the brain. Studies that address longevity and healthy brain function show the importance of having a loving and stimulating partner. Contrary to many beliefs, a relationship should not be hard work—this actually reduces brain function. If you are laboring to get along with your partner, it may be time for a healthy change.

9. *Live your passion*. Get in touch with what you really enjoy doing in life—and do it! Don't wait. And as much as possible, avoid doing things you don't do well. (Unless of course, it's something you really love, then learn how to do it well.) Many studies have shown how the brain lights up when doing something enjoyable.

10. *Get adequate sleep*. Most adults need at least seven hours of uninterrupted sleep each night. Children need ten to twelve or more. Create the best sleeping environment by eliminating noises, electronics, and lights in the bedroom. Have a healthy, comfortable bed and natural bedding. Keep the room a bit cooler and ensure enough humidity in the air. To better prepare for a good night, take a warm bath before bed. Avoid presleep bad habits: TV can negatively affect the brain, drinking alcohol within at least two hours before bed can disturb sleep, likewise with caf-

375

feinated drinks. And of course, avoid processed carbohydrates. And if you want to read late in the evening, do it on a couch or chair in the living room or study instead of in bed. One way to find out how much sleep you need is to avoid using an alarm clock. Go to bed when you feel tired and get out of bed when you wake up.

11. *Change routines.* While having a routine can make what you're doing more efficient, making changes will challenge the brain to grow and develop new pathways. Examples of changes include using a different hand for your computer mouse, taking a slightly different walking or driving route, and changing the décor, even just rearranging the furniture of your home or office with the seasons.

Too many people wait until their brain dysfunction becomes obvious before trying to do something about it. While much can be done for those with brain injury, the time to grow and improve the brain is the present.

ALZHEIMER'S DISEASE—IT'S PREVENTABLE AND WHY IT'S NOT A NORMAL PART OF AGING

Alzheimer's is defined as a progressive deterioration within the brain that can occur in middle or old age. The name itself refers to the German psychiatrist and pathologist Dr. Aloysius Alzheimer, who in 1901, observed that one of his patients at the Frankfurt Asylum, and only fifty-one years old, exhibited unusual behavioral symptoms, including short-term memory loss. After his patient's death, Alzheimer, along with other research specialists, dissected his brain and discovered amyloid plaques and neurofibrillary tangles. In a healthy brain, neurons connect and communicate with one another at locations called synapses. But these invasive plaques and tangles interfere with this process, causing permanent damage to the brain's communication network. In other words, healthy brain cells die off. By 1911, Alzheimer's description of the disease was being used by European physicians to diagnose patients.

Alzheimer's disease is the most common type of dementia, which is not merely a problem of memory loss but also refers to the inability to learn, reason, or have certain feelings. Other types of dementia include mild cognitive impairment, Parkinson's disease, Creutzfeldt-Jakob disease, and *dementia pugilistica*, which is caused by repetitive head trauma and is often seen in boxers and professional football players.

The changes that occur in someone with Alzheimer's adversely affect the parts of the brain that control thinking, decision making, moods, and memory. Once the classic behavioral symptoms develop, there's really no cure for the victim.

While Alzheimer's disease is considered the sixth leading cause of death in the United States, it's not fatal; but rather, the problem is often associated with other unhealthy conditions that can directly be a cause of death, especially pneumonia and other infectious diseases, dehydration, and malnutrition. This makes it difficult to determine whether or not Alzheimer's actually plays a direct role in the death. But the disease definitely affects quality of life.

Because Alzheimer's is a progressive condition, the dementia gradually worsens over the years. Those with Alzheimer's live an average of eight years after their symptoms become noticeable to oneself and others. Late-stage sufferers often require around-the-clock care and attention. They are as unprotected and defenseless as infants, placing a terrible strain on family members and finances. But given its aging baby boomer population, America is seeing a steady increase in those suffering from Alzheimer's. The disease currently affects five million Americans. The number is much higher for those with early onset or barely recognizable signs.

As Alzheimer's progresses, the brain produces less acetylcholine, a neurotransmitter important for many brain functions including memory. Acetylcholine is made in the body from the nutrient choline, found in the diet (it's especially high in egg yolks and in dietary supplement form). Phosphorus is another important neuronutrient (the Alzheimer's brain contains much less *phosphatides*, whose main component is phosphorus). This compound is important for the healthy function of synapses. Uridine monophosphate is one form found in foods that, in animal studies, has shown improvement in cognitive function. Broccoli, tomatoes, and organ meats are high sources in the diet. For many years, omega-3 fats have been shown to improve brain function, including learning and memory, and have a neuroprotective effect.

Alzheimer's disease is usually accompanied by oxidative stress as one of the primary mechanisms contributing to neurodegeneration and cognitive decline. The importance of antioxidants and phytonutrients to control oxidative stress and chronic inflammation was discussed in section 1 of this book. They play a role in the prevention of Alzheimer's and offer possible early treatment.

Unfortunately, research on nutrition and the brain is quite limited compared to funding for studies on gene and drug therapy. It's an issue of money—and corporate profits. There is no real financial return for companies and institutions to invest in researching various nutrients in a healthy diet—such as choline, omega-3 fats and antioxidant vitamins, minerals, and phytonutrients—that can help successfully prevent or treat Alzheimer's disease. Whereas investing millions to develop pharmaceuticals, which sometimes perform a very similar task, could bring billions in profits. Of course, the cost of these drugs to consumers will be high, adding to the existing health care burden, as will the potential of side effects. As big-pharma matters now stand, current FDA-approved Alzheimer's drugs have been shown to slow down the process of deterioration but only up to twelve months.

According to the Mayo Clinic, scientists believe that for most people, Alzheimer's disease results from a combination of genetic, lifestyle, and environmental factors that affect the brain. Less than 5 percent of the time, Alzheimer's is caused by specific genetic changes that will most likely guarantee a person will develop the disease.

Like virtually all other chronic illnesses, the condition starts long before the appearance of obvious symptoms. This "delay" provides the window of opportunity for prevention, when changes in lifestyles can influence the brain's physical and functional state. Unfortunately, most people wait for long after the arrival of symptoms before seeking help or asking, "Why am I always forgetting things?"

The early abnormal changes that take place in the brain, which include damage to certain neurons in particular areas, can sometimes be detected with positron-emission tomography (PET) scans and cerebrospinal fluid analysis. These initial abnormalities are now considered the *preclinical* stage of Alzheimer's. This first stage is only a category used for research purposes, as medicine has no preventative treatment. For patients who begin developing symptoms of memory loss, difficulty with new learning and finding words, this is the second stage of the disease, or called "mild cognitive impairment." Technically, it's not until the third stage, when symptoms worsen, that the term "Alzheimer's disease" is most often used.

However, categorizing Alzheimer's into distinct stages is quite irrelevant for the patient and those family members and friends affected by his or her condition. Moreover, changes in the brain observed in the first stage don't just appear overnight. There is a period before this occurs when the brain knows that it is being harmed—

so there really are four stages—the earliest being the most important and relevant since this is when individuals can protect their brains by being healthy and fit. This marks the time of true prevention.

Alzheimer's can strike even those in their forties and fifties, though the problem is more common in older individuals. The disease usually begins after age sixty and risk goes up with age. About 5 percent of men and women between ages sixty-five and seventy-four have Alzheimer's disease. This rate increases in the following years.

As mentioned earlier, genetics is not the sole cause of Alzheimer's disease. This condition appears clustered among family members or generations because individuals tend to adopt similar unhealthy lifestyles as their parents, siblings, and relatives, such as poor eating habits, obesity, and inactivity.

There are a variety of risk factors—more obvious indications of poor health—associated with Alzheimer's disease, and most of these are preventable too. For example, it's well-known that diabetes and hypertension are major risks. Likewise, cardiovascular disease, heart attack, and stroke are associated the onset of Alzheimer's disease. But if you step back and look at the big picture, it's clear that carbohydrate intolerance and chronic inflammation may both be a primary cause of the factors contributing to Alzheimer's disease.

Carbohydrate intolerance can also directly increase the risk of Alzheimer's disease. This occurs from the effects of chronically high levels of insulin in the blood that continually enter the brain. In addition, harmful chemicals called "advanced glycosylation end products" (AGEs) that result from carbohydrate intolerance accumulate in the brain and are also associated with the onset of Alzheimer's disease.

Chronic inflammation can negatively affect the brain, further increasing the chance of Alzheimer's. The "neuroinflammatory" process—inflammation in the brain—is related to various brain disorders, including stroke, a risk factor for dementia, and traumatic brain injury.

Increased physical activity is associated with a reduced probability of Alzheimer's disease. The best workouts may be easy aerobic activities, such as walking or other lower heart rate training. These activities directly and indirectly help the brain through improvements in circulation, immune function, and blood sugar control, and reduction in inflammation.

More Than Memory Loss

Memory loss is not necessarily the only symptom of Alzheimer's disease. According to the National Institute on Aging, someone with Alzheimer's disease may experience one or more of the following signs:

- Has difficulty with new learning and making new memories
- Has trouble finding words—may substitute or make up words that sound like or mean something like the forgotten word
- Loses spark or zest for life—does not start new projects
- Loses recent memory without a change in appearance or casual conversation
- Loses judgment about money
- Has shorter attention span and less motivation to stay with an activity
- Easily loses way going to familiar places
- Resists change or new things

- Has trouble organizing and thinking logically
- Asks repetitive questions
- Withdraws, loses interest, sudden mood changes, and uncharacteristically angry when frustrated or tired
- Takes longer to do routine chores and becomes upset if rushed or if something unexpected happens

Patients in the early stages of dementia, and especially family members and close friends seeking to help the patient find answers and treatment, often become frustrated and disillusioned because even the most respected specialists in this field have few answers and no overall cure. Like other modern diseases, the most potent remedy is prevention, and the time to start is the present. It only takes one short, easy walk or one healthy meal to start improving brain function.

CHAPTER 21

YOUR MUSCLES
Keeping Them in Balance to Prevent Aches, Pains, and Even Serious Injuries

One of the most common complaints in adults is discomfort, injury, or some other physical ailment causing aches and pains. Every day, millions of Americans treat these symptoms with aspirin, pain-relieving creams, gels, cold and hot packs, over-the-counter medication, and NSAIDs (nonsteroidal anti-inflammatory drugs) such as Advil, Tylenol, and Aleve. But many people do seek help for their aches and pains from their family doctors, chiropractors, osteopaths, physical therapists, massage therapists, and even surgeons.

While sometimes the problems are remedied quickly, many patients go from one specialist to another without resolution to their complaint. Usually underlying these physical problems is muscle imbalance. And yes, there are relatively simple ways to correct it.

Your body's muscles are a vital part of overall health and fitness. In total, the muscles are the body's largest organ, and they aren't just for lifting, pushing, carrying, moving, or sprinting to get out of the rain. They are responsible for other functions such as helping to pump blood through the body's miles of blood vessels, immune function, and burning body fat.

There are three different kinds of muscle in the human body, each with different functions:

- *Smooth muscle* makes up the walls of the arteries to control blood flow and surrounds the intestines from beginning to end to regulate the movement of food during digestion. These muscles are controlled to a great extent by the autonomic nervous system (the automatic or subconscious control of many body functions).
- *Cardiac muscle* is unique to the heart. While influenced by the brain and nervous system, as well as hormones, the heart also contains its own intrinsic mechanism, allowing it to beat independently.
- *Skeletal muscle* comprises the bulky muscular images we're so familiar with in fit-looking people. As discussed in chapter 13, most of these muscles are comprised of a variety of different fibers, primarily the aerobic and anaerobic types. While their basic movement is under conscious control from our brain (with many other

actions taking place we're not always aware of), you can also influence skeletal muscles significantly through exercise, diet, hormones, and therapies. Skeletal muscles are the focus of this chapter.

Unlike heart muscle, skeletal muscles work because the brain and nervous system control them; as such, it should be referred to as a "neuromuscular system," which includes the brain and spinal cord, the muscles, and the nerves that connect them.

In addition to their physical attributes, skeletal muscles influence many areas of metabolism, including fat storage, the liver, and the brain. Skeletal muscles also play a significant role in immune function because of their antioxidant capabilities; they are essentially home to much of our antioxidant protection, given a healthy diet and the intake of foods high in antioxidants. Muscles are even a major source of blood and lymph circulation. This occurs mostly in the red aerobic muscle fibers, which are well endowed with many miles of blood vessels.

The Full Spectrum of Muscle Function

A primary function of muscles is that they move bones and allow you to use your body for standing, walking, running, and every other physical action, including holding up this book. When muscles don't accomplish this task, it's typically due to some type of dysfunction. In general, the full spectrum of muscle function can range from very loose muscles that are grossly weak with no perceivable contraction to the other extreme of hypertonic or very tight, spastic muscles. Between these two extremes are a number of other important conditions. But before considering them, it's important to know how muscles normally work.

Normal Muscle Function

A muscle's normal activity is a combination of contraction and relaxation, technically referred to as "facilitation" and "inhibition," respectively. When walking, for example, contraction and relaxation occur continuously throughout the body. When muscles contract, they get moderately tighter while working harder; when relaxed, they have less force and also allow the opposite muscle to contract better.

The best way to explain normal muscle function is to feel it working. Let's use the biceps muscle on the front of the upper arm and the triceps muscle on the back of the arm. The contraction and relaxation of these two muscles, which usually work together to move the elbow, can provide an accurate view of how muscles normally work throughout the body. So try this experiment:

- First, in a relaxed, sitting position, with your left hand, feel your right biceps muscle on the front of your upper arm. Then feel the right triceps muscle on the back of your upper arm. At rest, they should both be relatively relaxed—firm but neither tight nor too loose.

- Next, place your right hand under your thigh, then pull upward as if trying to lift your thigh; in doing so, you contract the biceps muscle. Now feel the biceps muscle again with your left hand, and it should feel noticeably tighter. This is how a contracted muscle (one that is normally facilitated by the brain) feels.

- While continuing to lift up on your thigh, now feel the triceps muscle on the opposite side of the arm. This should feel much looser than the biceps and even a bit looser (depending on how much you pull up on your thigh) than when at rest. This is how a muscle relaxes itself more to allow the opposing muscle to contract. The biceps muscle is contracted (or facilitated), and the triceps is in a state of inhibition. In fact, without this extra relaxation (inhibition) by the triceps, the biceps could not properly contract.

During a walk, jog, or run, this same facilitation and inhibition takes place constantly in opposing muscles, just like the biceps and triceps. It occurs in the quadriceps (front of the thigh) and hamstrings (back of the thigh), the anterior tibialis muscle (front of the leg) and calf muscles (including the gastrocnemius and posterior tibialis), the pectoralis muscles (upper chest and front shoulder) and latissimus (back of shoulder and spine), and so on.

Normal muscle function is the optimal state of the neuromuscular system. It provides the best balance of the physical body—with the right combinations of inhibition and facilitation to produce the most effective physical activity.

Abnormal Muscle Function—Neuromuscular Imbalance

Understanding the normal function of muscles can also give you a better idea of the abnormal. The most common abnormal muscle condition in active and inactive people alike is muscle imbalance, which occurs when two or more muscles don't contract and relax as they should. This type of problem is referred to as "neuromuscular imbalance."

Using the example above, when you contracted the biceps and the triceps got looser, imagine if the biceps remained tight and the triceps remained loose even after you released your grip on your thigh. This is very much like the condition of muscle imbalance—except both muscles are in an abnormal state.

A muscle that stays too relaxed is referred to as "abnormal inhibition" and sometimes called "weak" (although this is not true weakness, which refers to the lack of power). This part of a muscle imbalance can be relatively minor, causing minimal impairment, or in some cases extreme to the point of causing severe pain in a joint controlled by that muscle. In most cases, this inhibition causes an opposite muscle to become too tight, a condition called "abnormal facilitation."

Together, these abnormal muscles—muscle imbalance—can adversely affect the joint(s) they control, the tendons they're attached to, and other muscles, ligaments, bones, and body areas (such as the pelvic, spine, or head) all over. This will also cause an imbalance in posture and an irregular gait.

The full spectrum of muscle function ranges from extreme weakness to extreme tightness, with normal in the middle (see chart below). The extremes are usually due to a brain or spinal cord injury; those with cerebral palsy, multiple sclerosis, or who've had a stroke typically have this type of muscle weakness and tightness.

The development of muscle imbalance may occur as follows:

- The abnormally inhibited muscle is lengthened and is often the starting point for many common physical ailments that are not induced by trauma such as falling or twisting your ankle. This muscle weakness itself is often silent. However, you might feel the lack of function produced by it, such as something not right in the knee joint while moving. And when the muscle doesn't properly control the movement of a nearby joint, it eventually causes that body part to become inflamed.
- Trauma—from a minor, seemingly innocuous muscle strain or a major hit or fall that directly injures the muscle—can result in the same abnormal muscle inhibition.

- The other side of abnormal muscle inhibition is tightness (abnormal facilitation). It often occurs as the body compensates to an abnormal inhibition that recently occurred. This tight muscle is often noticeably uncomfortable and sometimes painful, and it can impair movement by restricting flexibility. Tight muscles are shortened, making them candidates for mild, slow stretching; however, in most cases, this would be treating the secondary problem as the cause is usually the weak (inhibited) muscle. In addition, in attempting to loosen the tight muscles through stretching (which is not recommended), you risk weakening the inhibited muscle more (because it's already overstretched).

Two Types of Muscle Imbalance

Today, health care professionals, sports coaches, and athletes often use the term "muscle imbalance." Unfortunately, there is no consensus about how muscle imbalance is defined.

There are at least two different types of muscle imbalance:

- *Neuromuscular imbalance* was discussed above and involves the whole spectrum from brain and nervous system to the muscle itself.
- *Exercise imbalance* is generally a localized muscle problem, typically due to working one muscle or group much more than another, or using one muscle or group much less than another in daily life. (This is not to say that the brain and nervous system don't play a role in exercising a muscle, but the term "neuromuscular" differentiates the two types of muscle imbalance for convenience.)

Exercise Imbalance

It's not unusual for some individuals to define muscle balance and imbalance in terms of strength, making it more a local phenomenon because it reflects muscular exercise. In this case, the problem is too much or too little strength development in one muscle or muscle group compared to another. This can occur with lifting weights if the biceps muscle is used more than triceps exercises. The result is that the biceps becomes much stronger relative to the triceps. This could make the elbow or shoulder joint vulnerable to injury.

Full Spectrum of Muscle Function				
Gross weakness (little/no movement)	Abnormal inhibition (so-called weakness)	Normal	Abnormal facilitation (tight)	Gross tightness (hypertonic or spasm)

The cause of exercise imbalance can occur from improper weight workouts, performing one-sided-type sports such as tennis, or having a job that requires a high level of physical activity in only one muscle or muscle group. These are examples of using one while reducing the action of another muscle or muscle group causing imbalance. The lack of strength, typically from neglect or disuse, can also contribute to muscle imbalance.

Measuring Muscle Imbalance

Muscle imbalances can't be easily evaluated using X-rays, CAT scans, or other high-tech devices. But it's possible to measure the problem in other ways. In general, the "strong" muscle is measured against the "weaker" one:

- For neuromuscular imbalances, evaluations include testing a single muscle or muscle group to determine general contractibility.
- For exercise imbalances, specific measures of strength can be made.

Differentiating between normal deviations is important. The human body is not perfectly symmetrical, and therefore normal variations exist in muscle function and strength. The most common example is the expected difference between muscle strength on the left and right sides of the body—a right-handed person usually has more strength on the right side.

Observing posture and gait and considering the health and fitness history are two ways of observing both types of muscle imbalance.

Observing Posture and Gait

When working with patients to assess their muscle function, I would study their

Strength versus Power

It should be noted that strength and power are two terms often used together but should be defined differently:

- Strength is defined as the maximum force a muscle or muscle group can generate, such as in lifting a weight. Athlete A can bench-press 200 pounds and has twice the strength of athlete B, who can bench-press 100 pounds.
- Power incorporates a speed factor with strength. Athletes A and B can both lift 350 pounds, but athlete A has more power because he can lift this weight much quicker than athlete B.

The general terms "weak" and "strong" are usually associated with strength. However, these are vague meanings unless related to a previous muscle condition—for example, athlete A's leg muscles are stronger now that he is consistently exercising.

standing posture and gait. In fact, just moving around during a walk from the waiting area to my exam room, including the act of standing and sitting, provided valuable information about specific muscle dysfunction. Muscle imbalances are represented by excessive deviations in posture—curving of the spine, tilting of the head or pelvis, one-sided rotation of the upper body, or other distortions, some very subtle, others not. Expressing pain in a certain physical position also provides information about a muscle or muscles not supporting the body.

Irregularities in movement are more common with higher levels of activity, especially during exercise and in particular with running, which relies on more muscles. One just has to watch athletes on TV or the runners at the end of a marathon or long bike event to see the more exaggerated forms of imbalance: irregular movements and, in runners, even the erratic sounds of shoes hitting the pavement.

I recall my days as a student, learning about muscle imbalance and which muscles perform specific movements, and the imbalances that cause slight irregularities in gait. Some of my classmates and I would go to an indoor mall and watch people walk by, assessing them with our newfound understanding of human anatomy.

History

I found that the history of a person's pain or injury usually provides a significant amount of information regarding which muscles are imbalanced. In today's health care environment, however, taking down a patient's full history is a lost art. This is unfortunate since people knowingly and unknowingly provide many key clues by talking about their symptoms, and a good question-and-answer session may be the best assessment process that can uncover a hidden cause of a problem and lead to an effective therapy.

A person with knee pain who states he or she twisted an ankle a week before the onset of the problem is making an obvious statement about which muscles might be weak. In this case, one or more of the muscles that support the ankle that can also influence knee movement, such as the posterior tibialis, could be the cause of the knee pain.

Asking a patient a question such as "what movement causes pain" can provide important clues about which muscles are at fault. Difficulty with specific movements—for example, getting up from a chair, placing a hand on the low-back area, or combing hair—are associated with a particular muscle weakness.

Other assessment procedures are applicable to one type of muscle imbalance or the other as discussed next.

Testing Muscle Strength

Exercise imbalance can be measured in various ways. The simplest method is through observation. By comparing the bulk of the left and right sides of the thigh, one could sometimes see large differences in muscle mass. This might also include obtaining a measurement of muscle bulk, such as the size difference between left and right lower thigh just above the knee. While muscle bulk does not necessarily directly relate to strength, this provides a general measure of imbalance potentially caused by exercise or lifestyle factors—such as too much development in one muscle or muscle group compared to another. Left-right differences in the body usually exist but should not be significant. An example of a normal difference might be a right thigh measurement of 15 ½ inches and the left 15 inches.

Testing a muscle's strength is a simple way to measure individual muscles or muscle groups. If you can lift a fifty-pound weight fifteen times with your right biceps and seven times with your left, it shows you're much stronger on the right compared to the left. In this case, the difference is probably not within the normal variation of being right-handed. Using your left arm more in the course of daily living could eventually make up the deficit.

Information about muscle balance is sometimes evaluated on an electromyographic (EMG) device. This equipment measures the electrical activity of muscles at rest and during contraction. Studies using EMG are commonly used in research and by clinicians to treat various types of muscle problems. Like most other muscle evaluations, there are no clear standards for gathering and assessing different types of EMG findings.

Examples of Sports Medicine Measurements

Comparing the strength of certain flexor and extensor muscle groups is common in athletes. An example is the relative strength of the hamstrings on the back of the thigh in comparison to the quadriceps on the front can be measured. This hamstrings-quadriceps (H:Q) ratio is a common assessment. An H:Q ratio less than 0:6 is thought to be abnormal, and this imbalance in strength between the quadriceps and the hamstrings could potentially contribute to knee joint or hip injury.

Likewise, the ratio of biceps to triceps strength has also been used. Studies show that a ratio greater than 0:76 may predict elbow injuries, although this particular study was done observing baseball pitchers.

However, comparing before- and after-treatment measurements can be very useful to determine whether improvements are being made and which therapies may be most successful.

Testing Neuromuscular Function

Generally speaking, muscles involved in neuromuscular imbalance can sometimes be measured using some of the same methods as above. This includes posture and gait and a history. And more subtle neuromuscular imbalances are not as easy to observe compared to the significant weakness found in stroke patients.

The size of the muscle in relation to the body's left and right, or front and back, is not as relevant in the case of neuromuscular imbalances. In fact, strength and neuromuscular function in the same muscle sometimes don't correspond. A frail elderly person could have poor muscle strength but good neuromuscular function, and a person who regularly lifts at the gym could have neuromuscular imbalance contributing to an injury.

As part of an assessment process, EMG may be useful in evaluating neuromuscular imbalance. Some practitioners, however, also use it as part of their therapy and it is an example of biofeedback, defined here as a method of improving muscle function and correcting imbalance by consciously responding to the stimulation of pressure resistance by another person (such as a therapist) against a muscle.

Another form of biofeedback, manual muscle testing, is sometimes used with EMG but often performed separately as an assessment and at times part of the treatment. Muscle testing is often used before and after therapies such as muscle stimulation, manipulation, and massage to evaluate their efficacies.

Manual Muscle Testing

As a form of biofeedback, manual muscle testing is commonly used for the evaluation of muscle imbalance, most often employed to evaluate neuromuscular imbalance. It can also be used as therapy.

The first textbook on manual muscle testing appeared in 1949 to assess muscle weakness in polio patients, and gradually, muscle-testing techniques were improved for the evaluation of a full range of muscle dysfunction in all types of individuals. Today, various forms of manual muscle testing are used by tens of thousands of health care professionals worldwide. Manual muscle testing is also recommended by the American Medical Association's guidelines for physical impairment.

The objective of muscle testing differs considerably among its users. For example:

- Neurologists perform muscle testing to help evaluate brain and spinal cord function.
- A physical therapist may use muscle testing to rate a patient's level of disability.
- An athletic trainer may use muscle testing to assess a particular athletic injury.
- Chiropractors, osteopaths, and other medical doctors may use manual muscle testing as a form of assessment for neuromuscular imbalance.

Manual muscle testing involves physically evaluating individual muscles. This is accomplished by first positioning an arm, leg, or other body part associated with a particular muscle's action. In this position, the practitioner applies force against the patient's force from that particular muscle. Weakness due to abnormal inhibition may exist if the resistive force cannot properly be maintained, or sometimes if there is excessive pain.

Properly done, manual muscle testing can help differentiate between neuromuscular imbalance and exercise imbalance.

And it can eliminate the need for EMG and other tests, many of which are much more expensive.

Muscles attach to bones through tendons. So when a muscle is not functioning properly, the tendons don't either. Most tendon problems are secondary to muscles that don't work well. Likewise, ligaments connect bones to

TEN COMMON CAUSES OF MUSCLE IMBALANCE

1. Poor Muscle Development
   This can arise from chronic exercise imbalance (such as lifting weight with certain muscles and neglecting others), poor running gait (which can develop certain muscles more than others), or overtraining (too much workout time and or too much workout intensity).

2. Poor Lifestyle Habits
   This includes performing physical work requiring the use of certain muscles while neglecting others. Being overly right-handed while not using the left hand and being generally inactive (the couch potato) are two common examples.

3. Microtrauma
   These injuries may be less obvious, such as regularly wearing bad shoes, sitting at your desk or in your car too much, or chronic repetitive stresses such as typing.

4. Acute or Chronic Localized Injury
   These injuries are more obvious and include the common muscle strain, a twisted ankle, or traumatizing a muscle from a fall or whiplash-type injury in a car accident.

5. Chronic and Acute Illness
   Including diabetes (reduces neuromuscular function), sarcopenia (reduced muscle bulk with aging), chronic inflammation, and related conditions (arthritis, obesity, and many illnesses resulting in significantly reduced physical activity).

6. Neurological Disorders
   These include brain injuries (such as Parkinson's disease, stroke, birth trauma, head trauma) and spinal cord injuries (serious trauma that damages the spine affecting the spinal cord such as an auto, bike, or swimming accident).

7. Nutritional Factors
   This includes low dietary protein, dehydration, anemia, low blood sugar, and general malnutrition.
8. Pain
   Whether from unknown sources or chronic or acute pain from an injury or illness, the presence of pain itself can produce muscle imbalance maintaining a vicious cycle of cause and effect.
9. Aerobic Deficiency Syndrome (ADS)
   This important issue was addressed in chapter 10. Reduced aerobic muscle development can lower overall muscle function, causing an imbalance.
10. Stress
   As discussed in chapter 19, excess physical, chemical, and mental stress can directly and indirectly cause muscle imbalance through mechanical and chemical means.

other bones. And muscles have an important support relationship with both ligaments and bones, directly and indirectly. So when a ligament or bone problem exists, there is usually an associated muscle imbalance as well.

The cause of muscle imbalance must be addressed if normal muscle function is to be restored. Often, the body can accomplish this on its own, especially when it's fit and healthy. And as I reinforced throughout this book, being barefoot is a powerful physical activity that can help the body correct muscle imbalance.

In fact, the body is always self-correcting problems. Even without knowing it, the body is always working to restore muscle balance. During the process of correcting its own problems, the body may show relatively minor symptoms and often none at all. When your body can't fix a particular problem, that's when symptoms appear and an injury develops.

Self-care of Muscle Imbalance

While treatment by a health care professional is sometimes necessary, many people are able to correct their own muscle imbalances. There are a number of ways you can accomplish this. Furthermore, the following approaches to correcting muscle imbalance can also prevent a recurrence.

- First and foremost is to address the cause or causes of muscle imbalance.
- Second, allow your body to do the work. As I mentioned earlier, muscle imbalance

A HISTORICAL PERSPECTIVE OF MUSCLE IMBALANCE

A long history surrounds the concepts, theories, and practices that employ muscle imbalance. In brief, here are some of them:

- In 1741, French physician Nicolas Andre was one of the first to discuss muscle imbalance in his writings. He coined the term *orthopedia,* which means "straight child," and advanced the notion that scoliosis, abnormal curvatures of the spine, was due to muscle imbalance.

- In 1890, French scientist Étienne-Jules Marey made the first recording of a muscle's electrical activity and coined the term "electromyography." This would become a common instrument to measure muscle imbalance.

- In 1900, Nobel laureate Sir Charles Scott Sherrington, an English neurophysiologist, proposed his law of reciprocal innervation, which stated that muscle inhibition usually generates tightness in opposite (antagonist) muscles. Despite this notion, most of the therapies associated with muscle imbalance were directed at tight and painful muscles, which, within the tight/weak model of muscle imbalance, were the most symptomatic and easiest to detect. This involved using braces and surgery by many practitioners.

- In 1949, American physical therapists Henry and Florence Kendall's first textbook on manual muscle testing appeared, which evaluated weakness in polio patients. This marked a change in approach in treating muscle problems as both tight and weak muscles were observed and measured.

- In the early 1960s, clinical pioneers Dr. George Goodheart from the United States and Czechoslovakian Dr. Vladimir Janda took different paths in their pursuit of treating patients with muscle imbalance. Goodheart, influenced by Kendall's work, promoted the idea that muscle inhibition (weakness) was the primary cause of muscle imbalance associated with everyday aches and pain, along with more serious disabilities. This triggered a muscle-testing revolution among many clinicians seeking to find and fix mechanical dysfunction. Janda took the tight muscle road like some of his predecessors, directing therapy at the tight side of muscle imbalance. Both clinicians developed huge multidisciplinary followings that continue today.

- As the jogging and fitness boom of the 1970s evolved, strength exercises such as weight lifting and various workout machines became popular. One result is that many people developed muscle imbalance by creating too much strength in one muscle in relation to another.

  Today, there is usually a clear division among the many types of therapists who treat muscle imbalance. Some see the primary cause, and therefore direct their treatment to the tight side, while others focus on the weak muscles to correct the problem. On one hand, there are chiropractors, osteopaths, physical therapist, medical doctors, and massage therapists (to name a few) who evaluate and treat the tight part of muscle imbalance. While others in these same professions evaluate and treat weakness as the primary cause of muscle imbalance. I have always considered the weak muscle to be the primary problem in most cases, with the tightness a secondary problem.

will often correct itself naturally in a body that's most fit and healthy. This included the right exercise routine, a healthy diet, and proper management of stress.

- One powerful way to correct muscle problems is by developing a great aerobic system. In particular, the process of warming up before a workout and cooling down afterward can immediately correct many dysfunctional muscles.

- Spending more time being barefoot can encourage many muscles to function optimally, correcting imbalance. Since the muscles in the foot significantly influence bodywide posture, being barefoot can help all skeletal muscles.

- Eliminating chronic inflammation can correct muscle imbalance—as the body's natural anti-inflammatory chemicals are

also powerful regulators of muscle function.

- Since pain can cause muscle imbalance, finding the source of pain and eliminating it also can correct muscle problems.

- The application of cold (cryotherapy) can also help correct muscle imbalance. But extended, continued use of ice placed directly against the body must be pursued with discretion to prevent muscle damage.

Manual Biofeedback

Among the many tools I used in private practice to help correct muscle imbalance was manual biofeedback. It's a safe and effective and relatively easy approach for use by most health care professionals, with its basic techniques used by many laypeople as well.

NSAIDS AND INFLAMMATION CAN CAUSE MUSCLE IMBALANCE

Many people use NSAIDs when they have aches and pains, including aspirin, ibuprofen, Advil, Motrin, Nuprin, Naprosyn, and other prescription and over-the-counter drugs. But these can weaken muscles as one of their side effects. They can even worsen the problem despite providing symptomatic (and temporary) relief.

Recall the discussion about dietary fats and how they control inflammation from chapter 4. Conversion of the omega fats to inflammatory and anti-inflammatory chemicals relies on an important enzyme called cyclooxygenase, or COX. There are actually two COX enzymes, and many people are familiar with the term "COX-2 inhibitors." Aspirin and other NSAIDs temporarily block the COX enzymes so much less of the inflammatory chemicals are formed. While this reduces the inflammatory chemicals, it also lowers the beneficial anti-inflammatory ones. In addition, the cause of the problem—fat imbalance—goes untreated. So if taking NSAIDs makes you feel better, it usually indicates that your fats are not balanced. Here's a quick review on how to improve the balance of fats to control inflammation:

- First, eat approximately equal amounts of omega-6 and -3 fats. It does not necessarily have to be at each meal, but in the course of a day or week, strive for an overall balance. While this 1:1 ratio of -6 and -3 is ideal, the typical Western diet is often 5, 10, or even 20:1. It's no wonder there's an epidemic of chronic inflammation and pain! One reason for this is the high intakes of omega-6 vegetable oils such as corn, soy, safflower, canola, and peanut, and the low consumption of omega-3 fats, especially from wild fish, which is the best source, with beans, flaxseeds, and vegetables containing much smaller amounts.

- By eliminating vegetable oils (substitute olive or coconut) and taking fish oil capsules, which are high in the most potent omega-3 fat, EPA, the balance of fats can significantly improve. (The omega-3 flax oil is less effective.)

- Avoid refined carbohydrates, including sugar, which can increase the conversion of omega-6 oils to inflammatory chemicals.

- A number of other dietary factors can impair the production of anti-inflammatory hormones, thereby increasing the inflammatory ones: low levels of vitamins B_6, C, E, niacin; the minerals magnesium, calcium, and zinc (these should come from a healthy diet); trans fat; low protein intake; excess stress; and aging, which increases the risk of more inflammatory chemicals.

Other Types of Pain Drugs

In addition to NSAIDs for pain control, a second type of over-the-counter drug used for pain relief includes acetaminophen. The most popular nonprescription one is Tylenol, which doesn't act by reducing inflammation, and therefore is less likely to interfere with healing and recovery. In fact, it's not entirely clear how it works, but liver stress is among the side effects; the body needs to break down these drugs in the liver, which requires large amounts of the amino acid cysteine (best obtained in the diet from whey consumption).

Narcotics, such as opiates, are another type of pain reliever. These act in the brain to reduce the sensation of pain and also don't affect inflammation. However, they are easily addictive, and their use as a pain reliever wears off as the brain cells become desensitized. Common narcotics prescribed for pain include morphine and other opioid drugs such as codeine and oxycodone (OxyContin).

Yet another pain-relieving drug is THC, the active component in marijuana, which controls pain by stimulating certain receptors in the brain, similar to those that opiates act upon. THC can stimulate the brain's natural opiates, like endorphins. The only prescription form is the product Marinol, although many states now have medical marijuana laws.

Manual biofeedback helps the brain and body restore and balance muscle function. It addresses the problem of muscle imbalance that's due to a wide range of problems. It can be used in children and adults of all ages who have suffered minor local muscle injury to more serious brain and spinal cord injuries. This therapy helps restore muscle balance by strengthening weak muscles and relaxing tight ones. It's a simple hands-on system that requires no equipment.

Most people who have injuries associated with muscle imbalance fall into at least one of two categories:

- Local muscle injury is the most common cause of physical problems and is often associated with trauma to the muscle itself, such as the result of a fall, a so-called pulled muscle, a twisted ankle, or other injury. Microtrauma is even more widespread; it's the accumulation of minor physical stress in a muscle or joint, often unnoticed while it's happening, eventually causing a more obvious muscle problem. Daily living produces significant wear and tear on the body's mechanics—a stress that most people should adapt too well to. But often, this stress is not compensated for and muscle imbalance develops. In addition to exercise, too much sitting, repetitive motion injury, or walking in poor-fitting shoes often leads to microtrauma, which in turn ultimately causes muscle problems. Local muscle injuries can result in anything from minor annoying ache to a serious or chronic debilitating condition.

- Brain or spinal cord injury can occur at any age, even before birth, and usually milder forms can be found in many individuals who don't realize they have a relatively minor problem that still causes muscle imbalance. Trauma, infection, or reduced nutrient supply can easily cause brain or spinal cord damage resulting in poor muscle function. Many people are also involved in an auto accident or other trauma that can often sustain a brain or spinal cord injury—sometimes so apparently minor that many doctors or hospitals say you're fine, even after an MRI or CT scan.

MANUAL BIOFEEDBACK—IT CAN BE USED BY ANYONE

While health care professionals regularly apply the art and science of manual muscle testing, biofeedback, and other hands-on assessment and therapeutic activities, there are tens of thousands of other individuals who learn to use these important techniques every day. Almost everyone has used tweezers to take out a deep splinter (minor surgery), bandage an abrasion (emergency first aid), or in some instances even save a life by learning CPR (cardiopulmonary resuscitation). And it's not uncommon to see, in many public areas, including airplanes, restaurants, and malls, automatic cardiac resuscitators for emergency treatment in cases where a person's heart stops—complete with instructions for the average person to use to save a life.

Manual biofeedback is just as practical, if not easier, than some of these techniques, and its successful application to the majority of physical aches and pains can be surprisingly simple once a bit of experience is attained. Manual biofeedback can be used in the young and old, including children, athletes, and everyone else.

While traditional EMG biofeedback uses computer equipment, including mechanical sensors and electrodes attached to the skin, manual biofeedback does not use any equipment. Instead, it relies on the neurological sense of the person using manual biofeedback. This personal approach also allows for the recruitment of more brain-body stimulation with verbal, visual, tactile, and other sensory cues that further enlists the patient's participation and motivation. Like many forms of biofeedback, manual biofeedback relies on basic manual muscle testing.

While it takes another person to use manual muscle testing and the basic biofeedback therapies, with respiratory biofeedback, you can do it on yourself without assistance from others.

The Family Hope Center, which is based in Philadelphia, helps brain-injured children and teaches their parents how to apply many home therapies. A couple of years ago, the center asked me to make an instructional DVD on manual biofeedback. I was happy to be of assistance. The DVD and user's manual that I created contains an introduction to the concepts of muscle imbalance and how to remedy it, respiratory biofeedback, and proper breathing techniques. It also includes the detailed use of manual biofeedback and a library that demonstrates how to test and perform manual biofeedback on all the body's major muscles.

This DVD is now used by virtually all types of individuals dealing with sports injuries, common aches and pains, as well as improving brain function. For more information, go to my website—philmaffetone.com—and visit the "Manual Biofeedback" pages.

Manual biofeedback can help promote and restore muscle balance; it not only helps locomotion and posture but can improve brain function as well, including speech, vision, balance, memory, and even intellect. And because muscles have other important functions, such as energy production, circulation, and immune activity, increasing physical movement can improve overall health.

The Question of Pain

A pain symptom is a subjective yet important part of life. It's not a *sense*, but an emotion that the brain relies on for survival, telling one that there's a problem somewhere in the body and often forcing one to slow down or rest. While pain is felt in the brain, the body parts that produce it usually have either physical or chemical causes.

Pain is how the body tells you to take it easy so it can repair itself. Pain medications, which only treat the symptoms, not the cause, are among the best-selling prescription and over-the-counter drugs worldwide—the means most people suppress or mask the pain instead of finding its cause.

There are at least three possible causes of chronic pain:

- The problem that caused the pain is unresolved. For example, a muscle imbalance causing stress in the knee joint can cause inflammation and pain. Until the cause of the problem is corrected, inflammation and pain will continue.

- Even when the physical cause of the problem is corrected, the chemical imbalance associated with poor fat balance may still be present. Until this problem is corrected, pain-producing chemicals (including those of inflammation) can continually be produced.

- Certain types of brain cells, called glia, can become overactive following some injuries that have caused pain. These cells can continue to stimulate the pain in the brain even after the original cause of pain has resolved. And certain pain medications, especially morphine, seem to actually worsen this process. What triggers the glia to become overactive and act in this fashion is not well understood by scientists. Some substances can potentially turn off the overactive glia. These include THC, the active component in marijuana, and stronger prescription drugs (immune suppressant drugs such as etanercept and narcotic receptor blockers such as naloxone).

The process of pain starts in nerve endings found in the skin, blood vessels, nerve fibers, joints, and coverings of the bone. These nerve endings send messages through the nervous system to the emotional center of the brain (called the limbic system), where one interprets the feeling as pain. Call it an emotion, a feeling, or a mental state—it's simply a physical interaction between the body and the brain. This is why pain is relatively subjective, with no two people feeling it the same. If pain were a true sense—like smell, taste, vision, or hearing—it would be much more difficult, if not impossible, to control it with physical measures (applying cold), chemicals (taking aspirin), or mental measures (through hypnosis).

Once pain messages reach the brain, the brain sends information back to the source of pain in order to release natural analgesics such as endorphins. The spinal cord, comprised of nerves that go from the brain to the body, is the relay station for pain perception. This is one reason that "spinal blocks" can reduce pain symptoms.

The cause of a problem that produces pain is usually located where the injury occurred. But many times, pain is associated with problems elsewhere in the body or with problems that don't produce symptoms. An example is nontraumatic pain in or around the knee, the physical cause is likely due to muscle imbalance in the foot or ankle—and is often silent (asymptomatic). This is one reason so many knee problems never get fully corrected and become chronic; the true cause remains undetected and only the symptom is treated.

The gradual development of knee pain is a phenomenon I have seen and heard from countless patients who limped into my office. The chronology of a typical patient history went as follows: slow onset of knee pain that began as a mild ache, then after several weeks, increasing pain. Aspirin and other nonsteroidal anti-inflammatory drugs (NSAIDs) improved symptoms by reducing pain and inflammation somewhat, but the pain kept returning and led to restricted movement. Several other remedies were often tried to alleviate the knee pain—ice packs, analgesic lotions to dull the pain, rest, and even orthotics and different types of shoes. And if the pain disappeared, it would sometimes show up in another location around the knee or even in the hip joint.

Referred pain is neurologically different from, say, knee or foot discomfort. Referred pain is experienced in one location on the body while the cause is located elsewhere. One of the most common referred-pain patterns is in the case of a heart attack, where pain is felt in the lower neck, shoulder, and arm usually on the left side, while the problem is in the heart. Or pain in the middle of the spine may come from an irritation in the stomach. Referred pain occurs because signals from the heart, for example, and those from the skin in the arm (the referred-pain area) "cross" in the spinal cord, and when the message gets to the brain, it's impossible to differentiate between the signals' origins. That's why it's critically important to differentiate between arm pain that's due to a skeletal muscle problem and that from a heart attack.

Different types of pain such as throbbing or swelling have particular meaning. For example, physical pain can be associated with increased pressure, such as a swelling, typically from trauma. This type of pain is often

described as "stabbing" or "knifelike." Or if it's associated with blood vessels, sufferers experience it as "throbbing" or "pounding."

Chemical pain often comes from inflammation and muscle fatigue. This type of pain is often described as "burning" or "hot." Thermal pain from extreme cold or hot temperatures can also produce pain. This may be due to an ice pack left too long on the skin or sunburn. In fact, sunburn pain can come from all three types: thermal stress (hot sun), physical damage to skin, and chemical inflammation.

In addition to pain caused by muscle imbalance, other types of exercise-related muscle pain can occur. These include the following:

- Pain experienced during or immediately after physical activity may have a chemical origin. Lactic acid, produced from muscle activity, especially the anaerobic type, does not cause pain directly, but may be responsible for pH changes in the blood associated with pain. Reduced blood flow may also be linked to this type of muscle pain, which will subside quickly once activity is stopped.

- Delayed-onset muscle soreness usually develops within twenty-four to forty-eight hours after activity, with a peak in discomfort between forty-eight and seventy-two hours. This pain is usually associated with muscle damage such as microtearing in the fibers. Diminished ranges of motion accompany this pain pattern, and muscle dysfunction often continues long after pain has resolved.

Home treatment of pain associated with physical activity is best accomplished with cold stimulation—soaking the body area(s) in cold water for ten to fifteen minutes can be a wonderful remedy. Ice is not always needed; cold tap water works great and sometimes ice can cause excessive irritation by freezing the skin. Use cold stimulation two or three times the first day, once or twice the second. In most cases, this will significantly and quickly improve pain. Here are some other considerations:

- While the use of heat for pain is thought to be a common remedy, it can actually do more harm than good. Inflammation can be worsened with the application of heat. Unless you're quite sure an area is not inflamed, avoid using heat. Most areas of pain, including the joints associated with muscle imbalance, are accompanied by some degree of inflammation. Inflammatory pain occurs when fat imbalance produces more pain chemicals—balancing dietary fats helps prevent chronic inflammation.
- Low-fat diets can worsen pain and increase the risk of other muscular injury.
- Many people drink alcohol when pain is present, but this can just as easily amplify pain. The pain-reducing ability of alcohol occurs with high intake, something that also creates fat imbalance, ultimately increasing pain.
- Simple gentle rubbing of the skin, called tactile stimulation, can also control pain. This is accomplished by lightly stroking the skin at or near an area of pain. If you bump your head, you probably subconsciously rub the area. This stimulates large nerve endings in the skin that can help block pain sensation in the brain (the same mechanism as electrical nerve stimulation devices).

The most sensible remedy for pain is to find its cause, correct it, and prevent it from coming back.

Breathing Muscles

Of all the vital muscles necessary for optimal health and fitness, one of the most important is the diaphragm. This breathing muscle is located on top of your abdomen and under your lungs. The large flat muscle allows you to breathe by pulling in oxygenated air and expelling unwanted carbon dioxide. In many people, the breathing mechanism may be the weak link to improved overall function.

Poor diaphragm muscle function can lead to various problems such as general fatigue or poor function of many body areas due to reduced oxygenation. In this case, less air enters the lungs, and the blood does not receive the proper amount of oxygen. Moreover, poor exhalation does not eliminate the necessary amount of carbon dioxide.

Everyone can incorporate the actions of normal breathing into their day—not necessarily only during exercise but also during rest or downtime. This can help improve *one's* health and also repair muscle imbalance.

Normal Breathing

It's natural to take breathing for granted until you experience a breathing difficulty. But some people breathe improperly and don't even realize it, while many others could improve their breathing by controlling stress. Normal breathing is associated with proper muscle movement—the most important being the abdominal muscles in the front and sides of your abdomen and the diaphragm muscle. These muscles work together, allowing us to efficiently breathe in and out. Without normal breathing, the abdominal and diaphragm muscles may work improperly and even cause other muscles to not work. In this scenario, body movement—posture and gait, for example—can become impaired, oxygen can be reduced, and other problems can occur.

The abdominal muscles also help physically support your body structure—the spine, low back, pelvis, shoulders, and even the neck. The abdominals help you not only to walk, jog, play any sport like tennis or golf more efficiently but also to sit, stand, and even sleep properly. In some cases, improper breathing is the beginning of a complex set of imbalances, causing an injury to the low or middle back, hip, and shoulder.

Given the importance of the abdominal and diaphragm muscles, let's look more closely at the two components of normal breathing—inhalation and exhalation:

- During inhalation, the abdominal muscles relax and extend outward while the diaphragm muscle moves downward. This movement allows air to enter the lungs more easily and is accompanied by a slight whole-body backward extension, especially of the spine.
- During exhalation, the abdominal muscles contract and tighten and are gently pulled inward; the diaphragm muscle "relaxes" with an upward movement. This helps push air out of the lungs, with a slight whole-body flexion.

By watching another person's breathing, especially the belly moving out on inhalation and in on exhalation, one can often tell if it's correct. You can also evaluate your own breathing by feeling the muscles move. So try this quick experiment:

- Place the palm of one or both hands on the abdomen (over your belly button).
- Slowly breathe in and feel the abdominal muscles expand outward. Your belly should get bigger during inhalation.
- Slowly exhale and feel the abdominal muscles tighten and being pulled inward. The belly is more flat on exhalation.

401

During normal breathing, most movement occurs in the abdominal areas, and only slightly in the chest, which expands more with much deeper breathing.

Those who breathe improperly often move their muscles opposite that of normal—for example, they sometimes pull their belly inward on inhalation. In other cases, the chest is quickly and fully expanded and the abdominal area doesn't get a chance to move properly. These poor patterns of breathing can be caused by stress, the stigma of not showing their belly during inhalation. The use of so-called slimming garments that wrap around the belly can actually cause the abdominal muscle to weaken and therefore should be avoided. Even overexercising the abdominal muscles—typically with sit-ups or crunches—making them too tight to relax. In a real sense, poor breathing is the result of muscle imbalance—weak diaphragm and tight abdominal muscles are a common example.

It's particularly important to be aware of your breathing during times of stress, which is often when breathing can switch from normal to abnormal as you hold more tension in your abdominal and pelvic muscles.

If your breathing is abnormal or irregular, it's important to immediately retrain the breathing mechanism. This can be done using respiratory biofeedback (see chapter 20). The procedure is simple using the steps just outlined above for normal inhalation and exhalation.

Muscles and Bone Health

In general, by maintaining proper muscle balance and by being healthy and fit, you can significantly reduce the risk of bone problems, including fractures and osteoporosis—injuries that occur in both men and women.

There are a number of other factors that significantly influence bone strength, in particular, the proper mineralization of the bone. This is referred to as bone density. Your bones are not unlike muscles, intestines, skin, and other tissues throughout the body. They are full of life—living parts of us. As such, bones are always metabolically active. This means there is always an ongoing influx and output of nutrients—calcium, sodium, magnesium, zinc, protein, and others—which provide us with our level of bone density. If your bones lose more calcium, for example, than they take in, you risk weak bones vulnerable to injury and disease. Combine this with even minor muscle imbalance, and the risk of bone injury is high.

In addition to muscle balance, here are some other key factors that greatly influence bone health:

- Aerobic fitness: this helps maintain support of bones.
- Gravity stress: this is associated with physical activity that improves bone density. For example, someone who only bikes for exercise might add walking or jogging to their workout routine.

CRAMPS, SPASMS, AND SIDE STITCHES

These three problems are due to muscles not working correctly, and in a real sense also associated with muscle imbalance. A muscle cramp is a tight, suddenly contracted muscle that is overfacilitated. It usually occurs during physical activity such as running, paddling a canoe, or performing yard work, especially when you're too aggressive, such as sawing a tree limb. But waking in the middle of the night with foot or leg cramps is not uncommon. The exact cause of muscle cramps is often not fully known and may be very individual (one person's cramp may be caused by something different from another's cramp). Most important is this observation: Those with optimal health and fitness don't have complaints of muscle cramps, spasms, or side stitches.

A muscle cramp usually involves a single muscle or group of muscles. Possible causes might include dehydration, low levels of sodium or magnesium, an overworked muscle, or side effects from a prescription or over-the-counter drug. Muscle cramps generally last a relatively short time (unless you're having a bad one, then it feels like a long time). The terms "muscle cramps" and "spasms" are often used interchangeably as their definitions are somewhat scant. True muscle spasms are extremely tight and painful muscles that occur most often in people with neurological diseases such as multiple sclerosis and cerebral palsy and those with severe spinal cord injury.

Side stitches refer to pain typically in the side of the upper intestinal area; these usually occur during jogging and running. They may be directly or indirectly related to either the skeletal muscles such as the abdominals or the smooth muscle of the intestines.

Side stitches are also not well understood by physiologists, but they often appear to originate from the diaphragm or the intestines and usually just after fluid or other food is consumed during higher-intensity activity. They can not only be painful but also reduce your physical activity, often causing you to slow or stop. Bending forward while tightening abdominal muscles or breathing through pursed lips with increased lung volume can help reduce these painful stitches.

- Hormone balance: both estrogen and testosterone in particular help regulate bone mineralization as do adrenal hormones that regulate sodium.
- Adequate calorie intake: low-calorie diets can weaken bones.
- Proper fat and protein intake: both are necessary for bone health.
- Avoiding chronic inflammation: this problem can reduce bone density.
- Sun exposure: your main source of vitamin D, which regulates calcium.

When a bone is stressed, whether from physical strain, dietary or hormonal inadequacy, too little vitamin D, or disease, at least three types of injuries can result:

- A *stress reaction* is a subtle bone injury, microscopic in nature. It causes vague discomfort following physical activity, even just walking around. This problem can't be seen on an X-ray or other scan, making it somewhat elusive.
- A *stress fracture*, which is more painful and usually restricts activity, can occur if more stress affects the bone. It can often, but not always, be diagnosed with an X-ray. It is also an example of a microscopic bone injury.
- A *bone fracture* or break can occur with higher levels of stress. There are many different classifications of fractures depending on how extensive it is and where the break is located. While more serious fractures can require surgical repair, many others are capable of healing with just a cast or little or no support. In some cases, poor health is associated with bone injury, such as osteoporosis, where reduced bone density contributes to a compression fracture (collapsed vertebrae). Fractures are more obvious on X-ray.

If you experience trauma—a severe twisted ankle, a hard fall, or drop a heavy weight on your foot—and injure a bone, healing occurs much more rapidly if you have better muscle balance and are healthier overall. This is true even for an extreme case where surgical repair is necessary. Most importantly, whether a stress fracture from exercise or a more serious bone injury such as a broken hip from a fall, there are usually key causes of more severe health problems that need to be addressed.

Stress Fractures

The most common bone problem in active people is stress fracture. They can occur without obvious trauma and are often due to muscle imbalance interfering with weight bearing, gait, and other movement. While the bones in the legs (tibia and fibula) are common sites of stress fractures, they can also occur in the foot's metatarsal and navicular bones, the pelvis, and the wrist.

Pain from a stress fracture typically improves with rest and worsens with activity. There is often some swelling in the area, but sometimes it's not noticeable. The swelling around the site of fracture may prevent a proper diagnosis by X-ray if taken within the first two weeks of injury. Only after some healing has taken place will the X-ray show the problem. In these situations, a bone scan may help locate the stress fracture when the X-ray can't.

Most stress fractures will heal well in a healthy person without a major therapy. Rest, cooling the site of the fracture, cessation of weight-bearing exercise, and hard-soled flat shoes are often sufficient, but each case must be treated individually. *Aspirin and other NSAIDs must be avoided as they can delay bone healing.*

Just as important is the fact that something caused a stress fracture to occur; and that something—some imbalance in muscles, hormones, diet, or often a combination of problems—must be found and corrected. If this does not happen, you are vulnerable to future fractures.

A low-fat diet may be associated with a higher incidence of stress fractures—statistically more in physically active females. Fats are important for many aspects of health, with certain fats helping to carry calcium into the bones (and muscles).

The importance of optimal muscle function for bone health is often not addressed by health care professionals. However, this may be the most important contributing factor in stress fractures. Three muscle problems can exist in this context:

- Muscle imbalance can cause reduced support and increased stress on specific areas of the skeleton.
- Poor aerobic function, as seen in the aerobic deficiency syndrome, can result in the daily loss of bone support.
- Low muscle mass, such as that seen in sarcopenia, is associated with poor strength, loss of bone support, and increased vulnerability to falls and other injury.

Muscle balance is a key part of physical health and fitness. An imbalance of two or more muscles typically results in one being weaker, and often not symptomatic, and another too tight. This imbalance can be a primary cause of various aches and pains, some minor and merely annoying but others debilitating. Correcting muscle imbalance is something you can do—it's one of the jobs of a health and fit body. In some cases, finding a health care professional may be necessary to accomplish this task.

CHAPTER 22

THE GUT
Your Gastrointestinal Tract Is the Gateway to Good Health

I once had a patient whom I will name Cathy. She was diagnosed with ulcerative colitis more than ten years before coming to my clinic. This chronic inflammatory condition, including significant losses of blood, frequent diarrhea, and extreme fatigue, not only was a serious health problem but it was also wrecking her entire life. The medications that were keeping her alive had many side effects, and each year, on one or two occasions, she would get so ill that hospitalization was the only option. She resisted surgery, and as a last resort, she was willing to try a more natural approach one more time.

After extensive evaluations, I recommended that she strictly adhere to a healthy lifestyle to quickly pull her out of the vicious cycle she was in for most of her adult life. She made significant dietary changes beginning with the Two-Week Test. It was evident that Cathy had to eliminate all grains and starchy carbohydrates, eat smaller more frequent meals, and eliminate all processed and packaged foods. She started taking a number of supplements, including fish oil, L-glutamine, betaine hydrochloride, a natural form of folic acid, and probiotics. She listened to the music she loved whenever possible during the day and made a great effort to avoid the people and activities in her life that caused her stress.

Within a couple of weeks, her health was noticeably improved, and after a month, her intestinal function was significantly better. After another month, she quickly weaned off all medication. By six months, she claimed there were no symptoms of colitis—no discomfort, no bleeding, and normal bowel movements. A visit to her gastroenterologist showed significant healing of her colon, and blood tests were dramatically improved. She continued to see me about twice a year without return of any problems, except on occasion when she would eat improperly during travel or holidays—but eventually she was able to resolve these problems too.

Indigestion, upset stomach, heartburn, ulcer, gas, bloating, constipation, and irritable bowel syndrome are common complaints in today's modern, fast-paced society. Each year, about one hundred million people in the United States experience some kind of digestive disorder. While most of these ailments are temporary and not life-threatening, ten million people are hospitalized annually for evaluation and treatment of gastrointestinal, or GI, complaints. Health care costs exceed $40 billion annually for these patients, with new cases continuing to rise with an aging and increasingly overfat population. While digestive symptoms rise with old age, they can occur at any time, even in children. The

increase in GI problems as the decades march by in one's own lifetime is often due to a general decline in health, and by a reliance on over-the-counter and prescription medications. These drugs, taken regularly or in larger doses, especially to alleviate pain symptoms, further increases the risk of intestinal disturbances due to their side effects.

The GI tract—also called the gut—is a reflection of one's overall health. So let's take a closer look at what the gut does. It physically and chemically digests food into smaller pieces so these nutrients can be absorbed by the small intestine, with the unused matter eliminated from the body. We think of the gut as synonymous with the stomach and intestines, but that's not entirely the case. The gut actually begins in the mouth and continues through the digestive system into the esophagus, stomach, small intestine, large intestine (colon), and the rectum. Other organs that play a role in the function of the GI tract include the liver, gallbladder, and pancreas. The intestine is also home to a significant amount of an adult's immune system, and it is in constant and direct communication with the brain (consider where you first feel emotion—right there in your gut).

Gut problems are not just uncomfortable but an indication that the body may not be functioning properly. If this is the case, one may be unable to obtain all the nutrients from even a healthy diet. A faulty gut can also have a negative impact on immune, muscle, and brain function.

Even those without gut symptoms can have intestinal problems. An example is the individual who develops damage to the intestinal lining, such as from stress or too much alcohol. He or she might not even be aware of it, but small yet significant amounts of GI bleeding can occur without any symptoms being present, with blood in the stool not even noticeable.

A better understanding about the gut, and how different foods and stress affect it, is a first step in helping you correct many intestinal problems, leading to better absorption of nutrients.

The main function of the gut is the digestion of food and the absorption of nutrients. Most people are well aware of these activities, but the gut also assists the liver by eliminating toxins from the whole body. The gut produces vitamins and hormones and has its own extensive nervous system. So even if you eat the right foods, if they're not properly digested and the nutrients unabsorbed, nutritional imbalances can occur due to malabsorption. This could create a problem identical to those associated with not eating the right foods. Or a poor-functioning gut can reduce immune function, leading to more colds, flu, and allergies.

Common Gut Problems

Signs and symptoms of gut dysfunction are common in people of all ages. Among the biggest sellers of drugs, both over-the-counter and prescriptions, are those that cover the symptoms of an improperly functioning GI

tract. Most don't treat or correct the causes of the problems. But by being healthy and fit, most people with intestinal distress can significantly improve, and usually eliminate, their gut-related conditions.

Causes for many gut symptoms include poor diet, excess stress, hormone imbalance, and dehydration. Side effects of medication are frequent stresses for the intestines. Of particular concern are patients with arthritic conditions as more than fourteen million of them consume NSAIDs regularly. Up to 60 percent will have gastrointestinal side effects related to these drugs, and more than 10 percent will cease recommended medications because these symptoms are severe—they include intestinal upset and discomfort and GI bleeding.

Highly processed carbohydrates—including grains and other starches and sugars such as sucrose, maltose-based sugars, and corn sugars—can cause intestinal bloating and nausea. These problems can occur especially if food is not thoroughly chewed and mixed with saliva to assist in digestion.

Upper-gut symptoms include those that come from the stomach, such as nausea, cramping, vomiting, and discomfort sometimes felt upward into the chest and throat. Those specifically associated with lower intestinal stress are also common and include lower abdominal cramping and diarrhea, bloating and gas, and constipation.

The good news is that the majority of gut problems—from vague indigestion and acid reflux to ulcers and more serious conditions such as Crohn's disease and ulcerative colitis—can be significantly improved or eliminated by making the appropriate changes to improve your food intake, exercise habits, and other factors such as reducing physiological stresses. Let's consider each major area of the gut, its primary purpose, and how one can help it function better.

The Mouth

You use it for talking, singing, screaming, kissing, and even making odd noises. The mouth, however, serves another important function that many people neglect—helping to get more nutrients from your food and keeping the gut working well. Many intestinal problems begin in the mouth.

Gut symptoms often come from not properly chewing food or rushing through a meal. Problems with teeth, gums, or the jaw joint can affect chewing, due to discomfort or the bite being out of alignment. The chemistry of the mouth can also be a problem, such as low salivary pH, discussed below, which can contribute to poor use of digestive enzymes and related dental problems.

Chewing

In the 1890s, Russian physiologist Ivan Pavlov was fascinated by how dogs tended to salivate before food reached their mouths. His groundbreaking research into the timing and importance of saliva, chewing, and also human digestion later won him a Nobel Prize in 1904. After more than a century, physiologists continue building on that understanding.

Chewing helps the taste receptors on the tongue detect extremely small concentrations of substances within a fraction of a second of tasting it—one of the main reason humans love the taste of food. This stimulation elicits a variety of immediate responses throughout the body, including stimulating heat production and fat burning and improving digestion, absorption, and even the use of nutrients from foods. Chewing your food, called the "cephalic phase" of digestion because the brain immediately senses and responds to what's being consumed, can also help control blood sugar and insulin and control fluid and mineral balance. Most of us have experienced being ravenously hungry and even feeling weak, only to perk up the moment we started chewing on some food.

All food should be chewed for better digestion. But those that require the most chewing include concentrated carbohydrates—bread and other starchy grain products, including pasta, rice and beans, all cereals, starchy vegetables such as potatoes and corn, and most sugars. Of course, these processed foods should be avoided anyway.

A key enzyme in saliva is amylase. It starts the digestion of most carbohydrate foods, and without it, normal digestion of this food group may not properly occur, with the risk of producing gas, indigestion, and bloating. Most carbohydrates should be chewed

409

sufficiently and mixed with saliva for better digestion. Fruit and honey contain simple carbohydrates that don't require chemical digestion to obtain the important sugars they contain. However, fruit needs to be chewed into smaller pieces to help the intestine obtain the nutrients within, and chewing both brings out their wonderful tastes.

It is important to chew your food well. Keep matters simple: Rather than counting each mouthful, just chew and enjoy the tastes and textures of your food. Once it has turned into small pieces and is well moistened, swallow it and enjoy another bite. Rushing meals, eating while working at your desk or driving, and other poor dietary habits make it almost impossible to chew and digest well. Listening to enjoyable music during meals can help all phases of digestion.

Oral pH

The environment of the mouth is a critical part of its overall health, especially the acid-alkaline balance—the pH—of the saliva. And it can influence the rest of the gut. In addition, the pH in the mouth may reflect the body's overall fat-burning ability—those with lower pH levels typically have reduced fat burning frequently associated with low energy and increased body fat. As you improve your diet, build your aerobic system, and increase fat burning, your oral pH, among other things, should improve.

The acid-alkaline balance in saliva can be measured with a pH paper, available at a pharmacy, health store, or online. The pH of the mouth should be slightly alkaline, in the range of about 7.4 to 7.6 (slightly higher in children). You may hear or read that the mouth should be an acid pH, but this is confused with the fact that many people have a mouth with a pH in the acid range—6.0, 6.5, 6.8, and so forth. (A pH of 7.0 is neutral; above is alkaline and below is acid.)

Here's the procedure to test your pH:

- Wait about fifteen minutes after eating or drinking, or completely rinse your mouth with water and wait about five minutes.
- Use a small strip of pH paper, and thoroughly moisten it in your mouth for about five seconds.
- Immediately compare the color on your test strip with the color on the pH paper container to determine the approximate pH.

Initially, perform this test two or three times in one day, then again a few days later to establish your average pH level—although it should not vary by much if you follow the above procedure properly. If your pH is consistently too high (above 7.6), it may indicate a need to increase natural carbohydrates in the form of fruits. But if your pH is too low, it may indicate two things: You're eating too many carbohydrates, most likely the refined types, and you need to add more protein and fat to your diet. After making the appropriate dietary changes, check the pH twice a week to follow progress; improvements in pH could take up to a month or more.

In children and adults, low pH—less than 7.0—promotes tooth decay. While in practice I noticed those individuals with proper pH did not get cavities, but those who had tooth decay almost always had low pH.

Proper salivary pH is important to protect the environment of the mouth, especially the tooth's enamel and the regulation of healthy bacteria that normally reside there. Eating sugar-laden foods increases the risk of cavities. This occurs for two reasons. First, sugar and most carbohydrate foods trigger changes in the mouth that shift the environment, enabling unhealthy bacteria to reside there. Normally, healthy strains of bacteria reside in the mouth, but with poor diet, the unhealthy bacteria take over and convert some of the sugar to lactic acid, reducing the pH and promoting tooth decay. Second, consuming sugar and other high-glycemic foods affects the body's metabolism, reduces fat burning, and also lowers oral pH even when there is no sugar residue in the mouth—and even right after brushing. This lower pH environment is perfect for unhealthy bacteria to thrive and damage the teeth and gums.

The unhealthy bacteria in the oral cavity promote demineralization of the teeth—the loss of calcium. This can result in decay and loss of teeth and dislodging of old fillings.

In a healthy mouth, the normal bacteria include *Streptococcus sanguinis*, made up of a number of species. These bacteria are found in saliva and are also absorbed by dental plaque, where they modify the environment to make it less hospitable for the various strains of unhealthy *Streptococcus* that cause cavities.

Unfortunately, with the regular intake of refined carbohydrates, unhealthy bacteria are common. Once inside the plaque, the bacteria continue to maintain an acid environment, promoting tooth decay and demineralization.

The influence of fresh fruit on oral pH and bacterial is minimal because, with normal saliva production, the mouth is quickly cleared of these natural sugars. But with sucrose (white table sugar), which is the most common sugar consumed, and cooked starch (such as bread, pasta, and other grains), the mouth is unable to rapidly remove the residue due to the stickiness of these foods. This increases the risk for lower salivary pH.

A sufficient amount of chewing stimulates the increased production of saliva to help with the rinsing effect of the mouth and maintains a healthy pH. At the end of a meal, eating foods that raise oral pH can also help maintain the proper environment. A number of studies show that even a small serving of natural cheese works well.

Stomach

After entering the mouth, food is swallowed down a long muscular tube, the esophagus, into the stomach. The two most important aspects of digestion here are the physical mixing of food and the chemical action of hydrochloric acid, which is

PRACTICE GOOD ORAL HYGIENE

Going to see your dentist should be habit-forming. But we often leave the dentist chair armed with conflicting recommendations. A recent study published in the *International Journal of Paediatric Dentistry* found that "oral hygiene messages delivered by professional organizations showed inconsistencies and lacked scientific support." Much of this confusion is due to dental-based companies giving away free products such as that complimentary toothbrush or tube of toothpaste you receive after your visit.

The answer to dental problems is not simply brushing, using mouthwash, and flossing. Most people already do that and still have unhealthy teeth and gums.

The mouth is really no different from the rest of the body, with teeth, gums, and other living tissues relying on a healthy diet, optimal circulation, avoidance of chronic inflammation, and well-functioning immune system. So this is the place to start when it comes to the building and maintaining the best teeth and gums.

By avoiding poor health and chronic illness, you're more likely to have healthier teeth and gums. For example, more severe periodontal disease is higher in patients with heart disease.

Optimal pH is also one of the more important ways to better dental health.

Companies making unhealthy products have clearly infiltrated the dental profession, and it's often difficult to distinguish between safe recommendations and marketing hype. You should avoid toothpastes that are made with unhealthy ingredients such as fluoride, artificial sweeteners (including aspartame, saccharine, acesulfame-K, sucralose), sodium lauryl sulfate, and other artificial ingredients.

Also stay clear of mouthwashes with these and other unhealthy ingredients, including alcohol, which can dry out the mouth.

Brushing and a water pick are very effective at removing food particles and plaque, two important aspects of oral health.

Don't procrastinate either. Take care of dental problems if they develop—the sooner they are successfully treated, the better. However, finding the right dentist is equally important. When in doubt, don't hesitate to get a second opinion, especially if your dentist recommends seemingly more extreme or costly procedures.

Like other aspects of a healthy body, diet plays a key role in oral health. The single most important factor here is that by avoiding refined carbohydrates, your mouth will be significantly healthier. In fact, it's unlikely you'll have a healthy mouth long term no matter how often you brush, floss, and get cleanings and regular checkups if you continue eating refined carbohydrates.

produced in certain cells inside the stomach lining. Food is mixed with the help of three layers of smooth muscle that make up the stomach. This is the reason you may feel and hear normal noises from your gut—there's a lot of churning going on there, especially after a meal. It's much like your washing machine doing a load of clothes.

When food enters the stomach, hydrochloric acid is normally secreted and is vital to proper digestion, helping to make nutrients from foods available for absorption. This natural acid stimulates other enzymes, such as pepsin for the digestive of protein.

Hydrochloric acid helps make vitamins, minerals, and other nutrients more absorbable. It also kills bacteria, viruses, parasites, and other potentially harmful invaders that commonly enter through almost all foods. Reducing your hydrochloric acid with antacids can be detrimental for many reasons. First, protein digestion may be impaired and you may not absorb the much-needed amino acids. Undigested protein can get absorbed and trigger immune reactions, one common cause of allergies. Hydrochloric acid triggers the production of digestive enzymes in the small intestines and pancreas, which complete the digestion of protein and carbohydrate and prepare nutrients for absorption.

Taking antacids is not the only way to reduce levels of hydrochloric acid. As we age, there is often a lowering level of normal stomach acid. Excess stress can have the same effect since it typically reduces the stomach's acid, despite the common notion that stress overproduces acid—much of this myth comes from the marketing of popular antacids. Fewer people than one might think overproduce hydrochloric acid under stress. This usually happens between meals, where most have learned that eating a small amount of food reduces or eliminates the discomfort caused by too much acid.

Drinking liquids with meals may also dilute stomach acid and enzymes, resulting in less-efficient digestion. Drink all your water between meals, avoiding it about twenty minutes before and an hour or more after eating. Soda, milk, sports drinks, fruit juice, and other liquids are not part of a healthy diet and as such should be avoided. An exception to drinking liquids with meals is red or white wine, which can help digestion—not only can it relax you, it can also increase digestive enzymes. But drink in moderation.

For those with inadequate hydrochloric acid production, dietary supplements of betaine hydrochloride (a solid which turns to hydrochloric acid when swallowed) can be helpful. Common symptoms in people with low levels of normal stomach acid include belching and bloating after meals, bad breath, loss of appetite, and large amounts of foul-smelling gas. Those with reduced acid can develop abnormal fermentation in the stomach that produces other acids that are irritating, especially if they go upward into the esophagus, causing a burning feeling.

THE WONDERS OF SALIVA

Saliva more than moistens foods before swallowing. It plays an important role in the oral cavity against infections and in maintaining the overall health of the tongue, throat, and the other soft tissues in the mouth. That's because saliva has antibacterial, antifungal, and antiviral capacities—one reason why animals "lick" their wounds to help them heal faster (humans with proper oral pH can do this too). Saliva also assists in the actions of the many muscles in the mouth, including the tongue, which helps in chewing, swallowing, and speaking. (The mouth contains many muscles—there are eight within or that attach to the tongue, along with others, including the powerful jaw muscles.)

About 80 percent of the saliva stimulated throughout the day is accomplished by chewing, producing up to a quart or more, with a small amount produced during sleep. Most saliva is made in the three pairs of salivary glands—particularly in the large parotid in front of the ear and the sublingual under the tongue and the submandibular below the jaw bone. These glands also produce bicarbonate, which is how, in a healthy person, saliva maintains a relatively high pH.

Poor health can disturb the normal functioning of the nervous system, which specifically regulates salivation, often reducing its production. Those who have too little saliva are more vulnerable to oral health issues from cavities, demineralization of teeth, gingivitis, and infections from bacteria, viruses, and candida.

Xerostomia is a condition of reduced salivation—by about 50 percent—resulting in abnormal dryness of the mouth. In addition to an unhealthy body, it can be triggered by various medications, including antihistamines, antidepressants, diuretics, antihypertensives, and many others—ask your health care professional if this problem is affecting you. In addition, poor diet, dehydration, hormone imbalance, excess stress, and smoking can significantly reduce saliva production.

Low salivary production can contribute to inflammation and infection in the mouth and throat, chronic hoarseness, dry cough, and difficulty with speech. It can also reduce your sense of taste and smell, and in some cases, it is associated with reflux esophagitis, heartburn, and even constipation.

With higher levels of health, proper saliva production plays a primary role in oral health. Not only does it help rinse the mouth of food particles, control pH, and possess antiplaque and antimicrobial factors, but saliva contains important nutrients. These originate from the diet and are carried through the bloodstream to the salivary glands and are important for tooth mineralization. They include calcium, phosphates, sodium, fluoride, and protein.

A common condition called GERD—gastroesophageal reflux—has become a frequently diagnosed ailment. It is also a bonanza for drug companies. In true cases of GERD, stomach contents back up into the esophagus, causing irritation, with symptoms such as heartburn, indigestion, and discomfort occurring mostly after meals or when lying down or bending down. In severe cases, ulceration can occur in the esophagus. Most people with GERD have bloating due to gas. This often comes from eating starchy or processed carbohydrates, especially at the same time as eating dense proteins. Reducing or eliminating refined carbohydrates often eliminates the symptoms of GERD. In some individuals, eliminating lactose from dairy can do the same (lactose is a sugar that requires digestion). In other cases, poor stomach digestion, often from not enough stomach acid, causes GERD.

Small Intestine

After leaving the stomach, food passes into the small intestines for the completion of digestion and the absorption of nutrients. The small intestine, with its fingerlike projections called villi, is capable of pulling nutrients from the now-well-digested foods. Certain portions of the small intestine absorb specific nutrients as they pass. Once nutrients are made available through the action of digestion, they can now be absorbed into the bloodstream for transport to the liver and throughout the body.

While the villi are the structures that absorb nutrients, the overlapping factors of stress, poor digestion, or not eating (dieting, fasting, hospitalization) can significantly impair their function. In addition, the villi use an important amino acid, L-glutamine, as their energy source for the absorptive mechanism to function. Without adequate glutamine, absorption of nutrients can be impaired. Glutamine is a common amino acid found in meats and other proteins, but it is easily destroyed by heat (a reason to cook meat rare or medium rare, even medium-cooked meat can lose a significant amount of glutamine).

Once absorbed into the blood, nutrients are carried to the liver for processing. The liver acts like a manufacturing plant and distribution center. Some nutrients rely on others for their utilization. For example, calcium requires certain fats to be carried into bones and muscles. Other nutrients such as thiamin can go directly into cells to help generate energy.

The digestion of macronutrients—carbohydrates, fats, and proteins—into their basic respective components of glucose, small fat particles, and amino acids provides the raw materials for the body's energy needs. Once absorbed, glucose is acted upon by insulin and either used immediately for energy, stored as fat, or stored as glycogen. Fats are sent to storage until called for by the aerobic muscles for use as energy, and even amino acids are used to produce small amounts of energy.

INTESTINAL GAS

When too much gas accumulates in the intestine, it can cause more than discomfort. Pockets of gas anywhere in the gut can trigger a sympathetic nervous system response—a stress reaction. You could feel this anywhere in the gut. While small amounts are normal, larger volumes of gas are not, and usually indicate something is wrong with your diet or even the way you're eating. Here are the four most common causes of intestinal gas:

- A common cause is from eating starchy carbohydrates—bread, cereal, the many products made from wheat flour—and sugar. This includes milk sugar (lactose) from dairy products.
- Another common cause of intestinal gas is swallowing air. This occurs during eating and drinking liquids, especially water, as people tend to drink several ounces or more at one time. Drink liquids slowly to avoid swallowing air, and most importantly, keep your head more level—not tilted backward—to avoid swallowing air. In addition, chewing food and not rushing meals will help you avoid swallowing large amounts of air. Once air is swallowed, if it doesn't come back up soon as a burp, most of it must travel through the gut and come out the other end.
- Stomach dysfunction can cause of gas. This is typically due to low levels of hydrochloric acid.
- Large intestine dysfunction—often due to the wrong bacteria residing in the gut—can cause excess gas. This can also cause bad breath as some of this gas is absorbed into the blood and released through the lungs. (Some bad breath is due to local infections in the mouth.)

Other foods that promote gas include chewing gum, especially the sugar-free products containing sorbitol and other alcohol sugars. In addition, some individuals are sensitive to the natural sugar fructose found in fruits, and it is especially high in fruit juice.

Despite all their marketing hype, drugs to reduce gas simply don't work. The American College of Gastroenterology has reported, "Despite the many commercials and advertisements for medications which reduce gas pains and bloating, very few have any proven scientific value." If you have excess gas, addressing the causes as discussed here can usually significantly reduce the problem.

Large Intestine

After digestion and absorption of nutrients in the small intestines, the remainder of the food material passes into the large intestine or colon. Here, it's acted upon by healthy bacteria—microorganisms that humans have hosted for millions of years. An assortment of bacterial strains is normally present and varies with an individual's diet and lifestyle. These bacteria produce important nutrients, including vitamin K, some B vitamins, and biotin. Important end products produced by the bacteria are fatty acids, which help regulate the acid-alkaline balance in the large intestine and which in turn control the type of bacteria that thrives there. Some fatty acids also serve as an important energy source for the cells in the lower intestine. These microorganisms ferment some of the fiber from the diet, also improving the health of the intestine. Optimal large intestine function also impacts immune function.

Antibiotics, the lack of adequate dietary fiber, and excess carbohydrates are some reasons why bacteria in the large intestine change to a less friendly and often harmful type. These unhealthy bacteria and other microorganisms can produce metabolites that are absorbed into the bloodstream and can adversely affect brain and body function.

For those who have taken antibiotics, which quickly kill the natural gut bacteria, a dietary supplement containing live, freeze-dried friendly bacteria may be useful. Care must be taken when purchasing these products since many no longer contain live cultures. The best products are those that are refrigerated; contain six, eight, or more different strains of bacteria; and have bacterial counts in the billions, not millions. In addition, cultured foods, such as yogurt and kefir, may help accomplish the same task. However, avoid products containing added sugar and starch.

The bulk of the waste leaving the body is greatly influenced by gut bacteria. In some cases, up to 40 percent of waste volume can be attributed to bacteria. Reduced stool volume may be an indication of a poor microorganism population. Foul odor is another common sign. Likewise, reduction of odor and increased stool bulk would indicate an improved gut environment.

Balancing Overall Body pH

I mentioned the importance of proper pH, such as in the mouth. In fact, various areas of the gut maintain different pH values from an alkaline mouth, a high-acidic content of the stomach, a mildly alkaline small intestine, and a slightly acidic colon.

A healthy diet does more than provide you with many important nutrients. Through digestion of food, an important bodywide biochemical acid-alkaline balance occurs, which significantly helps maintain your overall health. In addition to the digestion of food affecting body pH, the kidneys play a vital role in this pH balance and require sufficient water for their action.

CONSTIPATION AND DIARRHEA

Constipation and diarrhea are two of the most common gut complaints. Most people can avoid or resolve these problems by being healthy and fit. Constipation technically refers to excess straining with bowel movements and the passage of small hard stools. It can occur when the waste (stool) moves too slowly through the lower gut. The most common causes include dehydration, changes in diet (this may occur initially, even when improving your diet), physical inactivity, and a variety of drugs. Treatment and prevention measures include sufficient water between meals, ten servings of vegetables and fruits (prunes are effective for stubborn cases, one to three per day with a large glass of water), psyllium (taken with a large glass of water), and easy physical activity (such as regular walking). In almost all cases, these habits will result in normal gut function (having at least one to three bowel movements a day). However, if more remedies are needed to treat constipation, it's best to see your doctor. The use of laxatives is usually not needed by those who follow a good diet and are healthy. The regular use of laxative can impair function of the whole gut and reduce your ability to have natural bowel movements (thereby being "addicted" to laxatives).

Diarrhea is an abnormal looseness of the stools, usually with increased frequency. Acute watery diarrhea is usually associated with some illness, accompanied by gas, cramping, and intestinal pain. When severe, it can lead to dehydration and dangerous losses of electrolytes (including sodium, potassium, calcium, and magnesium). Acute diarrhea is often caused by a viral infection and sometimes by drugs (especially antibiotics). Bacterial infections are sometimes the cause, especially when blood is present. Artificial sweeteners can also cause acute diarrhea (especially the alcohol sugars sorbitol, xylitol, and others that end in "ol"). Some people develop diarrhea under the stress of public speaking, travel, or staying away from home. These situations are usually associated with adrenal dysfunction. In addition, international travel can result in consumption of food and water containing bacteria your body is not familiar with, producing gut-related infections.

If you have serious acute diarrhea lasting more than ten days to two weeks, consider seeing your doctor as you could become depleted in electrolytes and water and there could be a more serious underlying health problem. When acute diarrhea becomes chronic, it may also be associated with more serious problems.

418

NSAIDs, antibiotics, and antacids can also cause chronic diarrhea, as can dairy foods and gluten-containing grains—especially wheat. Finding and eliminating the cause of the problem is the best remedy. In the meantime, keeping well hydrated is important; and pectin, best consumed from fresh apples or applesauce, can be effective as well.

An imbalance in the acid-alkaline state can seriously disrupt your health, not unlike too low a pH in the mouth causing tooth and gum problems or too high a pH in the stomach adversely affecting digestion.

The simple act of eating a healthy, balanced diet—as discussed throughout the first section of this book—accomplishes this pH control. The market is full of so-called miracle products that claim to fix your pH by making you alkaline, at ten times the cost of real food. But you can do it with a healthy diet without added costs.

For almost all of human existence, our diet has been slightly alkaline, which is considered to be optimal for the body's brain, muscles, and metabolism. With the agricultural revolution of the past ten thousand years came a dramatic rise in processed grain consumption, which significantly added more acid-producing foods to the diet, disturbing the delicate pH balance. Grain foods also replaced many vegetables and fruits in the diet, which were primarily those needed to maintain one's healthy alkaline state. Today, most "Westernized" diets are full of highly processed grains, especially wheat, which contribute to an over-

acid state. Excessive animal protein intake can also make the body more acidic.

Most food in the diet produces either an acid or alkaline residue. This affects the whole body via the bloodstream. Maintaining proper pH is vital because of the many systems affected by it.

The most potent foods that improve pH balance—keeping the body more alkaline—are vegetables and fruits and, to a lesser degree, nuts and seeds. The most dangerous foods are grains.

Below is a list of the key foods associated with pH balance.

Acid-producing foods, which lower pH, include the following:

- All grains, whether whole or refined
- Milk products, cheese, and all dairy
- Meats from all animals, including fish
- Eggs
- Salt

Alkaline foods, which raise pH, include the following:

- Vegetables

- Fruits
- Nuts and seeds

Fats and Legumes Are Neutral

These foods are not meant to be a list of "good" and "bad" but rather a way to relate to your diet. For example, if your meals are typically high in bread, pasta, cereal, rolls, and other grains, it can obviously be a problem for acid-alkaline balance. By eliminating refined carbohydrates and replacing them with vegetables and fruits, you'll quickly be on the way to better pH balance.

Eating too many acid-producing foods can result in a general bodywide imbalance—a state of chronic acidosis. This can cause bone and muscle problems such as fractures, osteoporosis, muscle weakness, and even muscle wasting. With aging, this increases the risk of falls, fractures, and disability and also leads to the loss of independence, all of which contribute to increased mortality rate and reduced quality of life. Many other problems can develop too, such as a kidney disease, high blood pressure, poor mineral balance (with significant loss of magnesium), asthma, cardiovascular disease, and other conditions. That is why maintaining proper pH will ensure better health and fitness in your later years.

The answer to the problem of acid-alkaline imbalance is not to create an opposite imbalance by overconsuming a high-alkaline product or eliminating all acid foods. Such is the case when high-quality animal protein is eliminated from the diet (which can actually worsen bone and muscle problems). Rather, establishing balance in the diet is a key to an optimal acid-alkaline state. It means eating sufficiently from both the healthy acid and the alkaline food groups. For many people, this means eating more fresh vegetables and fruits—ten servings a day for adults. It also means eliminating refined grain products. And this gives your kidneys an easier time at doing their job.

Kidney Control of pH

In addition to helping filter the blood and removing unwanted substances from the body through the urine, the kidneys also help maintain the correct body pH or biochemical acid-alkaline balance for your metabolism to function better.

The kidneys are bean-shaped organs, about the size of your fist, located just below the rib cage in the middle back, one on each side of the spine. Like the liver, the kidneys also filter the blood—about 200 quarts a day. From this, the kidneys filter out about two quarts or more of waste products, including extra water, which becomes urine. With rising rates of obesity and carbohydrate intolerance, there has been a dramatic increase in kidney disease.

The kidneys also produce hormones, some important ones include the following:

- EPO (erythropoietin) stimulates the bone marrow to make red blood cells.

- Rennin works with adrenal hormones to help regulate blood pressure by controlling sodium and water.

- Calcitriol continues the process of vitamin D production, which began in the skin with exposure to sunlight.

YOUR LIVELY LIVER

A healthy, fully functioning liver can make your life go much more smoothly. The largest of your internal organs, the glandlike liver is located under the front ribs on your right side. It weighs about three pounds, more in larger and less in smaller people. It performs thousands of important jobs for the body's metabolism. It maintains blood sugar during the night (by converting its stored glycogen to glucose), makes bile that's stored in the gallbladder for digestion of fats, produces most of the cholesterol in our blood (for use in cells throughout the body), and even manufactures the hormone somatomedin for building muscle and cartilage. One of the liver's most important tasks is removing toxins and waste products created naturally in your body during the course of normal metabolism and those unnatural ones taken in through food and air.

Like the kidneys, the liver also filters the blood, and by doing so, it breaks down and eliminates an untold number of chemical compounds. Some of these are normally produced within the body during metabolism while others are consumed in a healthy diet, with many more toxins in bad foods. In doing its job, the liver regulates hormones, cholesterol, fats, proteins, caffeine, sulfur (from cruciferous vegetables like broccoli and cabbage), various phytonutrients, iron, and many other compounds. Even healthy substances such as hormones and nutrients, when completing their tasks in the body, are disposed of by the liver. But if this does not happen, the continuous actions of hormones, for example, causes an imbalance—just as if there was too much production of that hormone. The brain also plays an important role in this regulation process by helping the liver decide how to regulate the breakdown of various substances.

Just as important, toxins that enter the body through food and our environment are filtered out and eliminated in the liver. These include pesticides and other toxic chemicals that find their way into our food and water, chemicals from air pollution (auto exhaust, cleaning products, perfumes, and toiletries), medications, and others. The liver accomplishes this through a complex process called detoxification. Once

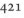

filtered, the liver disposes of all these substances, via the gallbladder, into the gut for removal from the body. Thus, optimal gut function also plays an important role in this process.

Liver Detox

To be successful with detoxification, the liver requires a variety of nutrients. Unfortunately, among the advocates of liver detox, many scams lure the public into buying their products by promising miracle cures. Most won't be as effective as eating real food because they contain synthetic vitamins and other chemicals—all of which must be broken down and eliminated by the liver. The very best way to promote healthy liver function comes from eating real food and avoiding environmental toxins as much as possible.

To obtain the many nutrients required for liver detox, focus on a regular diet full of a variety of organic, unprocessed foods—fresh vegetables and fruits, whole raw nuts and seeds, and high-quality protein (including whole eggs). Organic foods have more of these important nutrients and fewer toxins such as pesticides.

The signs and symptoms of poor liver detox may be subtle. So how do you know if your liver function needs more support? Ask yourself the following questions:

- Are you sensitive to caffeine (can consume only small amounts or none at all)?
- Are you sensitive to perfumes, paints, and other chemical smells?
- Are you sensitive to certain drugs: benzodiazepines (Valium, Ativan, Xanax), antihistimines (Benadryl, Claritin), certain antibiotics (Bactrim, erythromycin), and antifungals (Lotrimin)?
- Are you sensitive to certain foods: grapefruit, turmeric, curry, chili (capsaicin), or cloves?
- Do you eat less than two servings a day of animal protein (meat, fish, whole eggs)?
- Are you taking nonsteroidal anti-inflammatory drugs (Advil, Aleve)?
- Are you taking more than one dose of Tylenol or aspirin per week?
- Are you sensitive (even to the smell) to high-sulfur-containing foods such as egg yolks, onions, garlic, broccoli, or cabbage?
- Do you consume more than two alcoholic drinks per day?
- Do you eat less than about eight servings of vegetables and fruits per day?

If you answer yes to even one or two of these questions, it could indicate that your liver detoxification pathways are not as efficient as they should be. Liver function also slows down with age if we don't keep it going with adequate healthy food.

For ease of study, researchers and clinicians discuss liver detox as two different chemical pathways called phase I and phase II. Each is associated with specific toxins and nutrients. Through a careful evaluation of a patient, I could often determine which pathway needed more support, something difficult to do here. For simplicity, I have combined phases I and II together as one general category of liver detox. It is important to understand that too much of one nutrient may help one phase while hurting the other. This is another reason why many detox supplements can be harmful—they're too general and may not be specific for your needs. But a healthy diet will provide a natural balance of nutrients for the liver to use.

The most important compound for liver detox is a substance called glutathione. Fortunately, the body makes glutathione when we eat a variety of foods rich in specific nutrients. It's important to consume these foods regularly. Some of the key nutrients the body needs, and some foods containing them, to make glutathione include the following:

- Lipoic acid found in spinach, broccoli, peas, brussels sprouts, and many other bitter-tasting vegetables
- Sulforaphan from broccoli and kale (highest in broccoli sprouts)
- Gamma tocopherol and alpha-tocotrienol from fresh vegetables and raw nuts and seeds
- The amino acid cysteine, highest in certain animal proteins, especially whey

In addition, the process of detoxification normally produces large amounts of unstable chemicals called oxygen free radicals. A diet rich in antioxidants helps sweep up this radical "fallout" from liver detox. Potent antioxidants found in brightly colored vegetables and fruits—tomatoes, yellow summer and winter squash, cilantro, kale, carrots, melons, blueberries—include the carotenoids (lycopene, beta-carotene, zeaxanthin, lutein) and the full vitamin E complex, especially beta-, delta-, and gamma-tocopherol. Food doses of vitamin C (found in the white spongy material in red peppers and citrus and other vegetables and fruits) also work with other antioxidants.

To liven up your healthy meals, include foods rich in phytonutrients that also assist liver detox. These include citrus peel (make a citrus peel zest or a marmalade with honey), caraway seeds (grind them just before use), turmeric, ginger, garlic, and dill, just to name a few.

The liver detox pathways also require B vitamins, especially thiamin (B_1), niacin (B_3), and the folates. But avoid the synthetic forms because these have to be detoxed and eliminated through the liver too. Alcohol, in small amounts, such as red wine, may actually help liver detox. In moderation, alcohol is broken down in the liver (although the process starts in the stomach) but by a different mechanism that also requires B vitamins. But excessive alcohol taps into phase II detoxification, where it can cause significant stress.

If you have a history of liver problems, you should avoid certain foods and drugs. These include iron from dietary supplements, alcohol, and products containing acetaminophen (including Tylenol, Excedrin, and other aspirin-free products). Any drug, especially those taken by mouth (after absorption in the gut, they go directly to the liver) can be a problem. These substances can add significant chemical stress to the liver. In addition, avoid the foods that you know you're sensitive to and be especially aware of your caffeine tolerance. The liver is a powerfully amazing part of the human body—if a piece is surgically removed, it can even grow back. And many people won't get signs or symptoms that the liver isn't functioning well until a third or even half of its function is gone.

The liver makes bile to help carry toxins through the gallbladder and into the intestines for elimination. Dietary fats in the diet keep bile flowing properly, helping the liver do its job. These include olive oil, avocado, nuts and seeds, and other healthy fats and oils, including coconut. Extremely low-fat diets can reduce bile production and can be dangerous. Likewise, high-fat diets can overwork the gallbladder. (A variety of natural foods will also contain sufficient fiber to help remove the toxins from the gut.)

Improving liver function is a key to helping the entire intestine function in a normal, healthy way, especially the large intestine. The ability to detoxify many chemicals made in your body and taken in via the air, water, and food is one of the liver's important functions. This contributes significantly to improved fitness and health.

Avoid Special Detox Diets

Anyone eager to jump-start his or her way back to health and fitness might think, "Aha! Time for that two-week detoxification!" Would a juice or fasting diet be the best way to rid one's body of harmful toxins—the yucky sludge that resides deep inside the gut? Hollywood celebrities, for example, looking to lose weight before a movie often go on detox diets such as the Master Cleanse, which is a concoction of lemon juice, cayenne pepper, maple syrup, and water.

Some of these do-it-at-home detox regimens don't come cheap. The Fat Flush kit costs $112 and is made with herbs and nutrients like dandelion root, milk thistle, and Oregon grape root.

So what does the medical community think of these detox brews? Not much, actually. "It is the opinion of mainstream and state-of-the-art medicine and physiology that these [detox] claims are not only ludicrous but tantamount to fraud," Dr. Peter Pressman, an internist with the Naval Hospital in Jacksonville, Florida, told *The New York Times* in 2009. "The contents of what ends up being consumed during a 'detox' are essentially stimulants, laxatives, and diuretics. There is absolutely no scientific basis for the assertion that the regimens popularly defined as 'detox' will augment the body's own capacity for identifying and eliminating your own metabolic wastes or doing the same for environmental toxins." The fluids in your body constantly pass through the liver and kidneys; these organs serve as the primary heavy lifters when it comes to removing toxins and wastes.

Understandably, the public is always eager for a quick detox fix or the next superfood like the acai berry, whose health-curing properties have not been fully investigated. Fifty-four new food and beverage products debuted in 2008 with the word "detox" in their descriptions. Many of these fasting kits and juice regimens promote short-term weight loss because there are fewer calories being consumed, but the pounds usually return afterward. Some detoxers even believe that bowels should be irrigated several times a day and suggest colonics, enemas, and herbal laxatives to hurry things along. This practice, however, can cause long-term harm to one's gastrointestinal system.

Dr. Ronald Strum, medical director and founder of the Center for Integrative Health and Healing in Delmar, told *The New York Times* that "eating whole foods always trumps fasting or juice diets—and that education overrules everything." These whole foods include plenty of leafy green vegetables, especially spinach and kale, apples, onions, and carrots; and don't forget to drink a lot of water throughout the day, because the body needs fluid to transport toxins to the kidneys and liver for elimination.

Your body knows how to take care of itself; millions of years of evolution have seen to that. It's another reason why you need to stay away from the latest "gut-cleansing" fads or gimmicks. Just practice good nutrition instead.

425

Food Intolerance

I've discussed carbohydrate intolerance in great detail, but various other foods can also cause problems generally labeled as food intolerance. Symptoms come from various reactions in the body, although the gut is usually the main area of involvement; intestinal gas, nausea, diarrhea, and abdominal discomfort are the most common indications. More serious food intolerances can cause skin reactions such as a rash or welts; breathing difficulties such as wheezing and asthma symptoms; head and sinus problems including inflammation, runny eyes and nose, and headache; and whole body reactions such as edema (fluid retention) or even shock.

In addition to carbohydrates, including lactose (milk sugar), fructose, and the so-called sugar-free sugars sorbitol, mannitol, and xylitol, other foods can sometimes cause bad reactions. These include the following:

- Monosodium glutamate (MSG), commonly used in packed foods and in restaurants.
- Sulfites, which naturally occur in red wine, but are sometimes sprayed on vegetables and fruits (another reason to eat organic).
- Histamine-containing foods including cheese, eggplant, spinach, some fish (tuna and mackerel) and yeast
- A variety of additives and other agents used to make dietary supplements, medications, and cosmetics can also trigger reactions.

Your gut is truly a gateway to good health. By allowing it to function well—through better food choices and relaxed eating of regular meals—not only will the entire gastrointestinal track be happy, but also you'll reap untold benefits throughout your body.

CHAPTER 23

STOPPING CANCER THROUGH PREVENTION AND A HEALTHY LIFESTYLE

You may have read reports in newspapers and magazines that the war on cancer is gradually being won. Unfortunately, it's not. Each year, over a half million Americans die of cancer. The mortality rates for men have remained unchanged in recent years. Reductions in smoking as well as exposure to secondhand smoke have reduced lung cancer rates significantly, but there have been almost equal increases occurring for those of the kidney, pancreas, liver, and skin. Likewise among women, the rates for some cancers have been reduced, particularly for lung and breast (although still the most common form and cause of cancer deaths), while others are increasing, including kidney, pancreas, thyroid, white blood cells (leukemia), and skin (melanoma).

The treatment of cancer represents a huge financial strain on the health care system. The medical cost of the disease today is about $50 billion, about double that of 1987 figures. The reason for this increase is that more individuals are getting cancer, people are living longer, and more medical tests and high-tech screening procedures are employed.

The worldwide cancer epidemic is not a good picture either. The World Health Organization (WHO) estimates that by the year 2020, there will be a 50 percent increase in those diagnosed with cancer, bringing the annual number of patients to fifteen million. This does not include the significant number of those who don't have access to adequate care and never get a diagnosis of cancer. WHO also states that cancer has emerged as a major public health problem in developing countries, matching its effect in industrialized nations. But the organization also says that significant reductions could occur through a healthy diet and smoking cessation.

Just the word "cancer" strikes fear in most people. However, a better understanding of its earliest stages can help you prevent it—or more accurately slow down a process that everyone has to some degree. Putting this disease into proper perspective can help many people reduce their risk and, in fact, postpone a diagnosis of cancer in their lifetimes.

Detecting cancer in its earliest stages, then treating it through radical medical intervention such as chemotherapy, radiation, surgery, or some combination of these, has improved survival statistics of those diagnosed with cancer in recent decades. But this has done nothing to reduce actual rates at which people develop the disease.

One of the most important facts about cancer is often not emphasized: It's prevent-able through being healthy and fit. But when the term "prevention" comes up, most people, including health care professionals and those in insurance companies and government agencies, immediately think "screening" is the solution. But screening for cancer means looking for the existence of the disease—a tumor or other diagnosable form of cancer—so this concept is not one of prevention but of early detection.

Genetic factors play a role in cancer, but surprisingly, each of us also has significant control here too. Healthy dietary and environmental factors impact genes. Here's an example. Both fish oil and pectin (a fiber especially high in apples and other plants) can protect a person against colon cancer. These foods can "turn off" (called down regulation) the genetic signals that lead to cells becoming cancerous—just the opposite of what an unhealthy diet can do.

Screening and Early Detection

While early detection of cancer is important, it should not be the primary focus. Instead, the main concern should be improved lifestyle factors that prevent cancer in the first place. Going for your regular checkup for a cancer screening is akin to your doctor saying, "Tests show that you don't have cancer now, but come back next year for additional testing just to be safe."

The U.S. Preventative Services Task Force, an independent panel of medical experts in prevention and composed of primary health care providers, recommends the following cancer screenings:

- Men and women aged fifty to seventy-four years should be screened for colorectal cancer with any of the three tests—a fecal occult blood test every year, a flexible sigmoidoscopy every five years, or a colonoscopy every ten years.
- Women aged fifty to seventy-four years should be screened for breast cancer with mammography every two years.
- Women should begin screening for cervical cancer with the Pap test within three years of beginning sexual activity or at age twenty-one years (whichever comes first). Furthermore, women should be screened annually with three consecutive normal Pap tests and then at least every three years up to age sixty-four.

The Affordable Care Act (http://www. health care.gov/law/introduction/) provides insurance coverage of these recommended cancer screening tests by eliminating financial barriers such as copayments, which is an important first step to increase the number of people who can afford to receive these services.

Routine testing for disease is a hallmark of modern medicine, but it falls short of true prevention. By the time you test positive for a disease such as cancer, you've already had it for some time. For example, the diagnosis of melanoma on the skin of a fifty-year-old most likely began during childhood after a bad sunburn—the process of cancer was allowed to progress because the immune system and other natural defenses of the body were not healthy enough to slow or halt it.

Unfortunately, some screening tests themselves may pose additional serious health risks.

Potential Drawbacks to Screening

Certainly, finding cancer in its earliest stages increases the chance of a more successful treatment. But there are too many other times when the same type of evaluation can lead to unnecessary procedures, significant stress on the body, and even the increased risk of death. As an example, a suspicious growth in the lung could ultimately lead to unnecessary surgery, which may pose more risk of death than the growth itself, especially if it's benign, which is the case in most of these situations.

A hot topic of discussion is colonoscopy—a colon cancer screening procedure recommended by many health professionals and even the media and some celebrities. The colonoscopy bandwagon wants everyone to have regular colonoscopies.

Colonoscopy, like most other tests, is a valuable evaluation when matched with an individual's need. However, the risks that accompany colonoscopy are significant, a reason many health care professionals don't agree that everyone should have the procedure regularly. Perforation of the colon occurs in up to 30 of every 10,000 patients during this procedure, with death occurring in 1 in 10,000. But the mortality rate of colon cancer itself is only about 1.8 per 10,000. So the more people who undergo the procedure, the more complications can possibly ensue.

And just because a small patch of cancer cells is found in the colon or on your skin does not necessarily mean it would have quickly killed you—many people probably have cancer cells hanging around for decades but end up dying of other causes. In many cases, a better option than high-risk procedures such as surgery is to use low-risk, noninvasive screening practices such as blood, urine, and saliva tests to reveal risk factors or functional problems. There are virtually no health risks associated with these tests. By revealing imbalances that can be corrected before they become a full-blown disease, these tests are much more effective screening procedures than other high-risk invasive tests that are suited only for ruling out already-existing diseases. These might include a CBC blood test to assess both red and white blood cells and blood chemistry profiles that measure substances such as blood sugar (glucose), proteins (globulin and albumin), fats (cholesterol and triglycerides), minerals (sodium, potassium, calcium, iron), liver enzymes, vitamin D levels, and others. In addition, a simple blood test for C-reactive protein measures chronic inflammation, a precursor to diseases, including cancer. And salivary hormone tests can help reveal adrenal gland dysfunction.

If the need for testing, or additional evaluation, arises, be sure it's genuine; too many patients and doctors have the attitude that "insurance covers the cost." Matching your particular needs with a given test should be an important factor in determining to perform the test or not.

Cancer—It's Preventable

There's no question about it—most cancers are preventable. They're due to food and environmental factors, especially those associated with fat imbalance, chronic inflammation, chemical toxins, obesity, and even physical inactivity.

Your efforts are best directed at understanding how and where cancer begins, with the focus of slowing or blocking that process which occurs naturally in everyone. Fortunately, there's enough well-known information to form a logical plan for avoiding cancer by making the appropriate lifestyle changes.

Here are the four basic steps to avoiding cancer at the earliest stages:

1. The first is to avoid, as best as possible, the tidal wave of toxic chemicals in your environment. These contaminants trigger the production of oxygen free radicals in the body, which, associated with chronic inflammatory, are one of the primary causes of cancer. Environmental chemicals include the tens

of thousands of synthetic compounds used every day by unsuspecting men, women, and children. They're found in pesticides used on lawns, polishing compounds for cars, cleaning supplies for kitchen and bathroom sinks, and toiletries to make one presentable. We live in a world of harmful toxicity.

It's not possible to eliminate all these lethal chemicals because our air and water are polluted, but their presence can be significantly reduced by being healthy.

Once inside your body, many of these chemicals reside in body fat—so by reducing and maintaining body fat to healthy levels, you can eliminate their buildup in the body.

2. Another cause of cancer is chronic inflammation. Controlling it by balancing dietary fats as discussed throughout this book can significantly reduce the risk of cancer. (Toxic chemicals also can cause chronic inflammation.)

3. A common cause of cancer includes nitrogen-containing chemicals. These are often produced from foods during the cooking process such as barbecuing meat, but many foods produce these nitrogen compounds when cooked. Preventing overheating can easily be done—turning your steak every minute, avoiding very high heat, and not overcooking foods can prevent the formation of many of these chemicals.

4. The body can slow or halt the process of cancer when it has the many nutrients to accomplish the task. Eating raw fruits and vegetables is key. They also help control chronic inflammation, balance fats, and improve the immune system.

There are other triggers of cancer, ranging from household radon to synthetic hormones, found in the foods and prescription drugs (see also sidebar below on cell phone usage). But there remains the question of which came first or what part of the process do we blame. Let's look at an example of this process. Certain pesticides, commonly used throughout the United States, and chlorine, in the water supply, are two examples of chemicals that can disrupt the body's normal hormone balance. This imbalance can promote a cancer-causing process in hormone-dependent areas such as the woman's breasts and men's prostate. The most successful way to prevent these cancers is the following:

- Avoid exposure to the chemical triggers—by avoiding as much as possible pesticides and chlorinated water.
- Keeping body fat to healthy levels reduces the amounts of these chemicals in the body.
- And a nutrient-rich healthy diet encourages the slowing or stopping of the process of cancer in the breast and prostate.

431

Cell Phones and the Risk of Brain Cancer

From the earliest days of cell phone use, consumers, scientists, and health care professionals have been concerned about their harmful effects. Prolonged use is what worries everyone. Holding a phone by your ear appears innocent enough, but there's the health concern regarding long-term exposure to radio-frequency electromagnetic fields that are emitted by them.

With over five billion users worldwide, the World Health Organization (WHO) has recently classified cell phones as possible cancer-causing agents, adding them to a list that also includes lead, DDT, engine exhaust, and chloroform. The highest risk of brain tumors is found among the heaviest cell phone users.

The WHO cited a 40 percent increased risk for glioma, which is a malignant brain tumor, in the highest category of "heavy cell phone user"—those who averaged thirty minutes per day over a ten-year period.

If you rely on a cell phone to get through the day, the best recommendation is to avoid using it unless absolutely necessary and for as short a time as possible.

To further understand these ideas, it's helpful to know how cancer evolves from its onset to end-stage metastases.

Three Phases of Cancer

In most cases, regardless of what triggers cancer, there are three phases. In cancer's first initiation phase, a normal cell is changed to an altered cell through a process called mutation. Early in this first phase, free radicals can outweigh antioxidants, triggering DNA alterations. It is in this phase that a person may have the most control over the process by eating a healthy diet, avoiding toxic chemicals, and reducing chronic inflammation.

The next step is the proliferation phase, in which the cancer cells rapidly multiply, partly as a result of increased blood vessels that support such rapid cell growth. At this point, the affected area is referred to as a tumor. Free radicals and group 2 eicosanoids promote tumor growth; but antioxidants, the right balance of fats, and vitamin D, best obtained from exposed skin to sun, can impair it. In addition, carbohydrate intolerance can promote tumor growth through the action of excess insulin. Hormone imbalance can also contribute, such as when excess estrogens promote tumor growth.

These first two stages of cancer evolution are also termed precancerous or premalignant. While they are sometimes accompanied by signs or symptoms and discovered through medical tests, more often they are difficult to detect and usually go unnoticed.

Most people have these two phases going on all the time—a process that can last decades. During these two phases, your best chance to avoid cancer is through diet, nutrition, and lifestyle improvements. You have plenty of time to eat right and avoid chemical stresses if you start early.

With sufficient time in a less-than-healthy body, eventually a cancerous area enters the third step, the invasion phase. Here, tumor growth increases significantly and is typically accompanied by signs and symptoms—a growth felt under the skin, a rapidly growing ugly spot on your face, intestinal pain, or discomfort. At this point the cancer is relatively easy to diagnose. Also in this phase the cancer can metastasize—its cells can dislodge from the tumor and spread to other areas of the body. Unfortunately, this is the most common point that many people turn to nutrition for help, but it's also the phase in which this approach is least effective. Not that good nutrition can't help a person in this phase of cancer, but relative to how much benefit a person can obtain by eating well in phases 1 and 2, when the cancer can be avoided, it's the phase in which these measures have the least therapeutic value. Depending on the person, his or her overall level of health, age, and other factors, more radical therapy is usually necessary.

How Foods Can Prevent Cancer

We live in a "pill for every ill" world, and many people want to know which vitamin pill prevents cancer. But in fact, there is none. Pharmaceutical companies continue looking for this magic pill—a silver bullet to stop cancer in the early stages. If they find it, it will be something that already exists in foods that we should be eating regularly as part of a healthy diet.

Rather than any one nutrient that can be obtained from a pill, it's the combination of nutrients obtained by eating a variety of healthy foods that is by far the best protection to keep cancer from developing in the first place or slow the ongoing process. While billions of dollars are being spent on research each year to find "the cure for cancer," nature has always provided the ideal remedy. Here's just one example, which includes a group of phytonutrients called phenols. Researchers know these plant compounds have anticancer properties, probably through their antioxidant, antibacterial, anti-inflammatory actions, and have been shown to interfere with each step of carcinogenesis from initiation and proliferations to invasion.

Without question, the first place to start a cancer-prevention lifestyle is to eat a variety of vegetables and fruits. About 25 percent of those who eat the fewest fruits and vegetables have approximately double the cancer rate compared to those with the highest intake of these cancer-fighting foods. More frightening is that 80 percent of American children and adolescents, and almost 70 percent of adults, do not eat even five portions a day of these foods. The result is a significantly reduced

433

intake of key nutrients that help prevent cancer.

Key nutrients such as vitamins B_6, B_{12}, niacin and folate, vitamins C and E, and zinc, along with thousands of phytonutrients, are just some of nutrients that can prevent cancer. But don't look for the answer in the popular high-dose synthetic vitamins—they won't work like real food. In some cases, they can actually contribute to cancer promotion. As mentioned in our discussion of dietary supplements in chapter 9, common vitamin C products are one such example since these synthetic vitamins can cause the same type of DNA damage that leads to the development of cancer.

Remember that food and nutrition are not the only key factors in preventing cancer. Others include controlling certain lifestyle stresses such as smoking, poor aerobic function, high body fat, and excess hormones such as insulin and estrogens.

A Cancer-fighting Plan for Eating

A dietary plan that provides a balance of protein, carbohydrate, and fat as well as vitamins, minerals, and phytonutrients from vegetables, fruits, and other health-promoting foods can dramatically reduce the risk of cancer. It is important to obtain these nutrients from real foods or from supplements made from real foods, as it is the combined benefits of these items that reduce the risk rather than any single vitamin or mineral. So where do you begin with prevention? Here's a review:

- Consume antioxidant-rich foods. This should include ten servings of vegetables and fruits a day. Eat a rainbow variety of foods to ensure the presence of adequate micro- and phytonutrients to help control inflammation and provide antioxidants, fiber, and other anticancer substances. Regularly include cruciferous vegetables such as broccoli, cabbage, and brussels sprouts. Also choose vegetables and fruits with bright colors such as carrots, squash and tomatoes, and leafy greens for the wide range of folate compounds that are present in nature but not in synthetic-vitamin supplements. Berries and the whites of citrus are good sources of cancer-fighting natural substances too. Eat many of these foods in their raw state to avoid reducing the nutritional value.
- Include other raw antioxidant-rich foods such as almonds and cashews, sesame and flaxseeds, extra-virgin olive oil and garlic, turmeric, and ginger.
- Other foods include green and black tea and red wine as tolerated.
- Even real beef and other meats from grass-fed, organic animals contain important antioxidants.
- Consume anti-inflammatory food supplements as necessary. Most people can't get enough omega-3 fats to control inflamma-

434

tion, so a dietary supplement containing EPA from fish oil may be necessary.

- Eliminate refined carbohydrates and sugars—just one snack or meal with these foods can turn on genes that promote cancer.
- Avoid environmental chemicals at home and work. This includes chemicals from household cleaners, cosmetics and toiletries, paints, and other chemicals stored within your home.
- Control physical, chemical, and mental/emotional stress.
- Maintain proper levels of body fat.
- Maintain optimal aerobic fitness.
- Spend time in the sun!

Cancer, Vitamin D, and the Sun

Vitamin D is very important for skin health. But many people avoid the sun or use chemical sunscreens because they fear skin cancer. The use of sunscreen may actually contribute to cancer itself. The fact is, avoiding the sun, or the overuse of sunscreen, can leave you with low levels of vitamin D, putting you at risk for many types of cancer. Vitamin D can significantly help improve immune function, reduce chronic inflammation, slow the proliferation of cancer cells, and increase cancer cell death—all key aspects of cancer avoidance and prevention.

Research shows that reduced sun exposure poses a much more serious threat than skin cancer by dramatically increasing the risk of about twenty cancers, including those for breast, colon, ovarian, bladder, uterus, esophagus, and stomach. While studies show that naturally produced vitamin D from the sun protects against various cancers, vitamin D from supplements has not been shown to be as effective. This problem may partly be due to compliance (being inconsistent with taking supplements) and the fact that, in many individuals, supplementation does not raise blood levels of vitamin D sufficiently. In addition, there could be other health benefits from the sun, such as the effect on the brain.

While melanoma is the most talked-about skin cancer, it represents about 5 percent of cases, but is the most deadly form.

Melanoma

The relationship between sun exposure and melanoma is complex. Unfortunately, rather than understanding the scientific facts and the recent, up-to-date published research, many people fear the sun due to scare tactics used by companies selling sun protection products and the overall "sun is bad" campaign that's been going on for decades. Let's consider the latest objective information.

Melanoma is predominantly a cancer of pale-skinned people. Those individuals tend to burn more easily with increased sun exposure, placing them at higher risk for skin cancer. Those with naturally darker skin, and those with a recent history of moderate sun exposure and therefore more tanned, are more protected against sunburn and also have lower rates of melanoma and other cancers. There are two reasons why being tanned can help you. First, it provides great protection from overexposure, protecting the skin. Second, with all that sun, you most likely have higher levels of vitamin D, which helps the immune system protect against cancer. In fact, compared to those white-skinned individuals with moderate tans, those who are poorly tanned have three times the rate of melanoma. (Melanoma can occur in any area of the skin, not just areas of sun exposure, and can, on rare occasions, appear in the mouth or the colored part of the eye.)

While many health care organizations and government agencies promote avoidance of sun to prevent melanoma—and it's a common media mantra—studies with outdoor workers don't confirm this notion. In fact, occupational sun exposure might actually be associated with a lower risk of skin cancer. Instead of simply being exposed to sunshine, what the studies do show is that sunbathing and sunburn are both associated with the highest risk for melanoma. Overall sun exposure, including the regular sun exposure necessary to obtain and maintain a tan, is not associated with increased risk of melanoma in regions above the tropics, which includes the United States.

Perhaps the major environmental exposure associated with melanoma risk is what is called holiday sun exposure—after months of mostly indoor living, many people go on vacation in a sunny location and spend sig-

nificant time outdoors in the strong sun, often getting burned. However, those who are regularly exposed to moderate sun, including individuals venturing out in the sun mostly on weekends, are more protected against melanoma.

Despite the fact that sunburn is a major risk factor for skin cancer, significant numbers of people continue to overexpose themselves. In a study of over eight thousand people worldwide, Richard Bränström and colleagues at the Karolinska Institute, Stockholm, Sweden, found that half of the study's participants—and almost 30 percent of those with a history of melanoma—received at least one severe sunburn in the previous twelve months. Reported use of protective clothing, shading, and avoidance of midday sun exposure was more strongly related to reduced risk of sunburn than sunscreen use. (This study was published in the journal *Cancer Epidemiology, Biomarkers & Prevention*, September 2010.)

A poorly functioning immune system is associated with melanoma, like other cancers, and also a factor in the success in treating an existing melanoma. Natural (white blood) killer cells called lymphocytes are a critical component of healthy immunity. They are natural defenses against tumors and can differentiate between malignant cells and healthy ones. But in patients with melanoma, natural killer cells have poor function with impaired antitumor actions.

The immune system can be impaired by physical, chemical, and mental stresses, one being sunburned. The immune suppression associated with sunburn may be a mechanism making one at a higher risk for melanoma. Other factors that help immunity may also be important in the prevention and treatment of skin cancer, notably, the proper balance of fats to reduce the tumor-promoting eicosanoids—associated with chronic inflammation, another sunburn-related factor that raises melanoma risk—and the importance of antioxidant nutrients.

In addition to sunburn, another potent risk factor for melanoma is the presence of increased numbers of melanocytic nevi, a very common growth on the skin often referred to as a mole, birthmark, or beauty spot. These are also referred to as benign proliferations of skin cells—melanocytes. Typically, they may be the same color as the skin or darker brown, flat to dome shaped, and can appear anywhere on the skin. The average person has fifteen to twenty nevis. (Melanocytes produce a pigment called melanin that's responsible for skin and hair color. The penetration of ultraviolet rays into the skin results in the production of more melanin, darkening the skin to produce a tan.)

The presence of increased numbers of nevi raises one's risk for melanoma, with those having the highest number being five to ten times the risk as those with lower numbers. In addition, larger sizes (more than 5 millimeters in diameter) and atypical or irregular nevi can increase one's susceptibility to melanoma. The condition is now referred to as atypical mole syndrome and is more common in those regularly exposed to "holiday sun." The existence of these skin nevi, and whether they pose danger, is something a dermatologist can help identify.

Melanomas develop under what researchers called the "divergent pathway" model, two common but different ways. Most common are individuals who have a lower number of nevi, where melanomas develop only after significant sun exposure, especially a history of sunburn. These melanomas occur on exposed sites such as the head, neck, and arms (which is the same distribution pattern of other nonmelanoma skin cancers). A second pathway is found in members of the population with higher numbers of nevi. In these individuals, sun exposure is less of a factor, with the number of nevi the more important determinant of risk. The most common area of melanoma in these individuals is on the trunk.

In the most recent studies, dermatology professor Dr. Julia A. Newton-Bishop and colleagues of the Leeds Institute of Molecular Medicine, University of Leeds in England, where much of the modern melanoma studies originate, have extensively looked at the relationship between vitamin D, the sun, and melanoma. In summing up other recent work (in *Molecular Oncology*, February 3, 2011), they state, "A series of epidemiological studies have suggested that low vitamin D levels increase the risk of cancers," describing vitamin D's role in turning off cancer genes, its effect on impairing cancer proliferations and increasing apoptosis (cancer cell death). The research shows that the same benefits of the sun and vitamin D also apply to melanoma. And patients with melanoma have better therapeutic outcomes if their vitamin D levels are higher—which are also linked to be less severe, less deadly melanoma lesions—which increase their likelihood of surviving without a relapse.

How much vitamin D does the body need for these effects? These researchers state that "the data support the view that serum levels in the range 70–100 nmol/L might be a reasonable target for melanoma patients as much as for other members of the population." Many individuals have blood levels of vitamin D below the lower normal level of 50 nmol/L.

The researchers also state, "For white skinned people, there has been the view expressed that comparatively little sun exposure such as 5–15 min of exposure between 1000 and 1500 h [10:00 PM to 3:00 PM] during the spring, summer and autumn is usually enough sun exposure for individuals." But despite this seemingly short period of exposure, worldwide levels of vitamin D are frequently low in many people. In addition, the researchers state, "The high prevalence of sub-optimal levels might suggest that in real life rather than under laboratory conditions, rather more sun exposure is required. Furthermore, within white-skinned populations, somewhat surprisingly, we and others

have shown that in the very fair, vitamin D levels are actually lower than in brunettes for example, which is probably behavioral, related to the sun avoidance measures required to avoid sunburn. There may therefore be particular difficulties for fair-skinned peoples in achieving optimal vitamin D levels."

It's also possible that one's optimal levels are genetically determined. Those with an African ancestry, for example, have been shown to have lower vitamin D levels.

What does this mean for the population overall? Other studies project that Americans will experience 85,000 additional cases of all other cancers and 30,000 additional deaths in a single year that otherwise would be prevented if all residents received safe sun exposure to raise vitamin D levels. While this additional sunlight exposure would lead to 3,000 additional skin cancer deaths, it would result in 27,000 fewer cancer deaths overall. How many of these 3,000 deaths could be avoided by better health, including optimal vitamin D levels, is unknown. However, the Leeds University researchers state that increased vitamin D levels are associated with both "thinner tumors and better survival from melanoma" (thinner melanoma tumors are associated with reduced metastasis and better recovery and outcome).

While humans thrive in the sun, there are some commonsense ways to do so in a healthy manner—obtaining the cancer-protecting benefits while avoiding the risk of skin cancer.

First, avoid sunburn. This means limit exposure to the midday summer sun and avoid sunbathing.

Gradually build up your natural tan. Tanning is the body's natural defense against sunburn and skin cancer.

Be mindful of your diet, which contains nutrients to protect your skin against harmful reaction to the sun—a sort of natural, internal sunscreen that still allows you to obtain vitamin D. Certain antioxidants, phytonutrients, and oils have a profound effect on how your body reacts to sunshine. These nutrients include vitamins C and E, the carotenoids, selenium, and the phytonutrient lycopene. These nutrients will help protect not only the skin from sun damage but the eyes as well. Folate is also important since significant losses of this vitamin occur during sun exposure. (I must continue to emphasize that these same nutrients obtained from high-dose synthetic and isolated dietary supplements may not offer as much protection.)

There are also several factors to consider about dietary fats and sunshine. The most prevalent fat in the typical American diet is vegetable oil, including soy, corn, peanut, and safflower. These oils find their way into the skin and, with sun exposure, can cause excessive free radical stress—a key step in cancer formation. However, other fats have protective properties. Citrus peel oil, for example, contains limonene, a phytonutrient that has been shown to help prevent and treat skin cancer. In addition, omega-3 fats offer ultraviolet protection and can help control inflammation, which may be a trigger to skin cancer. Other phytonutrients contained in extra-virgin olive oil may also be protective—both through consumption and application to the skin.

Below are some important issues for women undergoing various treatments for breast cancer, but most of this discussion applies to almost all cancers in men, women, and children.

BREAST CANCER CONCERNS
BY CORALEE THOMPSON, MD

Two key factors for women undergoing medical treatment for breast cancer include reducing the common side effects and lowering your risk of future cancers.

All women are at risk for developing breast cancer. If a diagnosis has already been made, it's most likely you'll be undergoing one or more treatments that could include surgery, chemotherapy, hormone therapy, radiation, and biological (drug) therapy. Breast cancer therapies often come with significant side effects that can last a long time. These include nausea and other intestinal distress, hair loss, anemia, immune suppression, fatigue, skin changes, insomnia, depression and mood disorders, and others.

A variety of diet and lifestyle factors can help dramatically reduce or eliminate these signs and symptoms. In addition, recurrence of a cancer diagnosis is too common in many women, and these same diet and lifestyle factors can help reduce this risk.

Breast Cancer Risks

In recent years, the Centers for Disease Control and Prevention has finally started to move off their mainstream stance to publicize the following preventive measures for breast cancer:

- Stay physically active.
- Avoid being overweight (overfat).
- Avoid hormone replacement therapy (including oral contraceptives).
- Limit alcohol intake.

In addition to these, several other factors increase your personal risk of breast cancer:

- Aging
- Having no children or bearing children late
- No history of breast-feeding
- Early menses and/or late menopause
- Family history of breast cancer
- Rare genetic conditions and mutations
- Radiation treatment to the chest
- Having low vitamin D levels/poor sun exposure
- Reduced intake of vegetables and fruits

A Note on Genetics

While the issue of genetics often comes up whenever breast cancer is discussed, the existence of cancer genes does not mean one is powerless to fight back. Probably all women, and even men, have genes for breast cancer. This obviously does not mean one will automatically get the disease. If one's environment is not healthy—for example, improper food and nutrition, exposure to chemicals, increased stress—the breast cancer gene may be switched on, allowing the process of cancer to slowly evolve.

If you have specific cancer genes, called oncogenes, that have been identified, what you eat can turn on or turn off gene expression, even in one meal. Processed carbohydrates and sugar are the most dangerous when it comes to activating cancer genes. The HER2 oncogene (human epidermal growth factor receptor 2), which is often found in breast cancers (and those of the uterus, ovary, thyroid, and stomach and also in men with prostate cancer), can be activated by high levels of insulin (produced from eating refined carbohydrates including sugar) and suppressed by healthful fats such as those found in leafy greens and grass-fed animals.

For most women, quickly improving overall health can help combat the side effects of surgery, chemo, radiation, and other therapies and reduce the risk of a future cancer. This is best accomplished through specific lifestyle factors listed below.

Diet and Nutrition

Including at least ten plant foods in your daily diet—dark leafy greens (spinach, kale, chard, parsley, cilantro), bright orange and yellow (carrots, squash, mangos), red plants (tomatoes, ripe red peppers, grapes, radish), florets (broccoli, cauliflower), pods (green beans, peas, lentils), purple skinned (blueberries, eggplant, cabbage)—will provide you with abundant phytonutrients for many health-promoting actions that can help offset cancer therapy side effects and even reduce the ongoing process of cancer.

Use certified organic foods to avoid pesticides and other common chemicals, many of which may be carcinogenic.

It's especially important to build your immune system with foods that allow your body to make its most powerful of antioxidants, glutathione. In addition to ten servings of vegetables and fruits, eat these foods to help the body make more glutathione:

- Include cruciferous vegetables—broccoli, kale, cabbage, and others; the most potent is two-to-three-day-old broccoli sprouts (easy to grow yourself).

- Whey protein concentrate, which contains cysteine. (Avoid whey protein isolate and caseinates.) Cysteine is also important for liver detoxification of drugs and chemicals.
- Raw nuts (almonds, cashews) and raw seeds (sesame and flax), which contain tocotrienols and tocopherols.
- Organic lemon or lime skins (including the whites underneath) contain limonene, a phytonutrient that can help fight cancer cells. Consume just a small amount each day—use in cooking, salads, or just eat plain.
- Many foods and spices, for example, have powerful cell-saving properties: turmeric, cumin, ginger, garlic, chili, cinnamon, cloves, and coconut.
- Meat, eggs, and yogurt from grass-fed animals contain essential fatty acids that may enhance chemotherapy while protecting normal cells.
- The live cultures in yogurt and sour cream will help restore the loss of healthy gut bacteria.

Because digestion and intestinal function may be severely compromised, avoid foods that are difficult to digest even under normal circumstances, in particular, gluten-containing grains, especially wheat; even spelt, barley, oats, and rye are not well tolerated by many.

In addition to these specific recommendations, it's important to avoid all processed food, especially sugar, artificial additives, and preservatives. While diet and nutrition can be a complex subject, keep it simple. Eat real food in small quantities frequently throughout the day.

If you are overweight, even small amounts of weight loss can improve your surgical outcome and other therapies. Increased body fat is associated with two important issues: chronic inflammation, an important trigger for cancer, and higher levels of the hormone insulin, which stores fat and promotes inflammation. An effective way to address both problems is to eliminate all refined carbohydrates (white flour, corn and other processed products, sugar and sugar-containing foods, soft drinks, etc.). Performing the Two-Week Test (see chapter 2) previous to surgery may be the quickest way to prepare you if time is limited.

Dietary Supplements

The issue of dietary supplements is complex. Many products can be counterproductive to building health because they come with risks just like drugs. Popular supplements of vitamin E, vitamin C, and others should be avoided—instead, rely on vegetables, fruits, raw nuts, and seeds and other healthy food for these nutrients.

Consider the following dietary supplements to help counter side effects of surgery, chemo, and radiation:

- EPA from fish oil—can reduce inflammation, pain, and other common side effects of various cancer treatments.
- The amino acid L-glutamine—can help quickly restore normal intestinal function commonly impaired by cancer therapies (specifically helps absorb nutrients from food). The best dietary source of glutamine is red meat (cooked rare), and it's available in a safe dietary supplement form.
- Supplementing with extra fiber—plain, sugar-free psyllium may be best—can help prepare your intestinal tract for the traumatic stress of surgery, chemo, or other procedures associated with fasting and undernourishment.

Other Lifestyle Factors

Sleeping eight or more hours at night is a key feature for proper rest and recovery.

Check your vitamin D levels as soon as possible. Adequate vitamin D is vital for recovery, avoidance of side effect of therapy, and many studies show its importance in cancer prevention. Our primary source of vitamin D is the sun. Blood levels should be 50–80 ng/mL (or 125–200 nM/L) or higher year-round.

Reducing stress—not an easy task with a new diagnosis of breast cancer. But reducing stress in all areas of your life will help reduce the high levels of the stress hormone cortisol, which not only can contribute to chronic disease but also slow recovery. The quickest way to do this is by using the Five-Minute Power Break daily. Going for a very easy, short daily walk can also help, along with improving your heart, lung, and muscle function to enhance healing.

Treatments of Breast Cancer

Medical treatment for breast cancer is individualized. Common types of breast cancer include ductal carcinoma (the cells that line the milk ducts) and lobular carcinoma (the cells found in breast lobules). Uncommon types include inflammatory breast cancer and Paget's disease. Treatment options for these include surgery, chemotherapy and other biologics (specific types of drugs), hormonal therapy, and radiation. Various genetic markers make tailoring the right mix of therapy more specific than ever.

- *Surgery.* This may range from lumpectomy to complete mastectomy and reconstruction; preparing for surgery and recovering from it involves several important actions—all listed above. The healthier you are going into surgery, the better you'll recover.
- *Chemotherapy.* The side effects of chemotherapy are usually far worse than many surgical procedures. The drugs used in chemotherapy are designed to be toxic to cancer cells usually by inhibiting cell division or causing cell suicide (apoptosis). One major side effect is that healthy cells in the body are subject to the same toxic effects, especially those that are dividing quickly; intestinal cells, skin and hair, and blood cells, leading to side effects. High doses of some dietary supplements—typically folic acid and many forms of antioxidants—can inhibit the chemotherapy effect on the cancerous cells. It's very unlikely that eating these nutrients in real food will ever reach doses high enough to inhibit chemotherapy, and food doses of nutrients often work differently.
- *Hormonal therapy.* Also called anti-estrogen therapy and endocrine therapy, hormonal therapy has been used for over thirty years. With the discovery of estrogen-receptor positive breast cancers came agents to block estrogen's effects, including the drug tamoxifen. While blocking the effects of the woman's estrogen is important for treating estrogen-positive breast cancers, the healthy effects of estrogen in the rest of the body are also blocked. This produces common side effects such as hot flashes, vaginal changes, nausea, and reduced libido. Less common but serious side effects include blood clots and stroke, uterine cancer, and cataracts. The body's natural balance of other hormones is very important to maintain a better outcome of therapy, both short and long term. Two common hormone imbalances are elevations in cortisol (from stress) and insulin (by refined carbohydrates and sugar). Natural progesterone and fish oil are two supplements that can help reduce the unwanted side effects of hormone therapy and increase the effectiveness of tamoxifen-type drugs against breast cancer. Losing excess body fat is another way.
- *Biological therapies.* While "biological" therapies are designed to be more specific to cancer cells by working with your body's immune system, they are not without

risks. This is where understanding the genetic type of cancer can be very helpful in using targeted drugs called biological agents. The inherent risks of these "biologics" are that some cancers quickly develop resistance, which can also happen with chemotherapy. In addition, heart cells may be more susceptible to damage, and there is a slight increased risk of brain metastasis. Because of the concern of cardiac involvement, following a truly aerobic exercise routine is paramount. As for specific foods to eat (other than already mentioned), the purple pigments in plants contain flavonoids, phytonutrients that potentiate some biologics such as Herceptin.

- *Radiation.* Although the technical advances of radiation therapy allow for smaller and more targeted treatment, cells other than cancerous ones are damaged. All of the healthy lifestyle activities mentioned above will improve the recovery from radiation therapy.

Do Breast Cancer Patients Need Antidepressants?

For almost all women with a diagnosis of breast cancer, the mental and emotional stress can be significant. Whether real depression occurs in some women is a different topic and not discussed here, but the fact is that doctors often prescribe antidepressants. Reducing drugs and other chemical toxins from a woman's body is an important part of restoring health to help improve cancer treatment outcomes and avoid a future cancer diagnosis. A recent study of women whose cancer was treated with tamoxifen therapy and who were also taking the antidepressant paroxetine demonstrates the potential side effects of using these drugs: The patients increased their risk of death by 91 percent. A better understanding of breast cancer, the therapies and outcomes, diet and nutrition, and lifestyle factors, especially as they pertain to stress, is important for overall mental health.

If you are one of the many women with breast cancer, start improving your health right now. You can not only help yourself by avoiding side effects of medical treatment but also potentially prevent breast or other cancer recurrence. If you are one of many women without breast cancer, start improving your health today. You will not only help yourself through life but also potentially prevent chronic diseases such as breast and other cancers.

Understanding the power of a cancer cell is the first step in gaining control over it. This doesn't mean you will end up getting cancer. Those with a healthy immune system will be able to keep cancer cells at bay. By eating well, working out, and practicing effective stress management, you'll begin slowing or stopping the process of cancer in its earliest stages. The best treatment for cancer is preventing it altogether. It's really a lifestyle issue that often gets overlooked for years, but then when the test results come back negative, panic sets in. You don't have to wait. Take action now. The three best anticancer weapons to remember are good nutrition, regular exercise, and eliminating stress.

Sunscreen or Sunscam?

The use of sunscreen dates back at least to the ancient Greeks who used olive oil. Christopher Columbus observed natives in the New World painting their skin to protect it from the sun. In the 1930s, after getting sunburned, chemist Franz Greiter was inspired to develop one of the first commercial sunscreens. By 1962, Greiter created the "sun protection factor"—SPF—a rating of a sunscreen's ability to block the sun, which would become a worldwide standard in skin care and sunscreen products.

Studies of the relationship between cancer and the sun, and the importance of vitamin D, first occurred in 1941, in relation to death rates from breast and colon cancer. But by the post–World War II era, the sunscreen industry was about to explode, and talk about the good aspects of the sun and the importance of vitamin D to prevent cancer would be almost lost.

For decades, many people have used sunscreen with the notion that it will prevent cancer. And while many studies have attempted to show a relationship between reduced cancer rates and the use of sunscreen, they have all failed to do that. Instead, the use of sunscreen may increase your risk of cancer in three ways. First, using sunscreen gives many people the false sense that it's perfectly okay to stay in the sun for longer periods of time. Sunscreen won't block all the sun's rays, including the harmful cancer-causing UVA (ultraviolet) ray. As a result, increased exposure increases your risk of sun damage, raising cancer risks.

According to a 2011 published study of 292 national sunscreen brands and 1,700 products by the nonprofit Environmental Working Group (EWG), based in Washington DC, it found that over 50 percent of the sunscreens on the market do not provide adequate UVA protection. Many of them actually contained potentially harmful ingredients.

Second, there may be a relationship between the chemicals used in sunscreen and cancer development. Early formulations of sunscreens contained PABA (para-aminobenzoic acid) to absorb sunlight, but these sunscreens quietly disappeared from the market when it was learned that this substance causes DNA damage (which can trigger cancer). Subsequent products were found to promote free radicals, which also can contribute to cancer. The latest sunscreens contain elements such as titanium dioxide or zinc oxide to scatter or reflect sunlight, but unfortunately, these chemicals can also form free radicals on the skin; titanium dioxide has been linked to DNA damage as well.

The most popular chemical used in the majority of sunscreens since the early 1980s is oxybenzone (also called benzophenone-3). Absorption of this chemical occurs quickly through the skin, and its accumulation in the liver, heart, muscle, adrenal, and intestine has caused significant health concerns that range from allergy to hormone disturbances and breast cancer risk.

The EWG also urged sun-loving consumers to avoid retinyl palmitate, a form of synthetic vitamin A that is used in 30 percent of the sunscreens that were analyzed. In studies, this ingredient has shown higher rates of skin tumors.

Third, the proper use of sunscreen can reduce vitamin D production in the skin, and as discussed above, reduced levels of vitamin D can increase the risk of most cancers.

The next generation of sun protection products may simply be natural compounds such as antioxidants, carotenoids, flavonoids, phytonutrients, and essential fatty acids consumed through a healthy diet rather than placed on the skin. It's how the human skin has been protected for millions of years. My recommendation about sunscreen, like all other products used on your body, is this: Don't put anything on your skin you're not willing to eat (since it usually absorbs quickly into the body).

For most people with light and medium skin, reducing the risks of sunburn will significantly lower the risk of sun-related cancers. This can easily be accomplished by developing and maintaining a good tan, avoiding midday sun, especially in the summer months, and wearing protective clothing as needed, including a hat. In addition, maintaining adequate levels of vitamin D is key.

CHAPTER 24

HEALTHY HEART
Cardiovascular Disease Is Preventable

The average heart weighs just 1.2 pounds and beats 100,000 times a day and almost 40 million times a year to move 38.3 million gallons of blood during the average seventy-five-year lifetime. Now that we got those basic facts covered, here's the bad news: Heart disease is a leading cause of death in the United States and a major problem throughout the industrialized world. Chronic inflammation may be the most common precipitating factor for heart disease since there is a strong association between it and other cardiovascular problems, including sudden cardiac death, peripheral arterial disease, and stroke.

Other unhealthy lifestyle factors significantly increase the risk of heart disease. These include smoking, being overfat, and hypertension. Diabetes, an end-stage problem of carbohydrate intolerance, is a major risk element. Prolonged inactivity and no exercise also put you at nearly as great a risk for heart disease as smoking.

Heart disease is commonly known as cardiovascular disease. Both terms refer to conditions that involve narrowed or blocked blood vessels that can lead to a heart attack;

when it happens in the brain, it's called a stroke.

In the United States, heart attack and stroke accounts for more than 34 percent of all deaths each year, divided equally among men and women. Here are some other grim statistics:

- Over 80 million Americans have some form of cardiovascular disease—most are unaware of it.
- About 1.3 million Americans, equally among men and women, will have a heart attack this year, and about half will die. It will cost well over $300 billion to care for those who survive.
- About 800,000 strokes occur annually and about 150,000 of these results in death, slightly more women than men. Stroke is a leading cause of serious long-term disability, which costs about $70 billion each year.

Setting aside the rare cases of congenital cardiac conditions, almost all these heart attacks and strokes are preventable. How? Simply by following a healthy lifestyle that includes eating well and exercise.

Ask the average person, and even most physicians, what food group first comes to mind regarding cardiovascular disease, and the answer is usually fat. But despite the abundance of low-fat and low-cholesterol foods and diets, heart disease remains the most common cause of death. Researchers and mainstream medicine are quietly, and perhaps embarrassingly, moving away from the fat-and-heart disease camp.

While the four most common problems contributing to heart disease are an unhealthy diet, lack of exercise, being overweight, and smoking, there's a single factor involved in virtually all those with this condition. Chronic inflammation may be the most common cause of cardiovascular disease. If you have chronic inflammation, your risk for having a heart attack is doubled. Studies show that the more inflammation—as indicated with a simple blood test called C-reactive protein—the greater your risk of having a heart attack. Chronic inflammation is an easily preventable condition, and the food most often associated with it is refined carbohydrates.

Unhealthy conditions such as hypertension and diabetes, each a consequence of long-term carbohydrate intolerance, are traditionally seen as raising the risk for heart disease. This is due in large part to increased chronic inflammation.

Of course, other unhealthy factors coexist, which can increase the risk of cardiovascular disease. Among them is an imbalance of dietary fat, which also contributes to chronic inflammation. In other words, eating healthy foods such as olive oil, nuts and seeds, and wild fish can actually promote heart health.

Aerobic exercise is also obviously important for the heart; inactivity puts you at almost as great a risk as smoking. The heart is a muscle and, as such, requires physical activity

449

for optimal long-term function. Blood vessels also contain smooth muscle, which is "exercised" during the elevations in heart rate during regular workouts.

Cardiovascular Disease and Diet

The general public is understandably confused when it comes to the big three—cholesterol, fat, and salt—and their relationship to cardiovascular disease. Conflicting "news" articles and stories in the media do little to lessen the misunderstanding. So let's examine each of these dietary concerns.

For decades, the public was repeatedly told that cholesterol was viewed as the villainous cause of heart disease, so it stayed away from high-cholesterol foods, particularly egg yolks. Moreover, food companies began coming out with "low" or "no-cholesterol" products, ranging from TV dinners and dishes one could microwave to instant packaged food eaten out of the box or by just adding water. But by the 1970s, it was clear to me and many other clinicians around the world that cholesterol is not the culprit. Yet simple cholesterol blood tests for total cholesterol—often done inside shopping malls—frightened millions of people away from eating eggs for breakfast, despite the research showing that eating them won't raise blood cholesterol. Instead, people switched to a breakfast of processed cereal, which has been shown to contribute to the overfat epidemic and a much greater risk for heart disease.

Abnormally high levels of cholesterol can be a risk factor for heart disease, although your total cholesterol is not the best—or only—measure for heart disease risk. Many people who have heart attacks or strokes also have normal total cholesterol numbers, and many with high cholesterol never develop a cardiovascular disease.

Perhaps the greatest misconception about cholesterol is that eating foods containing it significantly raises levels in the blood. In truth, most studies have shown that eating cholesterol does not alone substantially increase blood cholesterol levels. Moreover, some studies show that not eating cholesterol can prompt your body to make more—and that eating eggs can improve your cholesterol numbers! (This is because eating egg yolks can raise the "good" HDL cholesterol, which lowers your ratio and risk.)

While there is a correlation between higher total cholesterol in the blood and incidences of heart attacks, evaluating cardiac risk calls for a complete fasting blood lipid profile that measures at least total HDL and LDL cholesterol and triglycerides.

The most important thing to know about cholesterol is that, by itself, it isn't "bad," but rather something to be kept in balance. It's also important to understand that most of the cholesterol in the bloodstream is actually made by your liver. If you eat more cholesterol, your body prompts the liver to make less of it. But if you take in less, your liver makes more.

That's why many people on a low-cholesterol diet still have high blood cholesterol levels.

Actually, all cells in the body—including those of the heart—make cholesterol every day. That's because cholesterol is necessary for many essential processes that keeps one healthy. For example, the outer surfaces of cells contain cholesterol, which helps regulate which chemicals enter and exit. And cholesterol is used to make many hormones, including sex hormones and those that control stress. Cholesterol is also a key component of the brain and nerve structure throughout the body and a key compound in the skin, allowing one to make vitamin D from the sun. As you can see, cholesterol is necessary—and good—for optimal health. It's only bad when out of balance.

The Good Cholesterol

HDL cholesterol—high-density lipoprotein—is called "good" cholesterol because it protects against disease by removing accumulated deposits of cholesterol and transporting them back to the liver for disposal (through the gut). So higher HDL numbers

---

BYPASSING BYPASS SURGERY

A healthy and fit body has arteries that are flexible, strong, and elastic. With poor health, the arteries can become stiff with buildup of plaque, which restricts blood flow to your organs, glands, and other tissues, including the heart. This process is called arteriosclerosis, or hardening of the arteries.

Atherosclerosis, a specific type of arteriosclerosis (the terms are sometimes used interchangeably), refers to the buildup of fats in and on an artery's walls—called plaque. It hardens as calcium deposits with the fat. This can restrict blood flow.

In the heart, restricted blood flow can cause reduced pumping of the heart, chest pain (called angina), and lead to death. A common treatment of this end-result problem is bypass surgery. In this procedure, narrowed, diseased arteries are replaced by vessels that are taken from other parts of the body. These and similar surgeries are performed on over a million Americans annually, with an individual cost of up to $50,000 (over $50 billion nationwide with much higher costs being incurred for long-term follow-up care).

Plaque can also burst, causing a blood clot affecting arteries elsewhere in the body, including the brain, resulting in a stroke.

Atherosclerosis, like other cardiovascular conditions, is a preventable condition—as this chapter discusses. Its risk increases with unhealthy aging, especially when other problems exist, such as high blood pressure, obesity, and smoking.

are generally healthier. It's best if you can divide your total cholesterol figure by your HDL number and get a ratio below 4:0, which is about the average risk for heart disease. Aerobic exercise, monounsaturated fats, fish oil, and moderate alcohol can increase HDL. Excess stress and anaerobic exercise, hydrogenated fats and excess consumption of saturated fats, and refined carbohydrates lower it.

More importantly, the recommendation that people substitute polyunsaturated fats for saturated can be devastating for HDL levels. If the ratio of polyunsaturated fat to saturated fat exceeds 2 (a ration of 2:1), HDL levels usually diminish, raising your cardiac risk. If your A, B, and C fats are balanced, as discussed in chapter x, you avoid disturbing this ratio. Due to the heavy marketing of poly-unsaturated oils since the 1970s, American diets now contain twice the polyunsaturated oil compared to diets of the 1950s and '60s. In addition, body fat samples today show that levels of linoleic acid (an A fat) are at twice what they were forty years ago.

The "Bad" Cholesterol

LDL cholesterol—low-density lipopro-tein—is known as the "bad" cholesterol. A recent trend in preventative medicine is to stress-lowering LDL cholesterol with drugs. But it's really not the LDL itself that causes the potential harm or risk. It's only when LDL oxidizes that it deposits in your arteries. Oxidation of LDL results from free radicals, in much the same way that iron rusts. While

lowering LDL levels can make less of it avail-able for oxidation, antioxidants from vegeta-bles and fruits can help prevent oxidation. In addition, many of the factors just mentioned that raise HDL also lower LDL, the reason these foods can significantly lower your risk of heart disease. LDL is best measured when blood is drawn after a twelve-hour fast for an accurate evaluation.

Excess dietary carbohydrates can espe-cially adversely affect LDL levels. This is due to excess triglycerides from carbohydrates producing more, smaller, dense LDL par-ticles, which are even more likely to clog arteries.

In addition, a lower intake of dietary cho-lesterol is linked to an increase of these more dangerous LDL particles. And to make mat-ters worse, these types of LDL particles are also associated with the inability to tolerate moderate to high levels of dietary carbohy-drates (i.e., insulin resistance) even in rela-tively healthy individuals.

Factors That Affect Cholesterol Ratios

One of the worst scenarios for your cho-lesterol is if the HDL is lowered and the LDL and total cholesterol are elevated. Hydroge-nated and partially hydrogenated fats (trans fat) do this, and the reason trans fat is a risk factor for heart disease. So read labels and avoid all products containing this dangerous substance.

Eating too much saturated fat can raise LDL and total cholesterol levels. An excess intake of dairy foods such as butter, cream, cheese, and milk may be the worse offender. Red meat such as beef, while it does contain saturated fat, can actually improve cholesterol levels. This is partly because, just as in eggs, about half the fat in beef is monounsaturated. Grass-fed beef has the best balance of fats compared to most beef, which is corn fed and contains higher levels of stearic acid, a saturated fatty acid that won't raise cholesterol and may actually help reduce it.

The Fiber-Cholesterol Connection

Fiber and fiberlike substances are also an important factor in decreasing total cholesterol and improving total cholesterol/HDL ratios. Most people don't eat enough fiber, especially from fresh vegetables and fruits. Eating at least one large raw salad daily in addition to other raw and cooked vegetables and one to three servings of fresh fruit or berries—totaling ten servings—will provide significant amounts of fiber. These foods also provide natural phytosterols, which help reduce cholesterol and may be the reason early humans, who ate very large amounts of saturated fat, may have been well protected.

Studies also demonstrate that more-frequent eating lowers blood cholesterol, specifically LDL cholesterol. This means eating healthy snacks.

One of my patients, Fred, had a long history of high blood cholesterol. At forty-eight years old, he was an engineer for the phone company. His blood tests revealed some interesting numbers. When he was first tested several years prior to seeing me, his total cholesterol was 288 and his HDL was 52. That's a ratio of 5:5—too high a risk factor. Fred tried lowering his dietary cholesterol for six months and then had his cholesterol tested again. This time, the total was very similar, 276, but the HDL diminished too much, down to 41. That drastically increased his risk to 6:7. His doctor recommended taking a cholesterol-lowering drug, which he did. Six months later, the tests showed his total cholesterol down to 213, along with his HDL, which decreased to 31. Now his risk was even worse, with a ratio of about 6:9. Fred was finally convinced to try another approach and stopped his medication. He started a program of easy aerobic exercise, walking each morning, lowering his carbohydrate intake, essentially eliminating all refined carbohydrates, and eating healthy fats, including eggs and olive oil. After six months, his blood test showed total cholesterol of 191, and HDL of 58, giving a much better ratio of 3:3. A year later, maintaining his healthy habits, Fred's test was even slightly better.

Eating Eggs

Most people love the taste of eggs, whether scrambled, poached, soft- or hard-boiled, or in a fancy soufflé. As I discussed in chapter 6, eggs are one of the best sources of quality protein and also contain a wide variety of other important nutrients, including choline, important to help control stress (another risk for heart disease). But egg yolks contain

453

Cholesterol-lowering Drugs and Inflammation

Studies show that some cholesterol-lowering drugs (the statins) can reduce inflammation. But considering the potential side effects of these drugs and their high cost, statins are an inefficient way to lower cardiac risk by reducing inflammation. The study found the popular drugs Pravachol, Zocor, and Lipitor significantly reduced inflammation, thereby reducing the risk of heart attack and stroke.

However, the long list of side effects for these drugs include liver damage and problems with neurological, intestinal, and muscular function, to name just some. In addition, patients must take this medication for many years and avoid alcohol. These drugs are also contraindicated for children, nursing mothers, and women of childbearing age.

The irony is that the anti-inflammatory actions of these drugs may be more important than lowering cholesterol. It's a lot less expensive and safer to use appropriate dietary and lifestyle adjustments in combination with omega-3 fat supplementation to reduce inflammation. Indeed, the American Heart Association recommends first using more conservative means before prescribing medication, including the right foods, balanced nutrition, and exercise.

cholesterol. Today, most experts agree that for most people, eating eggs every day is not going to worsen blood cholesterol. (If you're one of a very small number of people who can't metabolize cholesterol, it could be a problem. But if that's the case, most likely you already know your cholesterol is too high—above 250 or 300.)

After decades of medical research, studies have never linked egg consumption to heart disease. Stephen Kritchevsky, PhD, director of the J. Paul Sticht Center on Aging at Wake Forest University, states, "People should feel secure with the knowledge that the [medical] literature shows regular egg consumption does not have a measurable impact on heart disease risk for healthy adults. In fact, many countries with high egg consumption are notable for low rates of heart disease."

In most healthy people, the body normally compensates to keep cholesterol in balance, even when you eat whole eggs every day. In fact, as you eat more cholesterol, your body absorbs a smaller percentage.

Consider these other points about consumption of eggs and other foods high in cholesterol:

- Data from the Framingham Study revealed no relationship between cholesterol consumption and blood levels in sixteen thousand participants tracked over the course of six years.
- The fat in egg yolks is nearly a perfect balance, containing mostly monounsaturated

fats and about 36 percent saturated fat. Monounsaturated fat has been shown to raise HDL cholesterol levels. Studies published in the *New England Journal of Medicine* and the *Journal of Internal Medicine* indicate that eating whole eggs daily significantly raised the good HDL cholesterol.

- Egg yolks contain linoleic and linolenic acids, which are as important as all other vitamins and minerals and are crucial in the regulation of cholesterol. The study also showed that without these fats in your diet, your risk for heart disease is increased.

- Egg yolks are high in lecithin, which assists the action of bile from the gallbladder in regulating cholesterol. Cholesterase, an important enzyme in egg yolks, may also help control cholesterol.

With all this scientific evidence, there seems to be little logical reason to avoid eating eggs. But if that's insufficient proof for you, consider the clinical case of the Egg Man. As reported in the *New England Journal of Medicine* and on popular talk shows a number of years ago, an eighty-eight-year-old man with a documented history of eating twenty-five eggs per day was evaluated and found to be in excellent health, including normal weight and no signs, symptoms, or history of heart disease, stroke, or gallbladder problems. His serum cholesterol over the years has ranged from 150 to 200, despite the fact that he eats about 5,000 mg of cholesterol per day! He is an example of the fact that increasing cholesterol intake, even by significant amounts, may not affect serum cholesterol levels.

Will egg phobia end soon? More people are realizing that eating eggs doesn't raise their cholesterol and that consuming too many carbohydrates and trans fats can be much more of a risk factor for cardiovascular disease. For those who still want more information, visit the Egg Nutrition Center's website at www.incredibleegg.org.

Triglycerides

Another fat that's just as important to measure is the level of triglycerides in the blood. High levels can significantly increase the risk of cardiovascular disease. Some studies show that the increase in heart disease risk from elevated triglycerides may rival that of LDL cholesterol.

Triglycerides come from the conversion of carbohydrates into fat. Normally, 40 percent or more of carbohydrates are converted to fat. Some of these triglycerides end up stored as plaque on your artery walls. Many people focus on eliminating saturated fat and are unaware that eating too many carbohydrates is also associated with a higher risk for heart disease.

Triglycerides, like LDL cholesterol, must be measured in the fasting state for accuracy. Levels ideally should be under 100 mg/dl, though 150 is considered normal by most labs. If your triglyceride level is above 100, and especially 150, there's a good chance you're carbohydrate intolerant and need to cut back on eating these types of foods, especially those made with refined flour and highly processed sugars. Those with very high triglycerides often will see a dramatic reduction, sometimes to normal, after a successful Two-Week Test. (See chapter 2.)

Hypertension

One factor associated with cardiovascular disease is high blood pressure, or hypertension. It's not only a risk factor for heart disease, but overall mortality. Hypertension is generally defined as blood pressures above about 140/90 (the first number is the systolic pressure, and the second diastolic, as measured in millimeters of mercury or mm Hg).

Intense marketing of hypertension drugs, corresponding with newer definitions of hypertension, has resulted in more people being medicated and even those with normal blood pressure being told they are in a prehypertensive state. Indeed, doctors are now reading in medical journals that cardiovascular risk begins with blood pressures as low as 115/75 and that the blood pressure classification of prehypertension is a systolic pressure between 120–139 and diastolic between 80–89 mm Hg.

To make matters worse, most patients are prescribed medication for hypertension without seeking the cause of the problem. And most patients are not given appropriate diet and lifestyle guidelines that may reduce

their blood pressure to the point where medication may no longer be needed.

Among the problems that may contribute to hypertension is carbohydrate intolerance due to its influence of raising insulin levels. During the Two-Week Test it was recommended that if your blood pressure is high, have it evaluated before, during, and after the test. That's because for many people, significantly reducing refined carbohydrates and sugars, which reduces insulin levels, will lower blood pressure—often dramatically. As a result, if you're taking medication to control blood pressure, your doctor may need to reduce or even eliminate it.

The vast majority of hypertensive patients I initially saw in practice were able to reduce their blood pressure significantly just by strictly avoiding refined carbohydrates and sugars, especially when easy aerobic exercise was implemented. Most of these patients were able to eliminate their medication. Other important factors include balancing fats, various nutrients that can be obtained from a healthy diet, and controlling stress.

Poor aerobic conditioning can also contribute to hypertension. Recall that those who are inactive have a significant number of blood vessels shut down (these are the vessels in the aerobic muscle fibers). Aerobic exercise is an important factor in both prevention and treatment of hypertension. Even one easy aerobic workout can reduce blood pressure for up to twenty-four hours. Anaerobic exercise may not be nearly as effective and could even aggravate high blood pressure. It's important to discuss your particular exercise needs with a health care professional—especially one who is aware of the potential benefits of food, nutrition, and exercise.

Other dietary factors that can prevent or help hypertension include eating sufficient amounts of vegetables and fruits. When certain nutrients are low, such as calcium and vitamins A and C, the blood pressure may elevate. Basically, by increasing overall fitness and health, blood pressure can be normalized in the majority of people.

It's also important to look at the whole person, as hypertension often means other problems exist. For example, kidney problems and narrowed or clogged arteries are commonly associated with hypertension.

Sodium and BP

A common notion about high blood pressure is that sodium causes it. In some people with existing high blood pressure, too much dietary sodium—above an individual level—can magnify the problem. And that amount is very individual. About 30 to 40 percent of those with hypertension are sodium sensitive. For these individuals, even moderate amounts of sodium can increase their blood pressure further. Obviously, these patients should regulate their sodium intake, which is most easily done by avoiding packaged and processed foods and maintaining a diet high in fresh fruits and vegetables and other

natural items. But salt modification for those who have normal blood pressure is not necessary as sodium will not raise blood pressure in healthy individuals.

Sodium is a necessary nutrient, essential for good health. One-third of the body's sodium is contained in the bones, and most of the remaining two-thirds surrounds the cells throughout the rest of the body, where this mineral is a major player in their regulation. Balanced with potassium, sodium acts as an "electrochemical pump" in accomplishing this remarkable feat. Sodium also helps regulate the acid/alkaline balance, water balance, the heartbeat and other muscle contractions, sugar metabolism, and even blood-pressure balance.

In a study on salt and the heart, Jan A. Staessen, MD, PhD, and colleagues from the University of Leuven in Belgium reported in the May 4, 2011, issue of the *Journal of the American Medical Association* that higher sodium intakes did not translate into a greater risk of hypertension or cardiovascular disease. In fact, their study showed that those with lower sodium had an increased risk of cardiovascular mortality. They studied 3,681 men and women, and after about eight years, there were fifty deaths in the low-sodium group and ten deaths in the high-sodium group. The authors state, "Our current findings refute the estimates of computer models of lives saved and health care costs reduced with lower salt intake" and that they do not support the popular recommendations of a

457

HYPOTENSION—LOW BLOOD PRESSURE

Low blood pressure is called hypotension and is abnormal and unhealthy. It results in less blood getting to the heart muscle, brain, intestine, and virtually all the body's cells. Low blood pressure is considered below 90/60 mm Hg, but many individuals have signs and symptoms when systolic pressure falls under 100.

Hypotension can cause muscle weakness, sleepiness, fatigue, and dizziness and even fainting. In severe cases, low blood pressure can cause blurry vision, confusion, and be life-threatening.

Hypotension could be caused by various drugs, including alcohol, antidepressants and antianxiety medications, painkillers, and diuretics. In addition, dehydration, diabetes, certain heart problems like arrhythmias, and fainting can cause low blood pressure.

A specific type of low blood pressure is called orthostatic hypotension. It occurs following a sudden change in body position, most often from lying down to standing, although sometimes sitting up after lying down or just bending over to pick something off the floor while standing can trigger it. Symptoms include dizziness and light-headedness that usually lasts only a few seconds or minutes. Technically, orthostatic hypotension occurs with a pressure drop of 20 mm Hg or more, but many patients get symptoms with much less of a drop in blood pressure. (Postural hypotension that occurs after eating is called postprandial orthostatic hypotension.)

An imbalance in the nervous system (autonomic dysfunction) and poor adrenal function can also contribute to hypotension, especially the orthostatic type. Treatment involves finding the cause and eliminating it.

Following exercise of various intensity and duration, there is typically a normal drop in blood pressure into the lower ranges of normal. This postexercise hypotension is defined as a pressure that is lower than the pre-exercise value and can persist for minutes or hours after an exercise session. This phenomenon is one of the reasons exercise can help improve the health of those with cardiovascular disease.

generalized and indiscriminate reduction of salt intake. These so-called recommendations come from the American Heart Association and the U.S. government.

Other Nutritional Factors

When the topic of nutrition and the heart comes up, many people still think taking a vitamin E (alpha-tocopherol) sup-

Normal Blood Pressure Variations

The force of blood pushing against the walls of the arteries as the heart pumps blood creates pressure. This blood pressure is always changing. It lowers during sleep and relaxation and rises when you're awake, stressed, and excited. It even changes slightly from minute to minute to compensate with the body's need for increased or decreased blood supply. During the course of a twenty-four-hour cycle—the circadian rhythm—blood pressure is usually lowest in the early-morning hours, rises to reach a peak in mid- to late afternoon, then gradually lowers.

Normally, the systolic blood pressure range can vary 10 to 15 mm Hg while the diastolic can vary from 5 to 10.

In those with hypertension, because the blood vessels are not healthy, wider ranges of blood pressure reading most often occur. This includes the condition called "white-coat hypertension," where the stress of a visit to the doctor's office causes an elevation in blood pressure. This can result in a normal blood pressure of, say, 120/8, to jump to 136/90, leading your doctor to claim you have "prehypertension."

Blood pressure tends to rise with age because in most individuals, overall health declines with passing decades. By remaining healthy and fit, you can maintain normal pressures.

plement is a healthy habit for their heart. But research shows that the typical dose of vitamin E, 400 IU, can significantly increase the risk of death, including those who die of cardiovascular disease! Like other nutrients, food doses of vitamin E are very important for the heart (and the whole body), but as part of the whole E complex, which includes three other tocopherols and four tocotrienols.

Lower levels of certain B vitamins can significantly increase your risk of heart disease. Inadequate folic acid especially, and also vitamins B_6 and B_{12}, can elevate homocysteine levels in the blood, itself a significant risk for

heart disease. High homocysteine reflects inadequate levels of these nutrients. Folic acid may be the most important, but many people are unable to benefit from synthetic folic acid and only respond to natural versions.

Vitamin D is also important for the heart, with low levels associated with an increased risk of heart disease. The best source of vitamin D is from the sun, with fortification of foods being quite inadequate.

Other nutrients are important for optimal heart function, including vitamins B_1 (thiamin) and B_2 (riboflavin), magnesium, and many others. I could make a good argument that all the vitamins and minerals have

LOW SODIUM: A SERIOUS PROBLEM

While health care organizations such as the American Heart Association encourage low-sodium intakes, millions of people are sodium depleted. It's a serious problem that can not only reduce quality of life but also contribute to death. And it's a very common problem. The condition is called hyponatremia and is associated with sodium levels that fall below 135 mmol/liter in a simple blood test. The cause is poor sodium regulation, controlled by the hormonal system, and could be aggravated by low-sodium intake. One particular hormone condition that most often causes hyponatremia is the syndrome of inappropriate secretion of the antidiuretic hormone—SIADH. Antidiuretic hormone (ADH) is secreted by the brain's pituitary gland and regulates water and sodium as does the adrenal gland hormone aldosterone.

In the United States, three to five million people are diagnosed with hyponatremia annually. Because many individuals with this condition are without significant symptoms, there could be millions more who are undiagnosed. Signs and symptoms can include muscle dysfunction, irregular gait, impaired cognitive (brain) function, and bone loss. As a result, the risk of falls is high, and since sodium plays an important role in bone health, osteoporosis is common. Even in those with mild hyponatremia, nausea, vomiting, and abdominal pain can result.

Infections (tuberculosis, pneumonia), brain injury, cancer, and prescription medications (antidepressants, antiepileptic drugs, diuretics, certain antihistamines) are common contributors to the type of hormone imbalance leading to increased sodium loss and hyponatremia.

While hospitalized patients with hyponatremia have significantly higher rates of mortality, the increased risk of death is also high in those with mild hyponatremia who are unaware of its existence.

While many cases of hyponatremia are found in those past middle age, young, seemingly healthy individuals can acutely develop hyponatremia as well, typically from excessive consumption of water.

The overconsumption of water can worsen hyponatremia and lead to water toxicity, a condition where the body is unable to eliminate excess water through the kidneys. This disorder is sometimes found in athletes, especially marathon runners, who become overhydrated by drinking too much water and sports drinks before and during competition. The lethal combination of hyponatremia and water toxicity can even lead to death. In recent years, more than a dozen endurance athletes have died from this condition.

WHEN FIT PEOPLE HAVE HEART ATTACKS

Tragically, an undetected heart problem can sometimes lurk as a ticking time bomb even inside an athlete's body. At the 2008 U.S. Olympic marathon trials, Ryan Shay, one of America's best runners at age twenty-eight, collapsed and died about five miles into the race. New York City's chief medical examiner said that Shay's death was caused by "cardiac arrhythmia due to cardiac hypertrophy with patchy fibrosis of undetermined etiology. Natural causes."

"Natural causes"? There's nothing natural about a twenty-eight-year-old elite athlete whose heart stops in the middle of competition. Shay's irregular heartbeat stemmed from an abnormally enlarged and scarred heart.

Media coverage of athletes dying in sports as diverse as basketball, football, tri-athlon, and running is not uncommon. While we take physical injury in sports as an intrinsic part of competition, we're bewildered when a seemingly healthy and active person drops dead.

Sudden cardiac arrest, for example, is the primary cause of death in triathlon; it usually strikes during the swim. In the span of three weeks in 2008, three male tri-athletes suffered fatal attacks during the swim. Their ages were sixty, fifty-two, and thirty-two.

There have been nearly thirty deaths in triathlons since 2004 as recorded by the national governing body USA Triathlon. Close to 80 percent of these fatalities occurred during the swim. The average age of those who died was forty-three years.

And therein lies the irony: Triathlon's popularity is driven by a continuing revolving door of new participants who are eager to prove to themselves, family, friends, and work colleagues that they are fit. Yet there's something markedly wrong with this scenario. First, the meaning of health is self-limiting and wrong if one only considers fitness as its sole criterion.

Additionally, neither youth nor middle-age athleticism automatically confers health. Death comes when things go terribly wrong inside the body—what caused the heart to stop or artery to clog? Second, these occurrences are preventable. Third, it is important to differentiate between those young athletes who die in their twenties and younger and those in their thirties, forties, and older age-groups who make up the majority of competitive endurance athletes. Fourth, whenever the issue of fatality surfaces following a sudden death in a marathon or triathlon, the lifestyle habits of the person are almost never mentioned as a possible cause—especially

461

those factors that can contribute to heart disease, including diet, stress, and over-training.

In a 2011 study in the *Journal of Applied Physiology*, researchers in Britain tested national and Olympic-level endurance athletes, comparing them to both age-matched controls and younger endurance athletes. Half of the top athletes had fibrosis in their hearts—a condition of scarring that could lead to pathological changes in the heart muscle, abnormal cardiac function, and even death. Both the control group and the younger endurance athletes were without fibrosis.

A new study by Dr. Beth Parker and her colleagues from Hartford Hospital in Connecticut that was published in the *Journal of Sports Medicine* in 2011 assessed Boston Marathon runners. They compared those who traveled to the race by air (four or more hours) and those who lived within two hours of the race and traveled by car. This study showed that those who had spent more time traveling had even higher cardiovascular risk.

Studies have also demonstrated that endurance exercise can trigger the development of inflammation in the heart. Inflammation is not just a localized concern when, say, the knee gets injured. In 2010, Laval University's Dr. Eric Larose presented his frightful research findings on the topic of endurance and inflammation at the Canadian Cardiovascular Congress 2010 in Montreal. He had followed a group of twenty marathoners—fourteen men and six women, ages twenty-one to fifty-five, before and after their race. He showed that racing was associated with an inflammatory condition that raised the risk of death by a factor of seven. Most of these runners had significant inflammation that reduced heart function, with dehydration exacerbating the problem. While these runners all recovered by their three-month follow-up evaluation, this appears to be an indication that many runners have serious inflammatory problems that's due to the stress of competition.

But not all endurance athletes experience this risk. In Larose's study, just one runner did not have the inflammatory problem. The reason for this was not known, but those with a better balance of fats generally have lower risks of chronic inflammation. This appears to be the same ratio in athletes that I examined during my many years of private practice—the vast majority had some level of abnormal inflammation when they first visited me. Fortunately, most were easily able to resolve the problem by improving their health, especially as it related to dietary fats and reduction of refined carbohydrates.

462

Immune dysfunction and oxidative stress are also associated with inflammation. Diets high in vegetables and fruits provide adequate antioxidants to control these potential imbalances. Instead, many athletes regularly take supplements in hopes of making up for a poor diet.

The answer to the apparent paradox—how can athletes be fit but unhealthy?—is one of taking personal responsibility, especially considering that most ill health, including athletic deaths, are preventable. In an ideal world, it's best for athletes to take responsibility for their own health to assure they lower their risk of serious illness and death, which, not coincidentally, will also help them reach their athletic potential.

While most of the deaths in endurance sports occur in those over the age of thirty, the situation is different for younger athletes. About 30 percent of the deaths of young athletes are due to a heart condition called hypertrophic cardiomyopathy (HCM). In the United States each year, several dozen young athletes die during training or competition from this problem (with another six thousand nonathlete deaths among the more than six hundred thousand people with HCM). Prevalence of HCM is significantly higher in dark-skinned individuals and in men, although African American female athletes have a relatively high incidence. These conditions are considered congenital, acquired before birth during heart development.

About half of the young athletes who die have some other type of unhealthy heart condition, which is also preventable. This includes coronary artery abnormalities, abnormally enlarged ventricles, myocarditis (inflammation of the heart), and coronary artery disease. A smaller number, probably less than 2 percent, die from asthma, with prescription and recreational drugs representing about 1 percent of the deaths.

Accidental death of young athletes that is not associated with disease occurs in about 20 percent of cases. These are mostly due to blunt force trauma to the chest, which can immediately stop the heart. This occurs when the chest is hit by a ball or other object, or by another person, at a very precise point in the cardiac cycle. Adhering to specific rules in every sport can reduce the incidence of death by blunt force trauma.

Electrocardiograms (ECGs) are simple and inexpensive tests that can help diagnose many potentially fatal heart problems. Abnormal ECGs are present in 40 percent of trained athletes, including those without detectable disease; they are also twice as common in men and are more prevalent in endurance athletes such as runners, swimmers, and cyclists. Most cardiologists would consider these heart abnormalities related to so-called normal physiological changes due to training. However, in some highly trained athletes, irregular ECGs are identical to nonathlete patients with heart conditions such as HCM and other abnormalities. Whether these changes are due to overtraining, poor lifestyle, or are actually normal may be determined by further evaluations.

Both the International Olympic Committee (IOC) and the European Society of Cardiology (ECS) have advocated that all young competitive athletes be screened routinely and completely (including an extensive history, physical exam, and 12-lead ECG). But the latest guidelines of the American Heart Association do not make this recommendation, saying there is no law in the United States defining legal require-ments of sports governing bodies and educational institutions with regard to the screening of competitive athletes. However, in some European countries, local law requires cardiovascular screening, and physicians are considered criminally negligent if they improperly clear an athlete with an undetected cardiovascular abnormality that ultimately leads to death. These strategies have been successful, with about a 90 percent reduction in death from heart disease in competitive athletes.

Many athletes fear cardiovascular screening because if a problem is found, they can be banned from competition. Twenty-three-year-old college basketball superstar Hank Gathers died during a game in March of 1990; the cause appeared to be myo-carditis. Writing in the *New England Journal of Medicine*, Dr. Barry Morano of the Min-neapolis Heart Institute Foundation, an expert in this field, stated, "It is possible that had Gathers been withdrawn from competitive sports, his heart disease might have resolved within six to twelve months, permitting him to return safely to competi-tion."

For athletes in their midthirties or older, and at every level of sport, sudden death is primarily due to atherosclerotic coronary artery disease—also known as clogged arteries. What's so remarkable is that this preventable condition can develop through a less-than-healthy lifestyle that begins during one's childhood. Triggers include poor diet, excess stress, and overtraining.

The aging process typically causes a buildup of plaque in the blood vessels—but this too can be remedied with a healthy lifestyle. Even in those with so-called genetic predispositions, lifestyle factors can turn on or turn off the gene for heart disease.

In addition, stress in its broadest definition can be a significant contributing factor in the development of heart disease. Stress can come from an imbalanced diet, from trying to squeeze too much training into a day that is also filled with work and family obligations, and from emotional pressures, including competition.

Overtraining causes an imbalance in the brain, nervous, and hormonal systems (through increased sympathetic activity); it can increase chronic inflammation as well. Any of these problems can contribute to heart disease and increased risk of death. Stress and abnormal cardiac changes can be measured in overtrained athletes, even in the early stages. These include peripheral vascular resistance, high blood pressure, high cortisol levels, and abnormal heart rate variability.

Heart rate variability is a measurement of the time between each heartbeat while resting and provides much more information than just knowing the resting rate. The heart, in fact, speeds up when you inhale and slows down when you exhale. A healthy, well-rested body will produce a larger gap and higher HRV than a stressed-out, overtrained body. While more detailed measurements of HRV (along with other factors) is best achieved by an ECG (electrocardiogram) evaluation by a cardiologist, anyone can measure HRV at home using a simple, practical, and useful method.

A new and relatively inexpensive device called the "ithlete" is compatible with iPhones and touch-screen iPods, allowing you to record your resting heart rate for one minute using a standard chest-strap heart monitor and accurately calculate your HRV. The device provides great animation of the heart and lungs in action, graphs of your results, stores your personal information, and allows for daily testing, comparing your weekly and monthly results. As such, it warns you if HRV worsens, indicating the need for additional rest that day or an easy rather than hard workout. (For more information on HRV and the ithlete, go to www.ithlete.net.)

Overtraining in its early stage, just beyond the normal overreaching aspect of training, can produce abnormalities; ironically, this can result in short-term improvements in athletic performance. Many athletes who experience this phenomenon continue pushing themselves, mistakenly thinking their training is successful. Continuing on this path brings further ill health, including clearer indications of overtraining. For example, abnormal blood markers (such as plasma cardiac troponin T and I) have been found in triathletes and marathon runners following long races. These tests are indicative of a transient myocardial problem—a heart injury. Experts say they are still unsure about the seriousness of this problem. Immune markers are also distorted in many athletes following competition and during periods of hard training, even following a single long training session. This is associated with an increased frequency of upper respiratory illness in athletes. Some have severely compromised immune function, making them vulnerable to more serious health problems. Overtraining ultimately results in a declining performance.

The acceptance of poor health, by both athletes and even their coaches, is well documented in all sports. This has led to an epidemic of physical injuries. There is even a name for athletic cardiac changes: athlete's heart. Other overtraining outcomes have special names too and are often glorified: runner's knee, swimmer's shoulder, and runner's anemia.

a significant impact on the heart and blood vessels.

When looking at the overall picture of maintaining good heart health, it's relatively simple: Get more healthy and fit and you'll significantly lower your risk for heart disease.

Three key issues that increase the risk of heart problems include carbohydrate intolerance, chronic inflammation, and low levels of physical activity. Like most other lifestyle factors, successfully managing these is entirely under your control. Don't procrastinate either.

HEART DISEASE AND THYROID DYSFUNCTION—A FREQUENTLY MISSED CONNECTION

The thyroid gland resides in the front of the neck and produces hormones important for regulating sugar and fat burning, protein and calcium, and other metabolic functions. Thyroid hormones are closely related to the function of the heart and blood vessels, affecting oxygen uptake, blood flow, heart contractions, and even blood volume. These factors are important for a healthy cardiovascular system. So it's no surprise that in patients with heart disease, there may be an accompanying thyroid condition that compounds the problem. Typically, this is hypothyroidism, and often it's subclinical, meaning that the problem is subtle and often missed by health care professionals in their assessment. Hypothyroidism is considered by many to be a risk factor for heart disease.

In hypothyroid patients, low levels of thyroid hormones can lead to an increased level of homocysteine, high blood pressure, and elevations in both LDL and total cholesterol, all of which can raise the risk of heart disease.

An overactive thyroid—hyperthyroidism—can induce a different kind of stress on the heart and blood vessels, including a faster resting and exercise heart rate and the risk of atrial fibrillation.

Thyroid dysfunction is relatively common, more so with advancing age. Hypothyroidism occurs in about 4.6 percent of U.S. adults (4.3 percent in the subclinical form). Hyperthyroidism is present in 1.3 percent of the population (the subclinical form in 0.7 percent).

Data from the Framingham Heart Study demonstrates that some degree of hypothyroidism, as evidenced by elevated serum thyroid-stimulating hormone (TSH) levels (>5 mU/L), is present in 10.3 percent of individuals over age sixty years, with a higher prevalence in women than in men—13.6 versus 5.7 percent. (In hyperthyroidism, TSH levels are below normal.)

Those individuals being evaluated for thyroid function should be tested for TSH (also called thyrotropin), a pituitary hormone that stimulates the thyroid to produce free thyroxine (T4) and free triiodothyronine (T3), an iodine-dependent hormone. TSH may be the best single blood test for thyroid dysfunction, with T4 and T3 also easily tested in the blood (although even in under- and overactive thyroid conditions, T4 and T3 levels are sometimes within normal ranges). The results of these blood tests can help determine (or rule out) four situations: hyperthyroidism or its subclinical form and hypothyroidism or its subclinical form.

If T3 or T4 levels are high, a more clear indication of hyperthryoidism, another test should be performed, that of thyroid antibodies (which could indicate an associated autoimmune condition). In patients with hypothyroidism, low body temperature is a common sign, with under-the-tongue levels well below the normal of 98.6°F, sometimes as low as 96°F.

CHAPTER 25

HEALTHY SEX
For as Long as You Want

Humans are sexual beings. Sex is obviously how we have evolved through the process of procreation. But the pleasures of sex are also an important aspect of life and intricately related to health and fitness. Most people know this, as sex is often on their mind, although it's usually not part of normal conversation for most individuals. Instead, when discussions about sex come up, they're usually related to prevention of pregnancy or sexually transmitted diseases and the use of condoms.

Throughout my years in practice, I'd list the following question on the health survey for adult patients: "Is your sexual desire reduced or lacking?" A large number would answer yes. Based on my own assessments, very few of these patients appeared to have deep-rooted psychological problems, so that meant that their sexual apathy was related to fatigue, metabolic imbalance, stress, and other physiological factors.

Yet a positive by-product of improving one's overall well-being is a better sex life. And a better sex life also translates into better health and fitness. It's a win-win scenario.

So what do we really mean by the term "healthy sex"? At which age? Duration or frequency of intercourse? Number of children resulting from procreation? Number of sexual partners in one's lifetime? Monogamy?

Fantasy role-playing? And what about bisexuality and homosexuality?

While a healthy and fit adult human is biologically primed for regular sexual activity, studies show that majority of men and women after age twenty-nine have considerably less sex with each passing year.

The data in the chart below was compiled from individuals with "active" sex lives—surveys of those engaged in intercourse during the previous month. The published study was performed by a group of scientists at Indiana University and appeared in the *Journal of Sex Medicine* in 2010.

"People are often curious about others' sex lives," said Dr. Debby Herbenick, one author of the study. "They want to know how often men and women in different age-groups have sex, the types of sex they engage in, and whether they are enjoying it or experiencing sexual difficulties. Our data provide answers to these common sex questions."

Percent of Men and Women in Different Age-Groups Engaged in Active Sex.

AGE-GROUP	MEN	WOMEN
18–19	31%	43%
20–24	52%	62%
25–29	74%	74%
30–39	71%	64%
40–49	61%	56%
50–59	44%	40%
60–69	39%	29%
70+	28%	12%

Perhaps the two most frequent causes of reduced sex, or the lack of it, are hormonal imbalance and stress—both can adversely affect the entire sexual act from arousal through orgasm. Poor aerobic function and physical pain are also causative factors. For most people, addressing the cause of the problem is the first step to a better sex life. As health increases, more interest and opportunities for having sex and an easier ability to engage in it typically follow.

The overfat epidemic has also affected sexual habits of both men and women. In general, studies show that overweight individuals have significantly less sex.

Overall, healthy individuals not only have more sex but also better quality sexual encounters. By engaging in activities that vary their sexual positions, for example, couples can increase pleasure and chances of one or more orgasm, especially in women, and reduce or eliminate discomfort. Various positions also help stimulate the brain with more sensory experiences—including sight, scent, taste, sound, and feel—that improve the pleasures of sex. The lack of sight—closing your eyes—can also enhance the sensual pleasures of sex because, without having to devote significant energy for the brain's vast vision centers, it can *focus* more on feeling through touch and other senses. (This is why many people close their eyes during sex, but it also works with other activities such as playing or listening to music or trying to imagine something abstract.)

All these factors help individuals enjoy and desire sex, reduce inhibition associated with past sexual failures, and increase ease of orgasm, an obvious end result of sexual activity for both partners. Research shows that sex without orgasm is not only unsatisfying but, as discussed later, may even negatively affect one's health.

In 2002, the World Health Organization (WHO) described sexual health as "a state of physical, emotional, mental and social well-being related to sexuality; it is not merely the absence of disease, dysfunction or infirmity. Sexual health requires a positive and respectful approach to sexuality and sexual responses, as well as the possibility of having pleasurable and safe sexual experiences, free of coercion, discrimination and violence." While this is a safe statement on sex, I would add that people should be free to decide just how they want to enjoy the pleasures of healthy sex.

A SHORT HISTORY OF SEX STUDIES

Perhaps the first scientific survey of human sexuality was conducted by Stanford University's Dr. Clelia Duel, a physician, hygienist, and women's health advocate, who, between 1892 and 1920, interviewed women about their sexuality. This was an era when talking about sex, let alone studying it, was practically taboo. One of Duel's studies involved menstruation, gathering data from 2,000 women over 12,000 menstrual cycles.

A cultural backlash and bashfulness about sex helps explain why Duel's data was never published while she was alive. She died in 1940. But her records were later discovered in Stanford's archives in 1973. Her notes described many intimate thoughts from women, mostly born before 1870, along with sexual habits and appetites, spousal relationships, and contraception. It appeared that Victorian women weren't all that prudish. Her findings were finally published in 1980.

Another female health care professional from England, Dr. Marie Carmichael Stopes, published a best-selling book on human sexuality called *Married Love, or Love in Marriage* in 1918. It provided much-needed information about sexuality and human sexual response for a population that knew little or nothing about it. Stopes was one of the earliest writers to emphasize that women should experience sexual desire, that the sexual response of women is different from men's, and that sexual intercourse should be a source of mutual pleasure for both sexes.

Beginning in the late 1930s in the United States, Dr. Alfred Kinsey and his research team at the University of Indiana performed their groundbreaking work on human sexuality. Until this time, little was known about what men or women actually did sexually. Kinsey's team conducted thousands of interviews in the 1930s and through the 1940s, objectively examining the least studied of all human biological functions—sex. The result was the first large-scale systematic body of research of human sexual behavior, and the findings were released in 1947. The first report was limited to men, but in 1953, a separate study highlighted sexual activity in women. Both studies were later turned into national best sellers, causing public shock and widespread moral outrage. Yet an important outcome of Kinsey's research was that it replaced ignorance about sex with facts. Kinsey's work helped usher in the sexual revolution of the 1960s and the new professional field of sex therapy.

Kinsey was far from being alone in placing sex under the microscope. Beginning in 1957, William Masters and Virginia Johnson pioneered research into the nature of human sexual response and the diagnosis and treatment of sexual disorders. Their work began in the Department of Obstetrics and Gynecology at Washington University in Saint Louis, and eventually they started a not-for-profit research institution, which was eventually named the Masters and Johnson Institute. Through direct observations in the laboratory, Masters and Johnson evaluated thousands of sexual responses in men and women. Among their many findings was that women were capable of being multiorgasmic, dispelling the long-standing misconception that they were not. Their books, *Human Sexual Response* in 1966 and *Human Sexual Inadequacy* in 1979, both became national best sellers.

In 2010, Indiana University's School of Health, Physical Education, and Recreation published a mammoth-size study on human sexual behavior. Its National Survey of Sexual Health and Behavior gathered data from the sexual experiences of 5,865 adolescents and adults ages fourteen to ninety-four. It provided an updated and much-needed snapshot of contemporary Americans' sexual behaviors, including a description of more than forty combinations of sex acts that people perform during sexual events.

These studies are not done just because men and women, and adolescents, are interested and curious about personal comparisons—knowing who does what sexually and how often. But rather, the many studies performed since Duel and Kinsey's research serve a more important purpose. They have relevance for the development of sex education for all ages, reproductive health, and potential treatments for sexual disorders.

Because research shows that partners who are healthy and fit have more sexual pleasures with less complications and are sexually active well into their later years of life, these reports may also help individuals with their own personal sex strategies. For couples in their sixties, seventies, and even beyond, sex can and should be a part of their lives.

The Physiology of Sex

It's normal for virtually all healthy people to desire sex. Of course, a stimulating partner and a loving relationship is important too. When the desire for sex is significantly reduced or lacking, it usually indicates some type of physiological imbalance. In smaller numbers of both men and women, certain primary psychological problems can reduce or eliminate sexual arousal or even cause sexual aversion disorders. Some of these problems may be secondary to physiological imbalances.

In both men and women, the sex act involves many physiological processes. These include the actions of both the brain and spinal cord, with the help of neurotransmitters. Hormone activity, blood circulation, and muscle function also play key roles. Dysfunction in any of these areas can impair sexual activity and enjoyment. The result can be poor arousal, physical discomfort or pain, inability to reach orgasm, or lack of erection in men and poor vaginal lubrication in women.

Benefits of Satisfying Sex

What's the best recipe for the realization of both physiological and psychological benefits from sex? The research is clear: Of the many forms of sexual activities couples can engage in, the combination of intercourse and orgasm is the most satisfying. Of course, the many forms of foreplay leading up to intercourse and orgasm are also important and contribute greatly to the pleasures of sex.

Studies also show that certain aspects of sex are associated with reduced benefits. One example is masturbation or "solo sex," as it's sometimes referred to in the medical journals. It's common in all age-groups of people, at times more often than partnered sex. While it may be satisfying to a degree, it's less so compared to when intercourse is part of the sex act.

The use of condoms and various types of oral sex have also been surveyed. Overall, studies show these activities, including when orgasms occur, are not as satisfying, nor are they as health promoting as intercourse with orgasm. Freud claimed that condom use during intercourse, like other sexual nonintercourse activities, can have a detrimental effect that "fueled the neuroses." Current research indicates that condom users do have poorer relationship quality with their partners. Other studies show the greater physiological benefit of orgasms with intercourse versus nonintercourse and orgasms with intercourse using condoms. (Of course, factors such as pregnancy and sexually transmitted diseases must be seriously considered in the context of intercourse without condoms.)

In 2010, Dr. Stuart Brody of the School of Social Sciences, University of the West of Scotland, conducted a research review of previous medical studies that addressed health benefits from sex. He analyzed 174 of the top studies on this subject and categorized the benefits as psychological and physiological. The chart below highlights some of these rewards:

Psychological benefits include the following:

- Increased satisfaction with one's mental health
- Increased feelings of intimacy, trust, passion, and love
- Increased marital happiness
- Improved perception, identification, and expression of emotions
- Improved ability to relate intimately with the opposite sex
- Reduced feelings of depression
- Reduced suicide attempts

Physiological benefits include the following:

- Improvement of prostate health
- Reduced risk of breast cancer
- General anesthesia effects in women
- Improvement of pelvic muscle function
- Improvement in gait
- Reduced body fat
- Improved metabolism
- Balanced autonomic nervous system
- Lower mortality
- Lower blood pressure
- Improved handling of and recovery from stress
- Reduced stress hormones
- Improved hormonal balance
- Improved cardiovascular system
- Improved testosterone levels
- Reduced hot flash symptoms during menopause
- Increased levels of brain dopamine
- Longer life expectancy

Aerobic Sex: Take Your Time Because It Can Be an Ideal Workout if Done Properly

Why do couples race through sex as if it's a sprint instead of a mutually satisfying long-distance event? The average time of intercourse was looked at in a 2009 study "Canadian and American Sex Therapists' Perceptions of Normal and Abnormal Ejaculatory Latencies: How Long Should Intercourse Last?" The researchers showed that coitus

473

lasted anywhere from three to seven minutes and found that "very few people have intercourse that goes longer than 12 minutes."

But if you look at the act of making love as an aerobic workout, you can see a truer picture of what is happening with the human body. If one partner is always too tired in the evening, the problem often is aerobic deficiency. This may be caused by eating too many sweets or carbohydrate snacks in the course of the evening or throughout the day.

Suppose the unresponsive partner isn't really tired. Perhaps that's the excuse used because he or she isn't especially aroused sexually. This aspect of lovemaking is, for the most part, hormonal in nature, and sex hormones are affected by stress. Estrogen, for example, plays important roles from arousal to lubrication. Testosterone also plays a vital role in sexual desire. Excess stress, a low-fat diet, or other factors can reduce these hormones and have a devastating effect.

It is no coincidence that complaints of a lack of interest in sex often coincide with high-stress states. In many people, this "sexual deficiency" then contributes even more to the already-high stress level and prevents the person from getting a much-needed stress reduction. Sexual activity can be very therapeutic. In the course of your day and week, all kinds of stress can accumulate. That tension, the increased sympathetic activity often associated with stress, if not balanced, can be harmful. The act of making love, specifically, having an orgasm, can help eliminate that tension.

What of the complaint, often heard from women, that "he never lasts long enough"? Among the factors associated with this occurrence is a lack of stamina. This translates to endurance, or the lack of it. The inability to endure sexually is another symptom of aerobic deficiency. Correcting this often eliminates these complaints.

Another factor associated with the person who "doesn't last long enough" is that he is usually not sufficiently warmed up. Many people, more often men, choose to make lovemaking a sprint rather than an endurance activity. A slow warm-up of activity is vital to any workout, including lovemaking. In this instance, the warm-up is very important and can be accomplished with foreplay. Spending enough time warming up will allow the hormonal system to properly evoke the normal, healthy response in both partners. Without a warm-up, you may not be ready to continue effective, enjoyable sexual activity.

Cooling down is another aspect of sex too often neglected, just as in exercise; it's vital to the complete workout. Like warming up, or foreplay, cooling down is essential and should include a slow winding down, with easy, light-touch activity that produces even more feelings of relaxation. With exercise as a pattern, making love requires the same elements: a slow increase in activity, followed by the peak of the workout, and ending with a cooldown.

There are a variety of dietary and nutritional factors that can help sexual performance. No, there's no magic pill despite

474

all the ads for such gimmicks. The factors that really work happen to be the same ones that help improve overall aerobic and hormonal function as discussed throughout this book. More importantly, there are a number of factors that can have a negative impact on sexual performance—the same factors that can inhibit aerobic function.

Fertility

One aspect of sexual performance worth mentioning here is that of fertility. This problem can affect both males and females as potential parents. Women who want to conceive but are unable often suffer from a tremendous amount of stress. The first step for a woman who cannot conceive (after several months of trying) is to be sure that ovulation is taking place and that intercourse is taking place at the same time as ovulation. This can be done using a kit available from drugstores. If that doesn't result in success, make sure both partners have been examined and all physical or chemical reasons have been eliminated. If there are clear problems, your doctor will most likely have some recommended therapy. If no clear problems exist, you may be on your own again, unless you are willing to undergo more extreme hormonal therapy. This type of therapy never made sense to me for two reasons: It's not very successful, and it's relatively easy to balance the hormonal status, often resulting in conception. If the more conservative approach fails, one still has the option to try more extreme measures.

The most common cause of infertility I have seen is carbohydrate intolerance, probably by reducing the important sex hormones estrogen and progesterone. Alleviating carbohydrate intolerance through dietary changes helps remove stress from the adrenal glands, which can increase DHEA and other sex hormones. Ultimately, this improves fertility, sometimes even in the most stubborn cases. (And sometimes when conception isn't wanted—so if you're of childbearing age doing the Two-Week Test, be careful.)

In the case where fertility takes place but maintaining pregnancy is difficult, similar problems may exist. The difference is in the hormones that are most deficient. In many cases of early miscarriage, progesterone is too low. The same dietary factors may be important, but in addition, a natural preparation of progesterone may also be needed.

Sexual function is a normal, natural, and healthy aspect of human performance, one that should take place all throughout life. Imbalances in the aerobic system or the adrenal glands can adversely affect the sex hormones, resulting in sexual problems. Many common side effects of aerobic or stress-related dysfunction such as fatigue, poor circulation, or depression can adversely affect sexual performance as well.

Sex is an endurance workout, not a sprint, so perform it that way. Warm up, slowly raise your heart rate, reach the peak of the workout, and then gently cool down. (A heart monitor is not required, but it's interesting to plot a sexual workout at least once.)

475

Can Sex Kill?

A recent study published in the *Journal of the American Medical Association* in 2011 showed that engaging in sex can significantly increase the risk of death during or just afterwards. It cited evidence that the act of sex can increase the risk of a heart attack by 2.7 times. This is a dilemma because having sex is great—and it's a fitness activity that also has potent health benefits—just like good aerobic training. The problem with this study is not the study, but how the media reported it. They made it seem like sex was to blame when, in fact, it's poor health and reduced aerobic fitness.

Having sex a few times a week can actually make it a legitimate part of your aerobic training. In fact, regular sexual activity can reduce the risk of death from a heart attack during or after sex. That's because, as the fine print of the study showed, those who are physically active don't have the high level of health risk as those who are inactive. And should these two sexually active individuals eat well and manage stress, their risks of death during sex would be further significantly lowered—more than inactive people.

Unfortunately, most major newspaper headlines read, "Yes, Sex Can Kill You, U.S. Study Shows." That's sufficient-enough misinformation to create additional mental and emotional stress (which becomes another risk factor) in some people having sex, which could actually further increase their chances of death even more. Another disservice is what the media reports don't say, sex doesn't kill, poor health does when triggered by any kind of exertion, whether it's sex, sprinting to get out of the rain, or climbing several flights of stairs.

Sex Biofeedback for Men and Women

Born in 1894, Dr. Arnold H. Kegel was an assistant professor of gynecology at the University of Southern California School of Medicine who later invented a series of exercises to help strengthen muscles of the lower pelvic region as a nonsurgical treatment of genital relaxation. Kegel first published his ideas in 1948. Today, Kegel exercises are commonly used as an early treatment for urinary stress incontinence and female genital prolapse, when a portion of the vaginal canal protrudes from the opening of the vagina. (The condition usually occurs when the pelvic floor collapses as a result of childbirth.)

Kegel exercises are really a form of biofeedback by helping to improve the function of the muscles that make up the bottom of the pelvis, often called pelvic floor muscles. They help support the bladder, lower intestine, and uterus. For men and women who have sexual dysfunction, these muscles may not work well, but improving their actions can increase sexual pleasure. For women, the exercises can help improve having an orgasm, and in men, it makes it easier to delay ejaculation. In fact, erectile dysfunction (ED) can be successfully

476

treated with Kegel exercises; it can also be more effective than taking Viagra.

The first step in using Kegel exercises is to feel the pelvic muscles contract. This can be accomplished while you're urinating. Squeeze your pelvic floor muscles to stop the flow of urine. Once you're able to accomplish this, perform it each time you urinate—stop the flow of urine for five to ten seconds and then release it. Another option is to contract the muscle when not urinating—just think about relaxing your pelvis as if you are urinating, then tighten the muscles to hold it for five to ten seconds. Perform these with the rest of your body relaxed, about five to ten times each day. Once you're able to contract these muscles, they will start functioning better. After a few weeks, improved pelvic floor muscles will be more evident because you'll easily be able to stop your urine flow at any time—and sexual function may improve.

For women who have a difficult time contracting these pelvic muscles, it's often recommended to insert a finger into the vagina and attempt to contract—trying to squeeze the surrounding muscles. You should feel your vagina tighten and your pelvic floor move upward.

For men and women, contracting the pelvic floor muscles during sex can be an additional pleasure. Have fun and experiment. Give it a try—it just might increase the quality, and quantity, of your sexual experience.

If you're unable to successfully contract the pelvic muscles or are not sure what to do, seek help from a reliable health care practitioner.

Female Infertility: It's Often Due to an Unhealthy Diet

In the early 1980s, while in private practice, it became evident that in the course of helping patients lose weight with my newly developed Two-Week Test, some women previously unable to conceive did just that. At first it appeared that, with better overall health, fertility improved in a small number of women. But it became apparent that by reducing high insulin levels, a balance of many hormones occurred, significantly increasing fertility. My first step was to add additional instructions to the test's list of dos and don'ts. In particular, that fertility may increase in women of childbearing age. While the Two-Week Test is a way to jump-start a patient's metabolism to help increase fat burning and weight loss and can help improve many other problems because high insulin levels are reduced through a reduction of high-glycemic refined carbohydrates, it's also an effective way to balance sex hormones. One problem in many women who can't easily conceive is hormone imbalance, which significantly influences ovulation. The Two-Week Test quickly became a very successful way to help many women conceive who could not do so through other means and who wanted to avoid using drugs. Ellen was one such patient.

477

Coming to my clinic at age thirty-nine, Ellen's main complaint was back pain and fatigue. During my assessment, it was evident that for the past ten years, many diet programs failed to help her lose those extra fifteen to twenty pounds. Ellen and her husband tried unsuccessfully to have children throughout their marriage of fifteen years, consulting a variety of specialists. They remained sexually active and hoped for the best, deciding to avoid the medical industry's high-tech procedures and fertility drugs, which not only had potentially serious side effects but were also only about 25 percent successful and whose high cost they could not afford.

It was clear to me that Ellen was carbohydrate intolerant, and this would be the first therapeutic recommendation to help improve her overall health. On her next office visit after two weeks, Ellen had lost seven pounds, had greatly improved energy, and her back pain was 75 percent better. I saw Ellen six weeks after that visit, and in addition to feeling great, she happily reported being pregnant. By this point, she had lost another five pounds, had high energy, and no back pain. Ellen would eventually have a problem-free pregnancy, delivering a healthy baby girl.

Several weeks after Ellen told me she had conceived, another patient who had recently had success with the Two-Week Test, Sally, age thirty-one, also reported being pregnant after several years of infertility and seeing specialists. In the next couple of weeks, I had two new patients referred by Ellen, and soon afterwards, one from Sally, all of whom were trying to conceive but could not. A year later, my small group of once-infertile patients all had healthy babies, and several others had conceived after long periods of infertility. Ellen conceived again when her little girl was about two years old and eventually had a healthy baby boy.

I searched through the medical literature for connections between diet and fertility. There was nothing of significance. While many millions of dollars are spent researching fertility drugs and procedures, there was essentially none spent on the relationships between diet and fertility.

As the years passed and more female patients were helped with their infertility, small published studies began to show what was clinically evident: that reducing high insulin levels through dietary changes could improve hormone balance and help some women who previously could not conceive and get pregnant. Eventually, the Nurses' Health Study, which began in 1989 and relied on 116,000 women, was conducted by Dr. Walter Willett of the Harvard School of Public Health. Many of these women had a common type of reproductive problem (ovulation and the hormonal problems associated with maturation of the egg) and would become pregnant through changes in diet—in particular by eliminating refined carbohydrates, including sugar. Dr. Willett, along with coresearcher Dr. Jorge Chavarro, wrote a book on the subject in 2007 called *The Fer-*

tility Diet. Their primary recommendations included avoiding refined carbohydrates and trans fats, and regular exercise. Losing weight, eating plenty of vegetables and fruits, and increased water intake were also key recommendations.

This should be great news for the millions of women who are infertile. A relatively simple change in diet could significantly improve fertility and reduce body fat for a more successful and healthy pregnancy and a healthier baby. While I'm not a fertility specialist, this appears to be one of the most common causes of infertility because it produces an imbalance in the important sex hormones estrogen and progesterone. Alleviating carbohydrate intolerance through dietary changes helps remove metabolic stress and improve hormone balance. Ultimately, this improves fertility, sometimes even in the most stubborn cases.

More Causes of Infertility for Both Women and Men

There are many reasons why couples can't conceive, with potential problems in either partner. Here are some statistics:

- About 30 to 40 percent of the time, the cause is due to problems in both male and female.
- In about 20 percent of cases, infertility is due to a cause involving only the male partner.

- And in 40 to 50 percent of cases, infertility is due entirely to a cause involving the female.

In couples unable to conceive, physical causes of infertility should be first ruled out. These may include fallopian tube damage or blockage and endometriosis in women and blocked ducts or low-sperm production in men. In addition, poor health can contribute—this can include many diseases such as diabetes and thyroid over- or underactivity as well as unhealthy habits like tobacco use, prescription and recreational drugs (such as cocaine), and excess alcohol and caffeine. Genetic disorders can also occur and are less common causes of fertility.

The most common cause of male infertility has to do with his sperm. This includes abnormally low sperm production, reduced function (such as poor sperm size or motility), or both. This can be caused by hormone imbalance, with low testosterone being a frequent problem. Environmental toxins can also contribute to infertility in men, including pesticides, herbicides, and others like BPA. These toxins can enter the body through air, water, and food.

In a recent study (*International Journal of Andrology*, March 2011), researchers in Finland demonstrated a trend toward lower sperm production in Finnish men, who normally have very high sperm counts. Even more concerning was that, as sperm counts went

479

down, rates of testicular cancer increased. The authors concluded, "These simultaneous and rapidly occurring adverse trends suggest that the underlying causes are environmental and, as such, preventable."

In addition to the accumulation of toxins, overheating the testicles in a hot tub or sauna before intercourse can reduce sperm counts and also impairs their function, diminishing the chances of conception.

In women, hormone imbalance may be the most common cause of infertility. The glands involved may be the pituitary, adrenals, ovaries, or thyroid or combinations of these. Because the liver indirectly regulates many hormones, dysfunction here can also be a factor.

The first step for a woman who cannot conceive is to be sure that ovulation is taking place and that intercourse occurs at this time. Ovulation can be measured using a kit available from drugstores. If ovulation and intercourse normally take place but conception does not occur after a few months of trying, both partners should be examined and all physical or chemical reasons should be eliminated.

Unfortunately, for many couples who are unable to conceive, ovulation and intercourse appear to be in sync, but no other fertility problems can be found. This is the point when referral to a fertility clinic is typically made— but it should be a time to carefully look at overall health and fitness. In fact, this should be done before a couple attempts to conceive. If these more conservative approaches of improving overall health do not result in conception, couples still have the option to try more extreme measures should they choose.

Erectile Dysfunction

Erectile dysfunction, or ED, is defined as a male difficulty in initiating or maintaining penile erection adequate for sexual relations. ED may be present in up to half of the male population over the age of forty years, affecting an estimated 150 million individuals worldwide.

While the inability for a man to have sex can be emotionally and morally devastating, ED is usually an indication that more serious health problems exist. Two common primary conditions are carbohydrate intolerance and chronic inflammation, with other secondary problems developing. These include hypertension, diabetes, obesity, cardiovascular disease, sleep apnea, and both over- and under-active thyroid conditions.

Clusters of signs and symptoms often include ED. A common example is that ED is frequently associated with both depression and heart disease.

ED is specifically associated with diminished blood flow (poor circulation)—not just into the penis but also elsewhere throughout the body, including the heart. An early sign of heart problems, as an example, is a reduction in penile hardness. Some men experience ED for several years prior to a first heart attack. Often, the reduction in blood flow—to the penis, heart, or brain—is due to chronic narrowing of the arteries from calcium or choles-terol deposits.

Separately, various types of drugs can contribute to ED. Alcohol abuse, illicit drug use, and prescription drugs such as beta-blockers, ACE inhibitors, diuretics, and anti-depressants may contribute to or cause the condition. In fact, up to 25 percent of newly diagnosed ED may be due to side effects of prescription drugs.

The inability to achieve penile erection can involve a combination of factors. These can be mental/emotional (such as depression or anxiety), neurological (autonomic imbal-ance), hormonal (adrenal and sex hormones, especially testosterone), and vascular (blood circulation). Any or all of these problems can stem from aerobic deficiency, poor stress reg-ulation, and improper diet.

Nutritional factors can directly contribute to ED, especially oxidative stress, which relies on dietary antioxidants. Balancing fats is also important as those with ED often have low levels of the 1 series eicosanoids (derived from A fats).

For most men, treating ED with a pre-scription drug is clearly not addressing the cause of the problem. Despite the multimil-lion-dollar ad campaigns, there is no magic pill for all patients with ED. The main ingre-dient in many of these ED drugs is sildenafil citrate—sold as Viagra, Revatio, and under

"NATURAL" MALE ENHANCEMENT PRODUCT SCAMS

As the problem of ED grows and prescription drug advertising continues to make men and women more aware of the disorder, many smaller companies have provided consumers with over-the-counter, and often online, products that claim to enhance sexual activity and performance. But most don't. Some of the products even appear in drugstores, making them seem more credible. These include nonprescription supplements such as herbal preparations, so-called natural alternatives, and similar products.

An example is a product that mimics Viagra (chemical name, sildenafil). An over-the-counter product, Best Enhancer, recently appeared whose ingredients included sulfoaildenafil—a similar chemical that could have life-threatening side effects. The unapproved drug was not even listed on the label, a reason why this illegal product was eventually recalled by the FDA.

The FDA's website on safety information and adverse drug effects, MedWatch, is www.fda.gov/Safety/MedWatch.

So stay away from all "male enhancement" products. In fact, they can lead to reduced fertility, lower sperm counts, and prostate problems.

various other trade names. But these drugs are not effective in all cases, including those with circulatory problems.

Sildenafil is not a magic bullet—a man must be sexually aroused for it to work. And this medication is ineffective unless taken on an empty stomach at least one hour before sexual activity. So this drug is not a treatment for low libido.

Reduced libido is not uncommon, often worsening with age. The use of testosterone replacement therapy is sometimes recommended for both men and women (this hormone is also important in women's libido). But this must be prescribed based on a proper evaluation, including a blood test that demonstrates low levels of testosterone and not just on the symptom of low libido.

Below are some common symptoms associated with abnormally low levels of testosterone in men:

- Decreased frequency of morning erection
- Decreased frequency of sexual thoughts

- Erectile dysfunction
- An inability to engage in physical activity such as walking or running for exercise or lifting heavy objects
- The inability to bend, kneel, or stoop during a typical day
- Sadness
- Fatigue

The incidence of ED is growing—not just because of an aging population but in younger men as well. Those who are healthy and fit generally don't have ED.

Sexual activity should be a normal, natural, and healthy part of your life. If sexual desire or performance begins to falter, don't panic or seek an answer in a pill. Imbalances in various systems—aerobic, hormonal, nervous, and muscular—can result in sexual dysfunction, including infertility or impotence. The wonderful thing about the pleasures of sex is that it actually enhances optimal health and fitness.

A WOMAN'S PERSPECTIVE

Sex. It would not be the same without a women's perspective. So I asked Dr. Coralee Thompson to contribute to this chapter. Below are her comments on particular items important for healthy sex.

- *Passion.* It builds the foundation for truly satisfying sex. While a couple may have disagreements from time to time, frequent arguing accompanied by anger and hurt chips away at passion and intimacy. Foreplay really does include the day-today actions of endearment and passion. Lovemaking begins in the morning with your first hello. The worst sex buster is to lose mutual tenderness. You've heard the saying it takes two to tango, so find your best-matched mate and dance regularly.

- *Stimulation.* It's simple. Take the time to stimulate your partner well and know where and how you like to be stimulated. Let that progress through the years. Normally, the type and degree of stimulation may vary through the relationship. In the beginning of a relationship, a simple touch can produce excitement and sexual arousal. If this electrical jolt from only a touch wanes, it doesn't mean that your sexual desire wanes. Be alert to what feels good and be willing to ask for it. Be aware and sensitive as to what makes your partner feel good and be willing to give it.

- *Lubrication.* It's a vital ingredient to great sex, though it may increase or decrease through a woman's life. Healthy vaginal secretions are triggered by arousal and hormonal balance. When everything seems right, but the vagina doesn't moisten normally, saliva is the next best thing. Avoid using lubricants that have chemicals or fragrances. There's no need to apply oil directly to the vagina, but warmed coconut oil works great for stimulating the penis, breasts, and other sensitive areas.

- *Sex during pregnancy.* This can add a new level of sexual pleasure that most women may not know. The uterine contractions during orgasm are not only good for preparing the uterus for labor but are also intensely pleasurable. (Of course, if the pregnancy is not stable, sex is not recommended.) Finding the most comfortable position is important. If intercourse is not comfortable, a combination of masturbation and partner stimulation may be best. As long as the pregnancy is going well, and the bag of water (the amniotic sac) is intact, sex is possible up to the point of labor. In fact, it can be a great way to naturally and safely induce labor at the right time.

- *Sex after pregnancy.* This is a much more delicate time. The vagina and uterus require a certain amount of healing. This may range from a few days to a couple of weeks for a healthy woman before intercourse begins again. But orgasms without intercourse may help the uterus heal more quickly. Nipple stimulation is particularly enjoyable and effective during this time since oxytocin is readily released during orgasm as it is during breast-feeding.

- *Sex during the perimenopausal years.* This offers yet another dimension of sexual pleasure and challenges. Taking time to get aroused and well lubricated is vital to full sexual enjoyment. Nipple stimulation may be even more important later in life than ever before. Including other areas of stimulation that promote the parasympathetic response such as perianal, suprapubic, and urethral areas enhance the climactic capacity. Maintaining good muscle tone of the pelvis and the surrounding muscle groups improves sexual endurance and orgasmic potential.
- *Exercising.* Working out together can be a great prelude to sexual intimacy. Furthermore, a healthy, fit body means that you'll feel sexy.

Be prepared with those extra things that make sex more comfortable and pleasing—oils, tissues, covers, fans, clean hair and body with natural soaps, trimmed nails, moist skin, and fresh breath.

Time of day matters—early afternoon is often the best time of the day for sex following a healthy lunch or light exercise and shower. With busy schedules and children in the home, scheduling sex may be necessary. While spontaneity can add to sexual arousal, it may also mean that many other parts of your daily life interfere with regular sex. Plan ahead.

CHAPTER 26

FINDING A HEALTH CARE PROFESSIONAL

S ometimes, despite all your good intentions, optimal diet, and exercise habits, controlling stress and an all-around healthy lifestyle, you may still need to consult a health care professional for additional help. When this happens, finding the expert who best matches your particular needs is critical. A variety of doctors, specialists, physical therapists, chiropractors, massage therapists, nutritionists, and others can successfully help you. So finding the right one is essential.

In the most favorable scenario, the health care professional you choose should be able to personally relate to you, your lifestyle, and your particular needs. These individuals are on your side; they don't look askew at holistic considerations. They are experts who address both the causes and the symptoms.

If you find the ideal health care professional close to home or work, you're fortunate. Many patients I worked with at my clinic would fly in from out of town. Some would stay for several days at a nearby motel and come to my office to be evaluated and receive treatment, go over diet and exercise, and receive other lifestyle recommendations.

The first thing to do when seeking a health care professional is to ask your friends, colleagues, and relatives who are already following a healthy lifestyle. Find out about their successes and experiences and whether they were treated as a person and not as an assembly-line patient. In addition, ask how much time the doctor or therapist spent with them during a first visit, and on subsequent visits, and whether the practitioner answered questions and explained what he or she was doing. Also seek out information about philosophical compatibility; you don't want a doctor who thinks eggs are bad, low fat is good, or orthotics are a wise choice.

Before making an appointment, don't be afraid to call the office for information about how this health care professional practices. This is not unlike a job interview: You want to know about someone before developing a professional relationship. He or she may have a website. Check that out as well.

Once you show up for your scheduled appointment, it's important that you provide a significant amount of information about your health and fitness. This is obtained through the doctor or therapist taking down your personal history, which usually requires a fair amount of time. In fact, I often spent up to two hours with some patients before treatment commenced. Some of this can be obtained from extensive questionnaires or surveys, much like those used throughout this book (many of which I developed and used during my years of practice and which I sent to patients before their first visit). Furthermore, a dietary analysis is usually necessary to evaluate your nutritional status. I used to ask patients to keep a food-intake diary for five to seven days.

Observe how the practitioner addresses your specific concerns. If you have a good feeling about your visit, plan another as necessary. But if you don't feel comfortable, whether or not you can fully articulate why, search for another health professional. It may take some time to find the right one, but it's worth the effort.

The biggest problem in our current health care system is that patients usually end up seeing a specialist. For example, if you visit an acupuncturist, you'll get acupuncture treatment; visit a chiropractor, you'll receive spinal manipulation; visit a dietician, you'll get diet advice. This is usually not the most holistic approach. What if you have both a spinal problem and nutritional needs for the same problem? It's uncommon to find a practitioner who can address all your needs, although these health care professionals do exist and are worth seeking out. Today, many therapists are trained beyond their particular specialty. So a chiropractor may also perform acupuncture and dietary analysis, or a podiatrist may have expertise in exercise training and treat back problems. This is why you must actively manage and be involved with the entire process.

Another critical factor is a practitioner's legal scope of practice. This is dictated by each state's (or country's) licensing board, which allows an individual to apply specific therapies within his or her discipline. Today, the scope of practice of many practitioners has widened especially as more nontraditional courses and topics are added to school curriculums and professional seminars.

There are times when a specialist is necessary. In these cases, a primary care physician or general practitioner (what used to be known as a family doctor) will usually refer you to the specialist for a particular problem. This might include scheduling an appointment with a surgeon, cardiologist, or neurologist. Unfortunately, the general practitioner is becoming increasingly scarce in today's specialty-oriented health care system. Gone are the days when a single doctor might have treated several generations from the same family.

Assessment Procedures

The foundation of effective health care is assessment. There are two main approaches. The first and most common is a symptom-based assessment, in which a specific treatment or remedy is given for a particular condition. In this approach, the patient who complains of low-back pain radiating into the thigh may be given a diagnosis of sciatica. An off-the-shelf treatment for sciatica is given, usually directed at the area of pain. This might include prescribing a painkiller or applying massaging or manipulating to the low back. But the fact remains that each and every patient with sciatic-type pain has a unique problem with specific needs.

A second method of assessment is based on a more complete evaluation, which takes into account the patient's symptoms but

The Practitioner and Patient

The best health care practitioner is one who is compassionate, understanding, honest, and skilled at evaluating your problems and symptoms. Because of today's broken, unreliable, and disease-care system, the best health care practitioner is not easy to find.

The worst practitioner does not have sufficient time for you and tightly clutches to his or her overpassionate conviction with tunnel vision. They seem unable to look at the big picture and are often unwilling to treat the patient as an individual—meaning you. They may even be unhealthy and burned-out.

The ideal patient offers respect and appreciates of the health care practitioner, but never worships this person. This patient is never impatient and is open, involved, and willing to seek self-improvement. On the other hand, the bad patient is indifferent, even apathetic, and accepts whatever a health care practitioner recommends as long as insurance, Medicaid or Medicare, or other payer covers the treatment. This patient is passive, dependent, suspicious, fearful, and often a constant complainer.

487

includes other tests that consider the function of the whole person. In this situation, the goal of the assessment process is not necessarily to find a name for the condition but to ascertain the cause(s) and which therapy or therapies are best. For example, someone with a diagnosis of sciatica might have different sets of problems and causes from another patient's with the same symptom. An examination is made not only in the area of pain but throughout the body. The practitioner may evaluate the function of the low back and pelvis, but also other structures such as the foot and ankle, including an evaluation of muscle balance that supports these areas. Then, the exercise history, along with other daily habits, such as sitting, driving, and sleeping, is considered. Treatment is directed at the areas that appear to be the cause of the symptoms, which may not necessarily be the site of the pain. An effective therapy results not only in the elimination of pain but also in the restoration of normal body function and other factors that help prevent the recurrence of the problem. These might include improper footwear since it can contribute to muscle imbalance that could trigger low-back stress causing sciatic pain.

Unfortunately, in the past couple of decades, both mainstream and alternative medicine approaches have turned into symptom-based treatments. The result is a movement away from holistic care, despite the liberal use of the word. Many practitioners use a wide variety of assessment methods, therapies, and lifestyle recommendations not typical of their particular profession, often using tools that at one time were found only in other disciplines. While this can be a positive aspect of a holistic practice, it sometimes appears difficult to know who's doing what. For example, I've known dentists who regularly employed diet, nutrition, and exercise remedies; podiatrists who treated not just the feet but also the whole body; chiropractors who were primarily nutritionists; and naturopaths who prescribed drugs. Even the differences between traditional mainstream medical doctors and so-called alternative practitioners—best referred to as "complementary" medicine—is a blur. Today, most of the medical community embrace many complementary therapies with more than half of medical schools and family practice residency programs now including their teaching as part of the curricula.

Despite this overlapping of practices and treatments, let's look at some of the common disciplines currently available to patients, especially in the United States, and a general description of their approaches. Not included here are medical specialists such as cardiologists or neurologists.

Biofeedback

For over thirty years, I have developed and used various forms of biofeedback in clinical practice for exercise training, evaluating and correcting muscle imbalances, and treating patients with brain and spinal cord injuries. These specific biofeedback approaches included the use of a heart rate monitor, manual muscle testing, and the use of electromyography (EMG) and electroencephalography (EEG).

Scientists who trained human subjects to consciously alter their body function through sensory input to the brain coined the term "biofeedback" in the 1960s. However, long before mechanical biofeedback techniques emerged, natural biofeedback mechanisms were built into our brains hundreds of thousands of years ago—a key feature in our development, with early humans using it instinctively for survival. For example, sensing uncomfortable temperatures, humans sought ways to adapt through clothing, shelter, and fire; and walking on rough surfaces led to the development of minimal protective footwear.

Because the human brain and body has this built-in capacity for biofeedback, developing various forms that were sensible and useful was relatively easy. This included biofeedback techniques that incorporated equipment such as heart rate monitoring and those that could be done manually where reliance on equipment is not necessary, including EMG- and EEG-type procedures in manual biofeedback.

While the goal of manual muscle testing is widely varied, there is one common feature among all those professionals using it: Manual muscle testing is an important form of biofeedback used to help evaluate neuromuscular function, especially in helping to determine muscle imbalance, a common cause of physical injury, disability, and common aches and pains.

Chiropractic

While manipulation of the spine has been used as therapy for many centuries, the chiropractic profession, specializing in this technique, dates back only to 1895. Many chiropractors believe that spinal vertebra misalignments, called subluxations, interfere with the normal communication between the brain and the body to cause physical, chemical, or mental and emotional imbalances. The chiropractic subluxation refers most often to a spinal joint that is causing problems in the spine or elsewhere in the body. Some chiropractors also address imbalances associated with other joints, including the temporomandibular joint and those in the feet, knees, wrists, and others. Chiropractors have successfully treated patients with conditions ranging from back and neck pain to intestinal disorders and allergies. In the United States, chiropractors must receive a doctorate degree (doctor of chiropractic, or DC) through a rigorous education, nearly identical to that of medical or osteopathic school except that it does not include studies in surgery. Many chiropractors are also trained in other complementary disciplines, including diet and nutrition, applied kinesiology, Chinese medicine, cranial-sacral technique, and others.

Over the past several decades, chiropractic sports medicine and rehabilitation have been emerging fields within complementary medicine. Many professional, collegiate, amateur, and Olympic teams, along with individual athletes, use chiropractic care as a major part of their sports programs.

Osteopathy

Traditional osteopathy is a manipulative-based therapy using a conservative nondrug approach. There is a stronger focus on the bones of the head and neck and the musculo-skeletal system in general. In addition, other therapies are often used by some osteopaths, including acupuncture, diet and nutrition, and biofeedback.

Osteopathy was first developed in the 1890s by Andrew Taylor Still, who founded the first college of osteopathic medicine. Still was an American medical doctor and surgeon during the Civil War. He later criticized medicine for the overuse of drugs and began using more holistic methods that included diet, prevention, and fitness. By the 1950s, the majority of osteopaths were incorporated into mainstream medicine. Today, most osteopaths in the country practice like medical doctors, no longer using their traditional techniques. Their doctor of osteopathy degree (DO) is nearly identical to a medical degree. In many parts of the world, especially Europe, many osteopaths have maintained their traditional roles, often using many complementary approaches.

Cranial osteopathy, developed in 1939 by Dr. William Sutherland, an osteopath, is a subspecialty within osteopathic manipulative medicine. A cranial osteopath focuses particularly on the movements of the bones in the skull and their relationships with the spine and sacrum. These cranial-sacral techniques are commonly taught to many different health care professionals, including chiropractors, massage therapists, and physical therapists.

The body's cranial movements are described as a dynamic force within the living human: the "energy" of the central nervous system. In particular, cranial-sacral movement is associated with the circulation of the cerebral spinal fluid, which bathes the brain and spinal cord. Osteopaths describe precise movements of all twenty-six cranial bones, which constitute a significant part of the body's self-healing mechanism. Cranial bone motion is associated with the movement of the breathing mechanism; certain bones move specifically with both inhalation and exhalation movement. The amount of movement is in the range of fractions of a millimeter.

Cranial osteopaths believe that any disruption in cranial movement may have an adverse effect on any area of the body, causing imbalances. Problems within the cranial-sacral mechanism can occur as a result of trauma (beginning with birth), daily micro-trauma, breathing irregularities, muscular imbalances, and other problems.

Assessment is done by palpation of the cranium, sacrum, and spine; by postural evaluation; by muscle testing; and by other approaches depending on the practitioner. Correction of cranial-sacral problems is accomplished manually by applying gentle pressures at certain points on the cranium and sacrum, often in conjunction with inhalation or exhalation or through manipulation of certain spinal vertebrae.

Massage Therapy (Therapeutic Massage)

The profession of massage therapy is comprised of trained, licensed practitioners who perform various types of massage techniques. Massage therapy, also many centuries old, is frequently recommended by both mainstream and complementary practitioners for patients who have physical injuries, such as muscle pain, and for prevention purposes. Massage focuses on increasing blood circulation and lymph flow, reducing muscle tension and spasm, improving the range of motion, and helping to reduce pain. Foot massage can also stimulate the communication between the feet and the brain, helping foot balance and other foot function.

Massage involves soft tissue manipulation of the body's muscles and aids in stress reduction. It can lower high cortisol levels to help reduce anxiety, improve the immune system and adrenal function, and help other dysfunction associated with high levels of this stress hormone. A variety of techniques are used, including effleurage, petrissage, and vibration. I have found Swedish massage

to be valuable for many patients, especially those with adrenal dysfunction.

Trigger-point massage has also become popular. This approach involves specific finger pressure into myofascial trigger points in muscles and connective tissues to reduce hypersensitivity and muscle spasms. Trigger points may cause restricted and painful movement of muscles, ligaments, and tendons. Pioneered by Dr. Janet Travell in the 1940s, this technique became popular with her treatment of President Kennedy when she was the White House physician. Today, many health care practitioners perform trigger-point therapy.

Nutrition and Diet

Various aspects of nutrition and diet are taken into account by so many different health care professionals that it is difficult to categorize. Many within the field do not consider it part of complementary medicine since nurses and dieticians who work in hospitals and other institutions have been applying a form of basic nutrition therapy for decades as part of mainstream medicine.

The differences between mainstream nutrition/diet therapy and the complementary approach are many. Most different is the philosophy of mainstream medicine that associates nutrition with particular deficiency states—for example, vitamin C prevents scurvy—and that of complementary medicine, which considers the natural foods and nutrients that may improve overall body function. (In doing so, this approach also prevents deficiency.)

Another clear division in the field of diet and nutrition is the recommendation to consume processed foods with fortified synthetic vitamins and other nutrients versus unprocessed natural foods containing thousands of naturally occurring nutrients.

The same division applies in the arena of dietary supplements. Many practitioners advise taking high-dose synthetic vitamins in the same manner as prescription drugs are used. Other practitioners, however, recommend natural products but primarily emphasize the importance of an optimal diet to provide most nutrients.

Homeopathy

The history of homeopathy begins with its founder, Samuel Hahnemann (1755–1843), a German physician who coined the word "homeopathy" (*homoios* in Greek means "similar"; *pathos* refers to suffering). Hahnemann developed the "law of similars" into a systematic medical art and science. Immunizations, allergy treatment, and other medical approaches are based on this "law," although homeopathy works in a very different way, using extremely low-dose substances to treat patients. In effect, the practitioner seeks to find a substance that, if given in overdose, would produce symptoms similar to those a sick person is experiencing. The most controversial aspect of homeopathy is the dosages. They are produced by a series of dilutions that

result in an exceedingly low-dose substance. Homeopaths have observed that the more a medicine has been diluted, the longer it generally acts and the fewer the doses needed to be effective.

More startling is the fact that while homeopaths and scientists agree that solutions diluted beyond 24X or 12C (dilution levels used in homeopathy) may not have any molecules of the original solution, they assert that something remains: the essence of the substance, its resonance, its energy. Many practitioners have difficulty accepting these theories considering their science-based education, while others only look at the end-result success of homeopathic treatments.

Homeopathy evolved in the United States through the work of Hans Gram, a Dutch homeopath who immigrated to the United States in 1825. Today, homeopathy is widespread throughout the world, especially in Europe, Asia, the Far East, Central and South America, Australia, and Russia.

Naturopathic Medicine

Naturopathy is the holistic practice of natural therapeutics, or natural medicine, which works with a variety of hands-on and lifestyle factors, including diet, nutrition, herbal medicine, homeopathy, acupuncture, and physical medicine. In addition to treating a variety of imbalances, the naturopath focuses on functional problems to prevent future illness and injury. These practitioners assess patients through physical examinations, blood and urine tests, nutritional and dietary evaluations, and other methods.

Naturopathy began in the United States in the early 1900s when many of the natural therapies that had previously existed were joined together into one approach. For unknown reasons, by the mid-1900s, naturopathy rapidly declined as mainstream medicine flourished. Today, the naturopathic physician must obtain an ND degree (naturopathic doctor) from a four-year graduate-level naturopathic college. In the United States, only thirteen states license naturopaths, but with the expansion of many complementary practices, naturopathy is once again growing as other professionals are adopting these approaches and as the natural therapies' movement continues to evolve.

Physical Therapy (PT)

Physical therapy (also called physiotherapy) is the treatment of physical dysfunction due to injuries, disabilities, or deformities—all of which can be the result of an inactive lifestyle or aging. A physical therapist's approach might include massage, heat and cryotherapy, electrotherapy, spinal and other joint manipulation, and a recommendation for light regular exercise. Physical therapists provide treatments to help functional movement of individuals to develop, maintain, and restore optimal posture and gait.

The ancient Greek healer Hippocrates is considered to have been the first physical therapist. He employed a variety of physical treatments, including water baths and massage. But the modern profession of physical therapy originated in 1813 when Per Henrik Ling, referred to as the Father of Swedish Gymnastics, founded the Royal Central Institute of Gymnastics, which included the use of physical manipulation, massage, and exercise (the Swedish word for "physical therapist" is *sjukgymnast*, which means "sick gymnast"). In the United States, the first school of physical therapy was established at Walter Reed Army Hospital in Washington DC during World War I, where therapists helped restore physical function to severely injured soldiers. The current educational requirements for physical therapists range from a minimal four-year degree, although today, most of these practitioners have master's degrees and PhD's.

Chinese Medicine

This approach is one of the oldest known systems of assessment and therapy, dating back five thousand years. Using perhaps the first true holistic approach, traditional Chinese medicine practitioners address every aspect of the patient's life, including physical, chemical, mental and emotional, spiritual, and social facets. Chinese medicine includes four main components: acupuncture, manipulation and massage, herbal and nutritional remedies, and exercise disciplines called qigong (the most popular form being tai chi).

An important focus in Chinese medicine is assessment, which relies heavily on observation of the person—especially the face, skin, and breath—and on palpation of the radial pulses on the wrist. According to a Chinese theory, twelve energy channels, called meridians, contain life's energy (called chi or qi), the reason why this approach is sometimes called meridian therapy. On each meridian, there are many different points that can be stimulated by manual pressure (acupressure), needles (acupuncture), heat (through the burning of the moxa herb, referred to as moxibustion), and in modern Chinese medicine, electricity (electroacupuncture), with laser treatment becoming popular. Chinese medicine also incorporates therapies such as herbal medicine, music and color therapy, and even psychology.

The basic theory in Chinese medicine is that an imbalance of qi—which consists of yin and yang energy—is the cause of dysfunction, injury, and ultimately disease. The balancing of yin and yang energy is therefore the goal of the practitioner, who may use any or all of the therapeutic tools to accomplish this depending on which is most applicable to the patient's needs based on assessment.

This balance does not stop with the individual but continues into society as a whole. The individual, as well as the surrounding society, is a delicate balance of yin and yang. Yin represents water, quiet, substance, and night; yang represents fire, noise, function, and day. The two are polar opposites, and therefore one of them must be present to allow the other to exist; for instance, how can you experience joy if you do not understand sorrow? More interesting is the fact that many ancient Chinese visited their practitioners when they were well, paying the practitioner a retainer to keep them healthy. If they became ill, they stopped paying until wellness returned.

Kinesiology

Kinesiology, the study of human movement, is common in the coursework of undergraduate and graduate degrees, and postdoctoral programs, with some universities offering PhD programs in this discipline. Those educated and trained in kinesiology generally work with health care practitioners in hospitals, on sports teams, and in other arenas to assist in sports training.

Those studying the clinical sciences with a goal of obtaining a doctorate degree in medicine, osteopathy, chiropractic, or other areas often study the same type of kinesiology with more emphasis on neuromuscular function and the use of manual muscle testing as an assessment tool. These individuals are usually health care professionals who use complementary medicine, with the name professional applied kinesiology (PAK) separating this clinical approach from kinesiology. (It should also be noted that a significant number of people, many of whom don't have college experience in this field, also employ types of kinesiology. These include those in Touch for Health and many other programs that teach laypeople certain techniques.)

494

Many health care professionals who use various forms of therapy with the name "kinesiology" have evolved in the last fifty years and have incorporated the use of manual muscle testing. Virtually all these different types of kinesiology today—there are dozens—came from applied kinesiology (AK), which was developed in the early 1960s by Dr. George Goodheart, a chiropractor who employed a wide range of complementary approaches, including Chinese medicine, osteopathy and chiropractic, diet and nutrition, and sports medicine. In 1980, he became the first official chiropractor on the U.S. Olympic medical team and in 2001 was on *Time* magazine's list of the Top 100 Alternative Medicine Innovators of the Twenty-First Century.

Much like Chinese medicine, applied kinesiology combines many existing therapies into one overall system. Applied kinesiology practitioners use manual muscle testing as part of a detailed assessment process that focuses on the physical, chemical, and mental and emotional state. This and other assessment tools help practitioners find the therapies that best match the patient's specific needs. These practitioners theorize that when there is an imbalance in the body, it is usually reflected as a specific muscle imbalance.

There is not a specific academic degree for applied kinesiology; rather, those licensed health care professionals use manual muscle testing as one of often several complementary medicine procedures. Various professional organizations such as the International College of Applied Kinesiology offer postdoctorate courses and certifications in professional applied kinesiology.

Part of the lifestyle choices you make regarding your own well-being might require help from health care professionals. This process of choosing the most appropriate person or persons is not easy considering the dysfunctional health care system. Nonetheless, finding the best doctor or therapist is like seeking out the most nutritious food or finding the exercise routine that best matches your particular needs. This may take time and effort, but do it right and you will be able to continue along the road to a fun, healthy, and fit life.

Potentially, any health care practitioners can play a vital role in helping you understand and balance physical, chemical, and mental function. A significant number of these doctors and therapists use many different forms of complementary and traditional medicine. Whether the one you visit uses Chinese medicine, biofeedback, applied kinesiology, or some combination of therapies, the two most important considerations are the following: Have you completely recovered from your injury or ill health? Has your overall health and fitness improved?

CHAPTER 27

HOW TO AGE GRACEFULLY
It's Much Easier Than You Think

Not long ago, I ran into someone whom I hadn't seen in over twenty years. "Wow," he said, "you haven't changed a bit!" My temptation was to say what I silently thought, that he looked much older than his age. But that wouldn't be fair to him. The real point I want to make is that we all age differently, but not randomly; we have a lot of influence about the process. I personally made the choice to follow a path of healthy aging, and my friend had taken a much different path.

Graceful aging can only occur in a healthy body. This is the answer to the age-old puzzle of restoring youth—it's also not to lose it so quickly. It's not just about wrinkles, but having healthy skin and hair, a youthful body full of vigor and a vibrant, alert brain. Yet the marketplace is full of antiaging scams: powders, pills, and potions that claim to stop aging, which, of course, can't be done. Cosmetic companies make products with chemi-cals that attempt to cover the effects of aging. These companies make billions of dollars on products that don't work. Instead, they actually can increase aging because of the body's insult to the dangerous synthetic compounds contained in virtually all of them.

Research shows that more than half of all babies born in non–third world countries since 2000 have an excellent chance of living to age one hundred. No doubt modern medicine is keeping people alive longer, but the problem is that not nearly as much attention is paid to quality of life along the way.

Healthy aging requires that your immune system is working well, since that helps prevent or slow the process of disease and regulates how fast or slow the aging process will proceed.

But the immune system is not like the muscles, hormones, or gut, which has well-defined physical and chemical parameters. The immune system is not isolated in a single organ, but is bodywide; the brain, gut, heart, muscles all play key roles as does stress. And so does food—carbohydrates, fats, and proteins to phytonutrients and eating patterns—play a key role in aging.

The Two Sides of Aging

There are two different ages. Chronological age refers to how young or old one is by the calendar; physiological age refers to how young or old one is relative to average chronological ages. When comparing a person's physiological with their chronological age, some are younger and others older than their age in years. No one can control the years as they pass, but one can control their physiological aging.

All the issues I've addressed in this book relate to physiological aging. The balance of fats, controlling chronic inflammation, adequate protein intake, aerobic fitness, and other issues all can keep one's physiological age much younger than what the calendar says.

Oxygen and Free Radicals

Overall, one of the most important ongoing issues regarding aging is oxygen. Too much of it, or too little, and you age faster. Most people are aware of oxygen's benefits, but many people don't realize its potential harm. It's in this simple chemistry lesson: the conversion of the stable O_2 molecule we take in during each breath to its very unstable and destructive cousin, the superoxide or free radical molecule. When this occurs inside the body, it can lead to serious health problems. Scientists now associate the destruction by oxygen free radicals—a process also called oxidative stress—as a contributor to every major chronic disease, including cancer, Alzheimer's, heart disease, and diabetes. Free radicals also play a major role in the aging process.

Aging is the result of continuous reactions of the body's cells with free radicals. It is important to become aware of these potentially harmful substances, what increases their production and how to control them, in order to reduce the devastating effects of disease and control the process of aging.

Normally, the body produces free radicals to protect against harmful bacteria, viruses, chemical pollutants, and even toxic substances produced within the body. However, in a chemical-saturated world, it is possible to produce too many free radicals. When this occurs, free radicals can react with and damage any cell in the body. The most vulnerable area of the cell is the part containing

SHOULD AGING BE VIEWED AS A DISEASE THAT CAN BE TREATED OR DELAYED?

This question may sound rather odd, but there are many scientists who have been addressing it for years, and most answer with a definitive yes. This same question is the title of a newly published editorial (in the journal *Frontiers in Aging Neuroscience*, February 2011) by Dr. Ruth Elaine Nieuwenhuis-Mark of the Department of Medical Psychology and Neuropsychology at Tilburg University, the Netherlands.

This groundswell of support for calling aging a "disease" is undergoing the process of re-educating both the public and health authorities. Many research specialists in aging are lobbying the world's biggest drug regulator, the U.S. Food and Drug Administration, to consider defining the process of aging as a disease. This will most likely take place because this has already happened with other conditions such as obesity, which is a preventable lifestyle problem and not a disease in the real sense of the word.

By considering aging a disease, researchers are making the claim that it can be treated and delayed. Most importantly, branding age as a disease would speed the development of new drugs that treat many of the effects of aging—including diabetes, cancer, heart disease, and Alzheimer's. Currently, scientists argue that they are being hampered in their efforts by the FDA, who approves drugs only for specific diseases, not for something as general, natural, or normal as aging.

Do we really need a whole new line of drugs that attempts to increase longevity?

Dr. Ruth Elaine Nieuwenhuis-Mark's editorial concludes by claiming that making the jump to call aging a disease is "at the very least, questionable, and indeed, worrisome." She asks, "Do we really need to feed the already negative stereotypes which exist of the elderly in society? Should we not be celebrating how much the old bring to the world and have still to offer not only to close family and friends but also to society at large?" She closes with, "Labeling aging as a disease may or may not help research funding but it can only hurt public opinion of what it means to age."

unstable polyunsaturated fatty acids, as these fats are easily destroyed by free radicals. This destruction is called lipid peroxidation, and it's particularly associated with chronic inflammation. Together this is the first step in the disease process for most chronic illness. For example, before LDL cholesterol can be stored in the coronary arteries, damage from lipid peroxidation first occurs. Lipid peroxidation can even produce toxins capable of traveling throughout the body, creating damage anywhere. These toxins are known to be carcinogenic and even have the potential to cause genetic mutations.

The damage from free radicals, oxidative stress, results in the negative signs of aging. This includes physically and mentally slowing down, loss of strength, and bone loss, to name a few problems. The more of this damage, the more physiologically older we become.

Fortunately, the body has an effective way to combat oxidative stress: our antioxidant system, which controls free radicals by chemically changing them to harmless compounds. This system has two important requirements. First, raw materials are needed to chemically reduce free radicals. These are the many nutritional antioxidants from healthy foods—the various vitamins, minerals, and phytonutrients previously discussed. Second, the process requires an effective location in the body to perform this task—the aerobic muscle fibers.

Too much free radical activity, too little antioxidant activity, or both speeds the aging process, sometimes significantly.

Antioxidants to the Rescue

Throughout this book I've mentioned the importance of antioxidants. They're sometimes called free radical scavengers because they gobble up, chemically speaking, dangerous oxygen compounds. There are two key groups of antioxidants that accomplish this task. The first group includes various vitamins, minerals, and phytonutrients—there are many, probably thousands, and scientists have yet to discover all of them. They include vitamins A, C and E, beta-carotene, selenium, the bioflavonoids, and groups of phytonutrients such as phenols. As powerful as these are, there's a more potent antioxidant: glutathione.

Glutathione is not found in food and can't be taken in a pill (it's broken down in the stomach), although now intravenous and transdermal (a patch) forms have been developed for use in research and hospitals for patients with circulatory disorders, tumors, and other inflammatory-related diseases. The very best way to get enough glutathione is to give your body the raw materials it needs to make it: certain other antioxidants from a healthy diet. These include the following:

- The amino acid cysteine found in animal protein (especially whey).
- The phytonutrient sulforaphane, high in cruciferous vegetables such as broccoli, kale, and brussels sprouts. The highest content is in young, two- to three-day-old broccoli sprouts (before their leaves turn green)—these you can sprout yourself.
- Lipoic acid is an important antioxidant found in many bitter-tasting dark vegetables (spinach, broccoli, brussels sprouts, whole peas) and even beef (lipoic acid can also be made in a healthy body with similar nutrients).

- Gamma-tocopherol and alpha-tocopherol, parts of the vitamin E complex. These are found in raw nuts (such as almonds and cashews) and seeds (such as sesame and flax) and, in smaller amounts, in many vegetables. (Beware: popular doses of alpha-tocopherol—such as 100 IU or more of vitamin E—can reduce the levels of these other vitamin E components.)
- Food sources of vitamin C that include a variety of vegetables and fruits.

Most Potent Antioxidants	
Sulforaphane	Lipoic acid
Cysteine	Alpha-tocotrienol
Gamma-tocopherol	Alpha-tocopherol
Vitamin C	Lycopene
Beta-tocopherol	Beta-carotene
Zeaxanthin	Delta-tocopherol
Lutein	Canthaxanthin
Astaxanthin	Quercetin
	Co-Q10

While antioxidants such as sulforaphane, lipoic acid, and cysteine head the list of potent glutathione precursors, many other popular antioxidants are less effective. The list at the top of the next column notes the most potent antioxidants in order of their effectiveness—the most powerful being those that help the body make glutathione. As you can see, these are not the most popular versions as companies making synthetic vitamin C, unnatural doses of vitamin E, and relatively low-potent antioxidants such as quercetin and Co-Q10 push their products to unsuspecting consumers.

It's not necessary to remember the names of these antioxidants, but you do need to remember to eat as many antioxidant-rich organic foods as possible. These include a wide variety of vegetables and fruits, including blueberries and other berries, sesame seeds, almonds, extra-virgin olive oil, green and black tea, and red wine are excellent sources of antioxidants. Meats, especially

beef, contain significant amounts of certain antioxidants as does whey. Of course there are now hundreds of antioxidant products available in pill, liquid, powder, and other forms. If needed, be sure to take only supplements made from real, raw foods.

Early signs and symptoms of the need for more antioxidants may include immune problems such as lingering cold or flu, sensitivity to chlorine or other chemicals, and chronic inflammation.

Poor immune function can be elusive, as evidenced in one of my former patients whom I will call Alice. Despite being in her midthirties, she had a variety of vague problems. One of her previous doctors told me that he thought Alice was a hypochondriac. She experienced joint pain, but only on some days; was sensitive to perfumes, soaps, and other substances containing certain chemicals; and when she got a cold, typically a half dozen of them a year, it would last two to three weeks. In addition, she had skin rashes that the dermatologist could not identify, burning eye pain several times each week, and looked about fifty years old.

Alice's diet was chronically void of fresh fruits and vegetables, except for a salad of mostly iceberg lettuce twice weekly. Her unusual history alone was enough to lead me to recommend increasing her antioxidants. My dietary recommendations included immediately eating six to eight servings of fresh vegetables and a couple of low-glycemic fresh fruits each day, including blueberries. Within ten days, Alice started feeling better. A year later, she reported only one cold, lasting three to four days. And her friends were telling her she looked much younger, and she certainly felt that way.

Exercise and Free Radicals

A well-developed aerobic system is a key to making your antioxidant system work best. Even if you obtain all the necessary antioxidants, they need a place to do their job—these are the aerobic muscle fibers. The free radical breakdown by antioxidants occurs in the cell's mitochondria (where fat burning occurs) contained within aerobic muscle fibers. Improved circulation that accompanies aerobic fitness is the vehicle that helps antioxidant activity—in particular, in getting these nutrients into the aerobic fibers. Therefore, people in better aerobic shape, who have more aerobic muscle fibers and mitochondria, are more capable of controlling free radicals compared to those who are out of shape.

But exercise itself produces free radicals. Different levels of exercise intensity can produce varying amounts of free radicals. Easy aerobic exercise, especially at the heart rate determined by the 180 formula, produces little or insignificant amounts of free radicals, and this smaller amount is most likely well controlled through the body's natural defense system, especially if enough antioxidants are present.

However, exercising at higher intensities or lifting weights—any anaerobic exercise—can have the opposite effect. Anaerobic activity can produce more oxidative stress—some studies show a 120 percent increase over resting levels. This is the result of physical damage to muscles, lactic acid production, and higher oxygen uptake, which may increase tenfold during the activity.

Reducing Your Exposure to Chemicals

In addition to eating foods that contain antioxidants and becoming aerobically fit, you can also reduce free radical production by simply avoiding exposure to certain toxic substances in your environment. Consuming chemical pollutants via your lungs, skin, or through food increases free radical production by the body. Keep your home and work environment as free from pollutants as possible. Here are some tips to accomplish this important task:

- New building or home furnishing materials, including carpet, can quickly pollute the indoor air you breathe. If you've just done some remodeling, redecorating, or if you have tightly sealed your home to save on heating or cooling costs (thereby sealing potential pollutants inside), keep two windows open (preferably on east and west sides of the home) just a bit to let in fresh air and vent your environment. Pay attention to the items you bring into your house—plastic bags, boxes, new building materials, etc.—they all probably contain chemicals that will gas out as part of the toxin-releasing process. Keep as many of these materials in an outdoor shed or other location.

- Clean out your attic, basement, closets, or other areas in which you may have stored potential pollutants such as old cans of paint, aerosols, and cleaners. There is constant leakage of vapors from these products. Store all needed chemical products in an outside detached garage or shed and discard the items you don't need or want and those too old to use.
- If your garage is attached to the house, try to vent it, or at least leave the door slightly open. Your car constantly leaks fumes from gasoline, oil, and other chemicals. In most homes, these chemicals from the garage can easily find their way into your living areas.
- In addition to proper ventilation, an effective method to filter your indoor air is nature's way—houseplants. Besides being attractive, they are effective at filtering the

air, often more so than any mechanical filtering device. Through photosynthesis, plants absorb carbon dioxide along with other gases, including the chemicals given off from furniture, cleaners, and insulation. The plant's leaves filter the air, and the roots break down toxic chemicals into less harmful ones with their natural bacteria and fungi. The best plants for the job include elephant ear and lacy tree philodendrons, golden pathos, and the spider plant. Any green plant will work well. About ten plants per 1,000 square feet of living space are adequate. That's one to three plants per room, depending on room and plant size.

- Dietary pollution is another factor to consider. Avoiding the use of processed and packaged foods usually reduces chemicals and other additives in these items. Buying organic does the same for fresh foods.
- Certain natural foods in large amounts can also increase free radical production. These include sassafras (used in root beer) and black pepper.
- Reduce—ideally eliminate—cosmetics and toiletries that contain fragrances (most are synthetic chemicals) and other potential toxins. These include most types of soaps in your house and office; deodorant; before-, during-, and after-shave lotions and foams; hair spray, and mouthwash. Use only plain organic soaps without fragrance.

Cleaning up your environment does not mean being obsessive, which can introduce even more stress to your life. Just do your best to make your environment clean and safe. This, coupled with adequate intake of antioxidants and a regular aerobic exercise program, will help keep oxidative stress from speeding up your aging process.

Keys to Successful Aging

Virtually all mammals on earth have a life span six times their skeletal maturity. If we apply this animal model to humans, who reach skeletal maturity at about age 20, one should expect to live, on average, to age 120. In fact, scientists have isolated the genetic blueprints that allow us to live into our hundreds. Following our understanding of gene expression, it may simply be that most individuals don't allow that particular gene to keep them alive because diet, exercise, stress, and other factors impair the genetic process.

In our society, the average human animal barely reaches four times his or her skeletal maturity. According to the U.S. Census Bureau, only about 23 out of each 100,000

Wearing Your Free Radicals

Among the most common toxic substances you may be regularly exposed to is the solvent used in dry cleaning. This chemical, tetrachloroethylene (also known as perchloroethylene, or perc), is classified as a hazardous air pollutant by the Environmental Protection Agency. It has been associated with cancer and kidney problems and has a detrimental effect on the nervous system. Wearing freshly dry-cleaned clothing can be a danger since the residue of this chemical can remain in your clothing long after you leave the dry cleaner. As such, you continue to inhale perc, and bringing home your newly dry-cleaned clothes brings perc into your house. This can be a significant free radical problem for your body.

To avoid exposure to perc, avoid dry cleaning whenever possible. Many garments that say DRY CLEAN ONLY can still be hand-washed. Buy clothes that don't require dry cleaning. If you must dry-clean, hang your garment outside for as long as possible—at least one or two days or more—to allow the perc to escape or until the dry-cleaning smell is gone. If you're lucky enough to have in your neighborhood a professional wet cleaner, which uses only detergents and water, use this alternative—it's the future of the cleaning industry. (Beware: perc is also used for metal degreasing and to make other chemicals and is used in some consumer products—read all ingredient lists and label warnings.)

503

Your Final Day: A Great Way to Go

An old proverb says we should approach death with dignity. While living a long and healthy life past age one hundred, your physical and mental activity should be relatively high right up to the time of death—an event that should also be optimal. Perhaps on that day, you wake with the sunrise to a freshly made cup of organic coffee. You settle in for a vegetable omelet and, after reading e-mail from your children, grandchildren, great-grandchildren and their younger ones, you correspond to all. You spend some time writing in your diary, then head out for a short hike through the woods. After returning for a healthy lunch, you nap for an hour or so. You dally in the garden that afternoon and follow that up with a short walk. You watch the sunset with your significant other during a fine dinner complemented by a glass or two of Bordeaux, then share a healthy but delicious homemade dessert. You head to bed, fall asleep by ten thirty. Just past midnight, you die peacefully during a sound sleep.

people reach birthday number 100. But with modern technology, natural hygiene, and the awareness of chemicals that speed the aging process, there will soon be hundreds of thousands of people in the United States over the age of 100. The bureau estimates that by 2050, there will be between 265,000 and possibly four million centenarians.

Will you be one of them? And if so, will you welcome it, considering what your quality of life might be? While there is a genetic aspect to how long you will live, there also are many lifestyle factors that may be even more important. How well you care for yourself from the earliest age has a significant impact on both the length and the quality of your life.

Unfortunately, most people don't think they'll live that long, and many actually hope they won't. Others, however, welcome the challenge and excitement of seeing a fifth-generation descendant graduate from some futuristic high school, perhaps home-schooled by a certain wise old great-great-great-grandparent.

But who wants to attend this celebration in a wheelchair, unaware of where you are, what the name of the descendant is, or who his or her parents are? If you do happen to live to 100—or 120 years young—you want to be fully functional. Throughout this book I have offered information and insight to help you improve and maintain health and fitness, to achieve optimal human performance, and to avoid or postpone disease. It's no coincidence that all of these concepts also apply to successful and healthy aging.

The term "successful" or "healthy" aging is not a catchy phrase or new program. It's a real concept with practical applications for people of all ages. Scientists note three common paths for people as they age. "Successful aging" results in a higher quality of life. "Usual aging" would be considered "average." Finally, "diseased aging" results in low quality of life and slow death. Average is unacceptable, and diseased is no way to live or to die. The better you age, the higher your quality of life, the more productive you are throughout life, and the less likely you will die a slow, lingering death.

The younger you are, physiologically, the more you can do to control how well you age.

The older you are, the more you want to control aging. Regardless of your age now, your current actions can have significant impact on the way you age.

In my years of practice and research, I have identified several key factors that can have a direct and powerful impact on how successfully you age. As you read this list, you'll notice it's a review of many concepts that I have put forth all throughout this book. Return to those chapters that address each item for a more complete picture of what you should consider for a "new you."

ON ETHICS AND DIGNITY AND TAKING CHARGE

In 2003, Frederick Fenech, director of the United Nations International Institute on Ageing, wrote in the journal *Clinical Medicine* that "persons over the age of eighty are the fastest growing age group in developed societies; this is the group where physical frailty and diminished mental capacity are common, rendering them most vulnerable to abuse and where ethical dilemmas related to death and dying are frequent. This decline in functional capacity may lead to inability to take responsible decisions. This might require another person to act as proxy with all the attendant moral responsibility. The most critical cases of proxy decision-making arise when withdrawal of life support is being contemplated. The overriding principle is for the proxy decision-maker to show the maximum possible respect for the known or likely wishes of the patient. The formulation of so-called living wills may be of great help in the exercise of proxy decision-making."

Chances are, you've been making these tough decisions for a long time. In particular, you make the important ones, often after gathering information from others who may have certain levels of expertise on a particular subject. You want to continue that process through your life to include the issues surrounding your death and even how your body will be treated. And even plan for the possibility that you'll be unable to make decisions for a time before you pass.

Everyone won't have an optimal death, where a person passes away during sleep. But you can plan for one by enjoying a healthy and fit life and make sure you leave instructions for your children or caretakers should you be unable to function like you want. It's important to create a legal document that takes effect if you are not able to effectively communicate your wishes directly. Otherwise, you may have no control over important decisions that may be required. This includes the use of life-support remedies to keep you from dying or strong medications for severe pain. It's nice to think your loved ones and doctors will know what you want and follow them, but this does not always happen. This is where a legal document is important.

A document that I'm referring to is beyond a living will. It addresses more than the medical and legal issues but covers how you will be cared for should you be unable to communicate your wants and desires—from the foods you're given to the place you live, other comforts, any spiritual issues, and memorial matters, all are addressed.

Consider addressing these important issues now, on paper, and update them as necessary. Make them available to those closest to you, especially children, health care professionals, a legal representative, and perhaps other caregivers.

These documents should be in original and copied formats, signed and witnessed.

It's important to include the people you trust the most. And the laws of each state vary, so be sure your directions abide by these laws. Over time, you may want to make changes to your document. When this happens, be sure to make a new document the same way and replace those that others have with the latest version and destroy all out-of-date copies.

Seven Factors for Healthy Aging

1. Brain nutrients and brain stimulation
2. Anti-inflammatory foods
3. Antioxidant foods
4. Blood sugar control (and avoiding refined carbohydrates and sugars)
5. Eating protein foods
6. Physical activity to get aerobically fit
7. Mental and emotional health—controlling stress

Successful aging also includes the issues involving a person's need to love, have fun, socialize, and feel good about life. While volumes have been written about this subject, my contention is that when people take the necessary steps to better health, they feel

506

better mentally and emotionally and tend to socialize and enjoy life more, which leads to better overall mental health.

Lynn Peters Adler, a former lawyer who founded and runs the National Centenarian Awareness Project, has been working with centenarians for twenty-five years and sees certain similarities among them, including the following:

- A positive but realistic attitude
- A love of life
- A sense of humor
- Spirituality
- Courage
- A remarkable ability to accept the losses that come with age but not be stopped by them

You can influence aging as much as you can influence disease prevention and most other factors associated with fitness and health. It's less about the information—there's enough in this book to keep you busy for some time—and more about another important factor: taking action. The first step in this whole process is entirely in your hands—you decide to increase your fitness and health or, often through inaction, decide not to pursue fitness and health. Yet it's my hope that you follow through on the affirmative. It's never too late to make important lifestyle and dietary changes. And once that decision is made, you will happily discover that you have only just begun the exciting journey through the rest of your life.

APPENDIX A
Healthy Meal Ideas

How you cook your healthy food is important since even the best-tasting, healthiest ingredients can be ruined through improper kitchen practices. The biggest problems are overcooking, using too-high heat, and overheating certain types of oils. Consider the following guidelines:

- Meats, fish, and poultry can be oven- or pan-roasted, quickly grilled, and often cooked in their own juices. Fish is especially healthy when lightly steamed or poached and, when fresh and wild, can be eaten raw. Less oil or butter is needed for pan-cooking meats because they often contain their own fats. It's also important to avoid using high heat for too long. For instance when grilling a steak or lamb, trim off as much fat as possible and turn it every minute or so to prevent the excess formation of chemicals that can be harmful to your health. When you are grilling vegetables, turn them often as well. Ground meat should be bought fresh and cooked thoroughly as soon as possible. Many meat departments grind meat in the morning, so buy ground meats early in the day and cook or freeze them right away.

- The worst method for cooking is deep-fat or high-heat frying using vegetable oils. Use monounsaturated and saturated fats for cooking as they are not sensitive to heat. Coconut oil and butter are the safest fats for cooking, followed by olive oil, lard, and duck fat; the last three contain some polyunsaturated fats, so care should be taken to not heat too high. Most other fats are high in polyunsaturated oils and very prone to oxidizing when exposed to heat, producing free radicals—avoid corn, safflower, sesame, peanut, and canola oils.

- Vegetables can be steamed, stir-fried in olive oil, roasted, baked, or grilled. Cook vegetables minimally to avoid destroying nutrients—they also taste better when not overcooked. If boiling or steaming, use as little water as possible to avoid the loss of nutrients through the water. Slow-cooked vegetable stews will contain much of the minerals and heat-resistant vitamins in the liquid while some heat-sensitive vitamins will be lost. Don't throw out the water from your steamed vegetables. Either drink it or use it for a soup base or in a smoothie.

- Eggs can be soft- or hard-boiled or cooked sunny-side up, over easy, poached, or lightly scrambled. Letting the yolk remain soft is not only tastier but is healthier because heat-sensitive compounds are retained. Make sure the egg white cooks slightly because it's better for the intestines.

The meal ideas below are typical of the ones I use daily. They are general guidelines. Each meal you prepare is not only a delicious nutritional feast, but should be relatively quick and easy to make. Food preparation is an art and science, so exact ingredient lists are unnecessary as each time you create the same dish, it will be a bit different—hopefully better. Enjoy!

Salads

A hearty salad can be a meal (just add protein) or a part of a healthy meal. Some of the best simple salads are very easy to make: Always keep a container of cleaned leaf lettuce, tomatoes, carrots, and other items in the refrigerator, so a salad can be made in minutes. Add your favorite homemade dressing or just olive oil and balsamic vinegar and salt. Below are some fancy, unique, yet simple salads.

Apples and Beets

Shred green tart apples and raw peeled beetroots in a food processor or with a mandolin slicer. Mix together and squeeze in some fresh lime. Add salt to taste. Shred in carrots and ginger for a variation.

Arugula and Pears

Mix fresh baby arugula and diced pears. Add pecans, salt, olive oil, and Parmesan, pecorino, or Gorgonzola cheese.

Arugula and Roasted Grape Tomatoes

On a flat pan, roast grape tomatoes with a touch of extra-virgin olive oil and salt in a single layer at 250°F for about four hours. Allow to cool, and mix with fresh baby arugula. Add crumbled goat cheese.

Asian Coleslaw

Shred carrots, daikon radish, cabbage, red peppers, and cucumbers in a food processor or with mandolin slicer. Make a dressing with raw sesame or olive oil, rice wine vinegar, salt, grated fresh ginger and garlic, fresh lime or lemon juice, and a bit of honey. Spice it up with cayenne pepper if desired. Add cilantro or fresh basil for even more exciting flavors.

A note about peppers: Before they ripen, peppers are green. When ripe, they turn a particular color, depending on the variety. Ripe peppers are red, purple, yellow, or orange. Avoid eating green peppers as they are difficult to digest and not as tasty.

BEETS AND GINGER

Steam or bake whole beetroots. Cool and dice into bite-size cubes. Marinate in lemon juice, grated or finely chopped fresh ginger root, salt, and a touch of honey.

BEETS AND MÂCHE GREENS

Dice cooked beets and add to fresh mâche or other garden greens. Top with olive oil, vinegar, and salt.

GRAPEFRUIT, AVOCADO, SPINACH

On a bed of fresh baby spinach, add grapefruit sections and diced avocados. Make a dressing of blended grapefruit sections, ginger, garlic, honey, salt, and olive oil.

GRAPEFRUIT AND POMEGRANATE SEEDS

Simply mix grapefruit sections with fresh pomegranate seeds.

APPLES AND FENNEL

Thinly slice apples and fennel bulbs. Dress with apple cider vinegar, honey, and salt.

ORANGE AND FENNEL

Mix orange sections with chopped fresh fennel. Sprinkle with unsweetened grated coconut. Add plain sheep or goat yogurt. Mix well and let sit in refrigerator to chill.

FRESH PICKLES

Slice cucumbers (the small seedless ones are best), and add thinly sliced or diced garlic, fresh dill, salt, a small amount of honey, and white wine vinegar for the pickle juice. For a variation, include wheat-free soy sauce and sesame seeds. Store in glass jar in refrigerator.

HERBS AND WATERMELON

Mix a variety of fresh herbs and baby greens (basil, mint, cilantro, tarragon, dill, arugula, chard, spinach, lettuce). Cut a small watermelon into cubes and add crumbled soft goat cheese. Toss with olive oil and salt.

Dressings and Sauces

The flavors of many foods can be heightened with a good dressing or sauce. Following are recipes for my favorite healthful salad dressings and stove-top sauces.

PHIL'S SALAD DRESSING

In a blender, mix 8 ounces extra-virgin olive oil, 2 cloves garlic, 2 ounces or more apple cider vinegar, 1 to 2 tablespoons fresh or dried parsley (or cilantro), 1 to 2 teaspoons sea salt, and ½ teaspoon mustard.

Options:

Add 1 to 2 tablespoons sheep or goat yogurt or cream.

Blend in 1 avocado, 1 tomato, 1 mango, or juice from half a lime (in place of the vinegar).

Use 4 ounces of sesame or walnut oil for variation in taste.

Once you find the best combinations, make a larger amount so you always have it available. Shake well before serving.

Spicy Sesame Ginger Dressing

Combine about 4 parts olive oil with 1 part rice wine vinegar. Add small amounts of honey, sesame tahini, miso, grated ginger, salt, and chopped garlic.

Basic Butter Sauce

The most basic of sauces is also the easiest to make—simply butter and sea salt. When you make your vegetables, put some sweet cream butter on the vegetables while still hot, along with some sea salt. (Sweet butter is made without salt—the cream used to make this butter is a higher quality and more tasty than that used for salted butter.) Even those who never liked vegetables will usually eat them with a butter sauce. Variation: sauté garlic or onions with or without some spices (tarragon works well) in butter and some olive oil.

Ghee or Clarified Butter

Melt one pound of sweet (unsalted) butter, and bring just to the point of low boil to allow separation of solids and fat. Skim off solids that rise to the top (this can be added to soups or vegetables). Use the clear butter (ghee) like any other butter. Ghee does not burn like butter and does not require refrigeration.

Basic Tomato Sauce

This is a quick and easy, tasty, and healthful all-around red sauce. Just put some chopped fresh tomatoes or whole canned tomatoes in an uncovered pot and boil fast (not a simmer) until desired consistency—this may take a couple of hours or more depending on the volume. Add salt. When cooked down to a thicker sauce, tomatoes take on a unique taste all their own. Even without adding any spices, you'll have a great-tasting sauce. You can freeze it in small glass containers. Once you have the basic sauce, add garlic, parsley, basil, turmeric, or your favorite spices.

Basic Cream Sauce

The fanciest basic sauce is the cream sauce, simply made from heavy cream, butter, psyllium, and salt. Use just less than the same amount of cream as the amount of sauce you want. For example, for about 2 cups of sauce, use a bit less than 2 cups of cream. Heat the cream to just before it simmers. In a separate pan, melt about a half stick (4 tablespoons) of sweet butter on low heat. With a whisk, slowly stir in about ½ teaspoon finely ground psyllium into the butter. Slowly add the hot cream while continuously stirring over low to medium heat, bringing to a simmer for 5 to 10 minutes. Add sea salt to taste.

Once you can make a good basic cream sauce quickly and easily, you can create a variety of different sauces almost as easily.

For example, adding some chopped onion or garlic, a bay leaf, tarragon, or other spices to the cream, after heating it, makes a different sauce. For a cheese sauce, add any type of cheese to the basic cream sauce.

SWEET BASIL PESTO

In a blender or food processor, mix fresh basil, garlic, extra-virgin olive oil, pine nuts, and sea salt.

Soups

Almost any food can be the base for a delicious soup. And it need not be a lengthy or difficult recipe. Use vegetables in your refrigerator that are getting too old to serve fresh (or freeze them and use later): salad greens and other vegetables, meat bones, chicken and turkey carcasses, and other flavorful foods that you might normally discard. Lightly sauté vegetables and meat scraps in olive oil or butter, cover with generous amount of water, and add salt and spices as desired. Simmer. Strain the broth when cool and store in glass quart-size jars. If freezing, allow at least an inch of space from the top of the jar. If you are making a vegetable soup from wilted vegetables, try blending the cooked vegetables with broth, salt, and other seasonings for bisquelike soup.

SHABU-SHABU

This traditional Japanese-style soup is fun and delicious. In a bowl, slice paper-thin, bit-sized pieces of steak (best done when steak is still slightly frozen), and add wheat-free soy sauce and sesame oil. Marinate at room temperature for about thirty minutes. In a large bowl, mix shredded cabbage and carrots, chopped green onions, and other vegetables, with kelp noodles, finely sliced mushrooms, garlic, and ginger. Add boiling water or broth to a pot that can be heated at the dinner table (either a candle warmer or electric hot plate). Keep the water or broth near boiling during dinner. First, add some of the vegetables and noodles to the broth and allow it to simmer. Then, dip a piece of beef into broth with chopsticks—just for a moment for rare beef or a bit longer for medium rare—picking up veggies and noodles with the beef. Keep adding vegetables and noodles throughout the dinner. When finished eating the beef (it will further make a delicious soup), serve the liquid stock in bowls for the end of the meal.

ZESTY COLD TOMATO SOUP

A quick, raw, delicious soup. Blend until smooth about 12 ounces of fresh or canned peeled whole tomatoes, 2 carrots, 1 to 2 cloves of garlic, ½ small onion, and fresh basil leaves. Add salt and spice to taste. Serve with a topping of sour cream, diced avocado, and sprigs of fresh cilantro.

TRADITIONAL TOMATO

In a large uncovered pot—and a rapid boil, not a simmer—cook down cut-up fresh or canned tomatoes to a thick consistency (this could take an hour or longer depending on the volume). Add sweet basil pesto (fresh basil, garlic, olive oil, pine nuts, salt), fresh ricotta, heavy cream, salt, or a pinch of cayenne pepper. (This is also an excellent sauce for grilled eggplant or zucchini, omelets, or many other dishes.)

COLD CUCUMBER SOUP

Peel off the skin from 1 to 3 young cucumbers (and/or zucchini) with the mandolin slicer to make julienne strips. Set aside for a separate salad (see below). Slice and blend remaining cucumbers with olive oil, fresh garlic, sea salt, and fresh dill. Top with sour cream, slices of avocado, or fresh tomato.

RAW CARROT SOUP

Blend well carrots, vegetable broth, ginger, small amount of stewed tomato, peeled cucumber, curry, and sea salt. Serve cold. This recipe also works well with cooked carrots and may be served hot.

MUSHROOM SOUP

Sauté favorite mushrooms in duck fat (see Roast Duck recipe below), olive oil, or butter, with onions or leeks. Salt to taste. Blend until desired consistency, chunky or smooth—you may need to add broth. Top with thin slices of fresh mushrooms.

LENTIL SOUP

Soak dried lentils for two days, rinsing thoroughly twice daily. Cook for 30 minutes or until just tender. Sauté onions, garlic, ginger, and carrots in olive oil, and season with curry, cardamom, chili, and cayenne pepper to taste. Add lentils and ½ cup unsweetened coconut milk, and simmer until flavors are richly mixed. Serve with fresh cilantro, grated coconut, chopped walnuts, and fine-chopped dates.

BUTTERNUT-SQUASH SOUP

Cut butternut squash into large pieces, removing the seeds, and steam. When tender, cool and remove the skin. Puree in blender with unsalted butter and some of the remaining water to desired soup consistency. Add sea salt to taste. Variations include using coconut milk and curry or other spices such as cayenne pepper or cinnamon. Top with cilantro leaves or fresh parsley, tarragon, toasted shredded coconut, browned thin slices of garlic, or caramelized onions.

BUTTERNUT TARRAGON

Steam and blend butternut squash as above. Add 1 teaspoon of salt, ½ teaspoon cinnamon, ⅛ teaspoon each of nutmeg, allspice, and cayenne. Simmer until hot. In a separate saucepan, warm 2 tablespoons of shelled pumpkin seeds with a bit of honey. Put seeds in a separate dish to be used later. Marinate fresh tarragon and ¼ cup white vinegar, and in the same saucepan, reduce (boil down) until almost all liquid is evaporated. Gently whisk in 1 to 2 tablespoons heavy cream to thicken into a tarragon cream. Pour soup into bowls, pour the tarragon cream in the center, and top with the sweet pumpkin seeds.

Egg-Drop Soup

Heat chicken broth in a wide saucepan or skillet to just before boiling. Turn off heat and slowly drop in raw eggs (whole or lightly beaten) while slowly mixing the soup (use one or two eggs per serving). Serve in a bowl with chopped fresh spinach. Top with Parmesan cheese and salt to taste. This also makes a wonderful wintertime breakfast.

Chicken or Turkey Soup

Simmer your favorite whole bird in salted water until almost done. Cool and remove bones and strain unwanted debris. Add chopped onions, zucchini, kale, spinach, carrots, peas, or other available vegetables, and simmer until done. Season with salt and your favorite spices. Try cinnamon, cloves, or cayenne pepper. Stir in some sour cream or yogurt for a creamy variation.

Pork-and-Ginger Soup

Brown ground pork with chopped ginger, garlic, and cabbage until done. Season with a bit of wheat-free soy sauce and salt to taste. Top with sesame seeds, cilantro, spring onions, or scrambled egg. Fresh mung bean sprouts add a terrific crunch to this flavorful Asian-style soup.

Beef Onion Soup

Sauté ground beef while covered to create a broth. Sauté sliced onions in olive oil and salt, then add to cooked beef. Add chopped kale and a bit more water to make a thick soup. Bring to a simmer until done.

Option: add fresh yogurt or crumbles of mild blue cheese.

Mediterranean Goulash

A great broth for this is made from organic grass-fed beef-marrow bones cooked in a Crock-Pot. Sauté sliced onions in olive oil, add to strained broth. Add halved cherry tomatoes, sliced Asian eggplant (or small bits of regular eggplant), cut green beans, fresh oregano, sea salt, ground turmeric, and cardamom.

Vegetables

Vegetables should be the bulk of most meals. From a simple dish such as steamed broccoli to fancy fare such as spinach soufflé, vegetables should be a healthy and delicious part of meals and even snacks.

Acorn Squash

Carefully cut squash crosswise, scoop out seeds, and trim ends slightly to create a flat bottom. Bake in a pan with large end down with about a quarter inch of water at 350°F for about 15 minutes. Turn over, add a small amount of butter to the squash, and continue baking until soft. Option: fill with sautéed diced apples, raisins, walnuts or pecans, and cinnamon in butter.

Artichokes

Select large bright green artichokes with the leaves tightly held together. Cut the thorny tips off with scissors. Slice down the center and through the stem, or boil whole in water and olive oil until leaves easily tear off. Serve hot or cold with garlic, salt and butter, and olive oil as the dip. (The thorny inside hairs of the artichoke heart can be easily scooped out with a spoon.)

ASPARAGUS

Spears should feel crisp and not limp. Cut or snap off the white ends (they tend to be woody and tough but can be used to flavor soups). Steam lightly and serve with a butter sauce. Or brush with olive oil and place a single layer on a baking sheet and broil until bright green. Leftover asparagus is great in soups, salads, or chopped egg dishes.

BOK CHOY

Baby bok choy is most tender and is becoming very popular and inexpensive in some Asian supermarkets. Remove the white tough stem from the green leaves. Sauté the chopped stem at a low temperature in olive oil, then add the chopped green leaves and stir until just barely wilted. Bok choy is also great in soups and egg dishes.

BROCCOLI

Buy heads that have tight florets and are bright green. Cut off heads, lightly steam, and serve with a butter sauce. They're also great with a garlic sauce or cold in salads. Save the stems and peel for soups by dicing them (like celery or potatoes). Leftover broccoli can be chopped and used in an egg frittata, soups, or other dishes.

BROCCOLI OR CAULIFLOWER SOUFFLÉ

Cut or peel the tough broccoli stems (or cut a head of cauliflower in quarters) and steam with a small amount of water. In a blender, combine 4 eggs, salt, and 2 to 4 ounces of white cheddar or swiss for the broccoli (or soft goat cheese for cauliflower). Pour into buttered pan and place in another pan of water to prevent browning. Bake at 350°F for 30 to 45 minutes.

BRUSSELS SPROUTS

Clean and halve brussels sprouts (or keep the smaller ones whole). Lightly steam until just tender. Serve plain or with a butter sauce. Option: make a dressing of raw sesame oil, wheat-free soy sauce, grated ginger, and garlic, and sprinkle with raw sesame seeds.

BUTTERNUT SQUASH

Cut lengthwise and remove the seeds. Steam until tender and remove skin. Mash with butter as vegetable side dish.

CABBAGE

Thinly slice or shred green cabbage. Use raw for salads or toss with apple cider vinegar and salt for coleslaw (marinate for a day or two in refrigerator). For a side dish, sauté on low heat with olive oil and add ground caraway seeds, butter, and sea salt.

CAULIFLOWER MASHED POTATOES

Lightly steam cauliflower, then mix in food processor with a small amount of butter, heavy cream, and sea salt. It can also be mixed by hand. It should be the consistency of mashed potatoes. Top with chopped chives or parsley, sour cream, or cheese.

EGGPLANT DIP (BABA GHANOUSH)

Cube eggplant and sauté in olive oil, whole garlic, and salt until well done. Thoroughly blend with 2 tablespoons tahini, 1 tablespoon lemon juice, and basil (dried or fresh). If too thick, add more olive oil. Eat as is, use on flax crackers, as a sauce for meat, or with salads. It's delicious warm or cold.

GRILLED EGGPLANT

Cut eggplant crosswise in quarter to half-inch slices. Place in a covered strainer for 2 to 3 days in the refrigerator to dehydrate. Brush both sides with olive oil and sprinkle with salt. Grill to desired doneness. Serve hot off the grill or cold the next day. For a side dish, add crumbled goat cheese and olive oil, or top with tomato sauce and ricotta cheese. It's also great as a base for lasagna in place of pasta.

SNAP PEAS

Buy in season. They should be crisp and without brown spots. Snap peas are great raw in salads. They can also be slightly steamed or very quickly sautéed in olive oil.

GREEN PEAS

Frozen organic tender peas can be used for many dishes. They can be quickly warmed and served with butter or served with mashed cauliflower (above). Leftover peas can be added to salads. Cooked peas can be whipped with olive oil for use in a soufflé. For an Indian dish, combine cooked peas with unsweetened coconut milk, ginger, garlic, and curry.

KALE AND GARLIC

Steam chopped kale and set aside. Sauté thinly sliced garlic in coconut oil until crispy. Pour over kale and salt to taste.

LEEKS

Buy leeks with fresh-looking green tops. Thinly sliced leeks are incredibly versatile and can be caramelized in butter or olive oil like onions, added to soups, and served alone or on the side of baked chicken or other meats.

MUSHROOM PÂTÉ

Sauté mushrooms, sliced onions, and whole garlic in duck fat (or butter) until soft. Remove from heat. Add coarsely ground pecans, cashews, and/or walnuts, sea salt, and favorite herbs. Blend in food processor to desired consistency and store in a pan refrigerated. This is great warm and cold.

ROASTED FENNEL

Buy fennel that is firm and not wilted. The tops are great cooked in soups and raw in salads (see above). The bulbs of fennel can be sliced thin and served raw. For roasted fennel, cut the bulb into quarters, lightly steam, and then slow-roast in a pan with olive oil and salt. For an Italian-style dish, serve roasted fennel with roasted red peppers, cherry tomatoes, and grilled egg-plant or zucchini.

SPAGHETTI SQUASH

Cut crosswise, remove seeds, and steam until just slightly tender. Larger squash may have to be quartered. When cool, use a fork to gently pull out the spaghetti-like threads. This is great just with butter and salt. Or use like spaghetti as the base for a tomato or meat sauce or in any other dish.

SPINACH

Baby spinach is best as a salad served with crumbled boiled eggs and thinly sliced onions. Or try it with strawberries, apples, or pears, with walnuts or pecans. Larger leaves of spinach can be chopped, lightly steamed, and served with a butter sauce. It's also great in soups, made into a soufflé (below), and used in many other dishes.

SPINACH SOUFFLÉ

Steam about 1 pound of fresh spinach, drain (save the water for soup), combine with 2 eggs, salt, 2 ounces mozzarella or cheddar cheese, and blend well. Bake in buttered dish (placed in another dish with small amount of water) at 350°F for 30 minutes (or until solid).

Option: combine with a carrot soufflé. This can be made by following the same recipe except substitute 2 medium carrots for spinach and add curry powder. Before baking, pour carrot mixture into dish first then care-fully pour the uncooked spinach soufflé on top. Bake as above until firm.

STRING BEANS

Buy crisp young string beans. Snap or cut off ends. Flash sauté in olive oil, keeping them crisp. They go well with toasted pine nuts, sau-téed onions and garlic, a dash of sesame seeds, and very lightly tossed in raw sesame oil.

TURNIPS

Young small turnips may be peeled, sliced, and served raw as part of a salad. Cooked tur-nips may be whipped and served like mashed potatoes. Roasted turnips are great with a pot roast, along with carrots and other root veg-etables.

WATERCRESS

Fresh watercress is great raw in salads. Watercress is delicious when lightly sautéed in olive oil with a dash of salt. It makes a great dish with sliced roast beef.

ZUCCHINI

Choose smaller-size zucchini for dicing or julienning. Use larger zucchini for stuffing, baking, or grilling.

Flash sauté julienned zucchini and then add a mixture of beaten eggs and cheese to make a delicious frittata. Turn once and lightly salt.

Diced zucchini is also great when added to lightly sautéed chopped onions and garlic.

Slice larger zucchini in long flat strips to grill outdoors or on stove-top iron grill. Align across the grooves in the grill to create dark stripes going across the length of the zucchini. Brush lightly with olive oil.

Very large zucchini are great stuffed and baked. Cut lengthwise, scoop out center, and mix with sautéed onions, garlic, and ground meat or cheese. Replace the stuffing in the center of the zucchini boats and bake at 450°F until tender. (If the zucchini is very hard, it should be slightly steamed before baking.)

Breakfast Ideas

No need to skip this most important meal.

No-Crust Quiche

Beat 12 eggs and 1 cup heavy cream until foamy. Stir in 1 ½ cups sheep or goat cheese, ½ cup cherry tomatoes halved, 1 ½ cup spinach, and season with sea salt. Pour into well-buttered pie plate and bake 30 to 40 minutes in a preheated oven at 350°F or until middle is set but still moist; do not overbake. Serve warm or cool. Add less cheese, more vegetables, or other variations.

Wheat-Free Oven Pancakes or Waffles

In a good blender, place ½ cup almonds, 3 eggs, 1 medium apple, ½ teaspoon salt, and blend until smooth. Pour into buttered pan and place in 400°F oven for 25 minutes or until firm. Option: top with berries or sliced fruit before baking.

Waffles! Use the same recipe, using a well-buttered waffle iron. These waffles store well in the refrigerator or freezer.

A note on maple syrup: avoid it. It's a very high-glycemic sugar. Instead, use a small amount of honey or prepare your own syrup by mixing honey with blueberries or other fruit. Or combine honey and frozen berries in a saucepan and heat to reduce to a thick syrup.

Basic Farm Biscuits

In a mixing bowl add 2 eggs and about ⅓ cup lard* and mix well. Add ½ cup of finely ground almonds, and ½ teaspoon salt. Mix all ingredients well and form small biscuits. Place on a buttered skillet or oven sheet. Bake for about 20 minutes at 350°F. (The dough can also be placed in a buttered dish and baked as above—remove from dish when cool and slice like bread.)

Homemade mango jam—combine frozen organic mango and honey, heat until thick (mash with a fork when cooking). Cool. Use other fruit as option.

*Make your own organic lard: Slowly cook a package of organic bacon. Pour off the fat through a strainer, and use for cooking.

Lunch and Dinner Entrées

Fish Marinade

Cut fresh wild salmon or dark tuna in ½-inch strips or keep whole. Marinate overnight in rice wine vinegar, grated ginger, sesame oil, wheat-free soy sauce, and sliced scallions. Lightly sauté the fish (rare is best), and serve on a bed of greens.

Baked Ocean Perch

Place ocean perch (or other small white fish like wild trout) in baking dish with crushed garlic, sliced lemon, and olive oil with a very small amount of water. Cover and bake at 450°F for 10 to 15 minutes.

Wild Salmon Alfredo

Cut slightly steamed salmon into small pieces, or use smoked salmon. Add a few tablespoons heavy cream. Slowly heat to a simmer. Pour on top of cooked spaghetti squash (see recipe above) or raw spiral-cut zucchini or yellow squash. Sprinkle with Parmesan cheese. Salt to taste (if you use smoked salmon, do not add salt).

Seared Tuna

Marinate tuna in wheat-free tamari, ginger, wasabi, green onions, and honey. Sear tuna lightly on grill (rare is best). Serve with sautéed ginger and onions.

Vegetable Spaghetti with Tomato Sauce

In a spiral vegetable slicer, prepare raw zucchini or small yellow squash. Or use cooked spaghetti squash. Lightly salt and top with hot tomato or meat sauce. Sprinkle with grated hard cheese. Option: add sliced pimento green olives.

Zucchini or Grilled Eggplant Lasagna

In a buttered baking dish, add sliced medium-size zucchini or eggplant (both should be previously grilled or steamed). Add a layer of tomato or meat sauce, then ricotta, another zucchini/eggplant layer, and top with tomato sauce and grated cheese. Bake at 375°F for about 20 minutes or until desired tenderness. Very nice when baked and served in individual-size baking dishes.

Lamb Patties

Combine fresh ground lamb with chopped onions, walnuts, mint leaves, and salt. Form into small patties and sauté over medium heat. Remove the lamb patties from the pan and mix 2 teaspoons sour cream into the pan to make a gravy topping.

Options:

- A cucumber-yogurt topping is great (see above).
- Lamb patties are also great grilled or steamed.
- For a great wrap, serve patties in steamed cabbage leaves or crispy romaine lettuce. To steam cabbage leaves, cut cabbage in half, remove the core, place flat side down in a covered pot with about a half inch of water, and steam until tender.
- Sliced tomatoes, grilled Halloumi (cheese), mint leaves, and even kiwi slices are terrific in this tasty combination of flavors.

Grilled Lamb Tenderloins

Lightly grill lamb (rare is best), then serve topped with mint pesto made by blending fresh mint leaves, garlic, olive oil, lemon juice, walnuts, and salt.

Roast Duck

Pierce the duck's skin all over with a sharp knife and salt generously. Place in large pot with 1 to 2 quarts of water (covering about ½ the duck). Boil 90 minutes to 2 hours depending on size. After boiling, remove duck from water (let cool and skim off fat for cooking, and use water for soup). Place duck in oven and roast for about 60 minutes at 350 to 400°F or until skin is brown and crispy. Serve with cherry sauce or cilantro and toasted pine nuts.

TURKEY

Follow the recipe for Roast Duck, but do not pierce the skin before boiling.

MEAT LOAF

Thoroughly mix about a pound of freshly ground beef with about 1 cup finely chopped vegetables (zucchini, kale, spinach, carrots, etc.), 3 to 4 stewed tomatoes, 1 chopped yellow onion, and 2 eggs. Bake at 350°F for about 60 to 90 minutes. (This is a very moist meat loaf and looks pink inside, so check temperature to make sure it has reached 180°F.)

SHEPHERD'S PIE

Use the Cauliflower Mashed Potatoes and Meat Loaf recipes listed above. In a shallow baking dish, cover cooked meat loaf with a layer of mashed cauliflower and top with Parmesan cheese. Bake until hot and cheese melts and browns slightly. (Single-serving baking dishes work great for this recipe.)

CRISPY CHEESE SHELL

Shred or thinly slice organic mozzarella cheese. Spread it out on a buttered flat pan, in whatever shape you want. Bake in 400°F until it starts to brown. Let cool slightly, and cut into chips or use as a taco shell (it will become solid if allowed to cool completely). Option: use a large lettuce leaf as a wrap, adding the cheese shell on the inside with guacamole, meat, tomatoes, salsa, and others.

Desserts

PECANDY

In a pan, melt 2 tablespoons butter, then toast ¼ cup coconut flakes. Turn down heat, and add 1 cup pecan pieces, ½ cup ground almonds, and ¼ teaspoon salt. Add ¼ cup honey and continue heating. Remove from heat and cool slightly, then add ¼ cup ground sesame seeds or tahini. Flatten and spread in pan or dish and when cool cut into squares.

Options:

- Toast shredded coconut before adding butter and pecans to have a crunchy coconut taste.
- Stir in chopped dates.
- Vary the type of nuts (walnuts, pistachios, hazels).
- Use pure cocoa butter instead of regular butter.

CHOCOLATE PECANDY

Lightly toast ¼ cup of coconut flakes in a skillet. Add 1 tablespoon of butter. Reduce heat and add ½ teaspoon of salt, ½ cup ground almonds, ½ cup of coarsely ground pecans, ½ cup of ground hazel (or other) nuts, ¼ cup of ground or cacao bean pieces (or cocoa powder). Add ¼ cup of honey and mix well. Turn off heat, and stir in ¼ cup of tahini. Press into a buttered pan, cool, and cut into bars.

IRISH POTATOES

Mix well 4 ounces cream cheese, 1 teaspoon vanilla, ¼ teaspoon cinnamon, ¼ cup honey, and ½ cup finely shredded coconut. Chill, form small balls, and sprinkle with cinnamon. Serve chilled.

COCONUT SNOWBALLS

Mix 1 cup unsweetened shredded coconut, ½ cup egg white powder, 2 tablespoons honey, a dash of vanilla, and 1 to 2 tablespoons heavy cream (or enough to make sticky balls). Roll in toasted shredded coconut. (To toast coconut, place in a dry skillet on medium heat, and stir frequently until slightly browned.)

BUTTERNUT-SQUASH PIE

This is tastier than pumpkin pie, and healthier too! Steam quartered butternut squash until tender; let cool enough to remove peel. Blend about 2 cups of butternut squash, 4 eggs, ½ teaspoon salt, 4 ounces cream cheese, ⅓ cup honey, and ½ teaspoon pumpkin pie spice or favorite blend of cinnamon and spices. Place in buttered baking dish (and place in another baking dish with ½ inch of water). Bake at 350°F. Allow to cool before serving. Serve plain, with whipped or sour cream, or top with chopped nuts and dates.

ALMOND BISCOTTI CAKE

Grind 1 cup almonds (with some course pieces remaining). Mix in 5 eggs, a pinch of salt, ⅓ cup heavy cream or coconut milk, and ⅓ cup honey. Pour into buttered dish and bake at 350°F for about 40 minutes.

FRIED BANANAS

Peel and slice small ripe bananas. Sauté in coconut oil until slightly brown and caramelized. Place in a bowl and sprinkle with coconut and a pinch of date sugar (or coconut sugar). Options: keep bananas whole, drizzle with cherry sauce, top with whipped cream, combine with other favorite fruit—mango is especially nice.

CREAMY AVOCADO PUDDING

Blend until smooth 1 large avocado, 3 tablespoons sour cream, 2 tablespoons honey, 2 to 3 tablespoons lemon or lime juice, and a bit of zest. Serve plain, or top with slices of mango, sprigs of cilantro, and lime peel.

VERY BERRY SAUCE

Heat to simmer frozen blueberries, raspberries, strawberries, or other berries. Reduce to desired thickness and remove from heat. Add honey to taste. Use on desserts, healthy waffles, or other foods. (Some prefer to press raspberries through a strainer to remove seeds.)

CREPES DE FRUTAS

For each person, beat 1 egg with ½ teaspoon honey and a teaspoon of heavy cream. Melt butter or olive oil in a small skillet on low temperature, and add a thin layer of egg

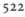

mixture. Slowly cook until surface is slightly sticky but firm. Remove from skillet to plate, and spread a thin layer of sour cream, and roll into logs. Top with Very Berry Sauce (above), fresh fruit, whipped cream, yogurt, or some other healthy topping of your choice.

Coconut Pound Cake

Melt 1 stick butter, mix in 4 egg yolks, ½ cup honey, 1 teaspoon vanilla, and ¼ teaspoon salt until creamy. Add 1 cup coconut flour and about 1 cup water, and mix well. Whip 4 egg whites until stiff, and fold into batter. Bake at 350°F for 20 to 30 minutes. Top with cherry sauce, Very Berry Sauce, or lemon-honey mixture.

Coralee's Carrot Cake

Blend until smooth 3 eggs, 1 cup almonds, ⅓ cup honey, 1 large carrot, 1 apple, 2 tablespoons butter, 1 teaspoon salt, and 1 teaspoon cinnamon. Bake 350°F for 35 minutes.

To make a quick frosting: mix about a half cup of cream cheese with about 2 tablespoons of honey. Option: add orange zest or orange extract or vanilla extract.

Banana Bread

Melt 4 tablespoons (½ stick) butter or coconut oil and stir in ⅓ cup honey and 4 beaten eggs until smooth. Add 1 teaspoon of vanilla and 3 mashed very ripe bananas. Add 1 cup finely ground almonds, ½ tea-

spoon cinnamon, and ½ teaspoon salt. Add water if needed to make a smooth cakelike batter. Option: mix in ½ cup chopped walnuts. Bake at 350°F for about 45 minutes.

Cashew Chews

Mix well 2 tablespoons cashew butter, 1 tablespoon sesame butter, 1 tablespoon egg white powder, 1 tablespoon honey, and 2 tablespoons dried coconut. Roll into bite-size balls and push a small date (or half a large date) into each center. Sprinkle with additional coconut.

Option: add unsweetened cocoa bits.

Mission Fig Mousse

Chop ripe mission figs and blend with a small amount of honey and heavy cream. Serve alone or on top of cheesecake, brownie, or other healthy dessert.

Variations: cut top of fig and carefully scoop out the center. Blend with 2 tablespoons of cream and about 1 tablespoon of honey for 6 figs. Spoon the fig mousse back into the skins. Top with tiny strips of fresh sweet basil (cut strips with scissors). Sprinkle with date sugar and a pinch of salt. (Option: a balsamic vinegar reduction decoratively poured over the top sets this off beautifully.)

Cheesecake

Blend well 1 cup sheep or goat yogurt or cream cheese, 1 cup ricotta cheese, 4 eggs, ⅓ cup honey, 1 teaspoon vanilla. Pour into buttered baking dish. Place in another dish with an inch of water. Bake 30 to 45 minutes at 350°F until firm. This is wonderful hot or cold. Top with your favorite fruit, shaved almonds, fruit sauce, or other healthy topping.

MANGO SORBET

Cut up a ripe mango and 1 or 2 small bananas, and freeze until firm (but not rock hard). Add to blender and mix well with ½ cup unsweetened coconut milk. Serve with colorful berries.

APPLE-PEAR CRISP

Slice 1 tart apple and 1 pear. Place in a baking dish alternating apple and pear slices. Mix ¼ cup ground almonds, ¼ cup ground whole oats (optional), ¼ cup butter, ¼ cup honey, and ½ teaspoon cinnamon and sprinkle on top. Bake 45 minutes at 350°F.

FAST APPLE-PEAR CRISP

Dice or slice apples or pears, and quickly sauté in butter until slightly browned. Place in serving dishes and sprinkle with cinnamon. Warm 1 tablespoon of honey and 1 tablespoon heavy cream in a sauce pan, mix well, and pour over fruit. Sprinkle with ground or chopped almonds. Option: top with whipped cream.

PHIL'S FUDGE

Mix ⅓ cup unsweetened cocoa powder and ⅓ cup egg white powder. Melt 2 tablespoons butter in a saucepan on low heat, then add ¼ cup honey. Mix in cocoa and egg powder mixture. The consistency should be like soft rubber. If it's too dry, add honey; if too wet, add cocoa or egg powder. Press into buttered glass pan and cut into squares. Keep refrigerated if you want them firm, or leave out to keep them soft.

Options:

- Add ¾ teaspoon of peppermint oil.
- Add almond, cashew, or peanut butter center (premix very small amount of honey with the nut butter and place between thin layers of chocolate).
- Add unsweetened shredded coconut—add to dry mix before blending.
- For white chocolate, use pure cocoa butter instead of butter and cocoa powder, and add ½ teaspoon of vanilla.

STUFFED MAJOOL DATES

Open date, remove pit, stuff with a small piece of blue cheese and butter, close date, eat, and enjoy!

FLAXSEED CRACKERS

Soak 1 cup of flax seeds in 1 cup of water for 6 to 8 hours. Add salt and other favorite seasonings and mix well. The flaxseeds release a very sticky substance that holds the mixture together, so wet your hands to work with the mixture easily. Place 1 to 2 tablespoons of mixture on parchment paper and flatten out like a thin cookie. Dehydrate the crackers in an oven set at 180°F, outside in the sun, or in a dehydrator, turning crackers over when top side is crispy. Dehydrate 4 to 8 hours until both sides are crispy.

INDEX

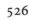

INDEX

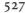

INDEX